Springer Texts in Statistics

Advisors:
George Casella   Stephen Fienberg   Ingram Olkin

Springer Science+Business Media, LLC

Springer Texts in Statistics

Alfred: Elements of Statistics for the Life and Social Sciences
Berger: An Introduction to Probability and Stochastic Processes
Bilodeau and Brenner: Theory of Multivariate Statistics
Blom: Probability and Statistics: Theory and Applications
Brockwell and Davis: Introduction to Times Series and Forecasting, Second Edition
Carmona: Statistical Analysis of Financial Data in S-Plus
Chow and Teicher: Probability Theory: Independence, Interchangeability, Martingales, Third Edition
Christensen: Advanced Linear Modeling: Multivariate, Time Series, and Spatial Data; Nonparametric Regression and Response Surface Maximization, Second Edition
Christensen: Log-Linear Models and Logistic Regression, Second Edition
Christensen: Plane Answers to Complex Questions: The Theory of Linear Models, Third Edition
Creighton: A First Course in Probability Models and Statistical Inference
Davis: Statistical Methods for the Analysis of Repeated Measurements
Dean and Voss: Design and Analysis of Experiments
du Toit, Steyn, and Stumpf: Graphical Exploratory Data Analysis
Durrett: Essentials of Stochastic Processes
Edwards: Introduction to Graphical Modelling, Second Edition
Finkelstein and Levin: Statistics for Lawyers
Flury: A First Course in Multivariate Statistics
Heiberger and Holland: Statistical Analysis and Data Display: An Intermediate Course with Examples in S-PLUS, R, and SAS
Jobson: Applied Multivariate Data Analysis, Volume I: Regression and Experimental Design
Jobson: Applied Multivariate Data Analysis, Volume II: Categorical and Multivariate Methods
Kalbfleisch: Probability and Statistical Inference, Volume I: Probability, Second Edition
Kalbfleisch: Probability and Statistical Inference, Volume II: Statistical Inference, Second Edition
Karr: Probability
Keyfitz: Applied Mathematical Demography, Second Edition
Kiefer: Introduction to Statistical Inference
Kokoska and Nevison: Statistical Tables and Formulae
Kulkarni: Modeling, Analysis, Design, and Control of Stochastic Systems
Lange: Applied Probability
Lange: Optimization
Lehmann: Elements of Large-Sample Theory

(continued after index)

Charles S. Davis

Statistical Methods for the Analysis of Repeated Measurements

With 20 Illustrations

Springer

Charles S. Davis
Senior Director, Biometrics
Elan Pharmaceuticals
7475 Lusk Boulevard
San Diego, CA 92121
USA
Chuck.Davis@elan.com

Additional materials for the book can be downloaded at www.springer.com. In the following, it is referred to as "website.zip (data files and SAS programs)".

Library of Congress Cataloging-in-Publication Data
Davis, Charles S. (Charles Shaw), 1952–
Statistical methods for the analysis of repeated measurements/Charles S. Davis.
p. cm.— (Springer texts in statistics)
Includes bibliographical references and index.
ISBN 978-1-4419-2976-1 ISBN 978-0-387-21573-0 (eBook)
DOI 10.1007/978-0-387-21573-0

1. Multivariate analysis. 2. Experimental design. I. Title. III. Series.
QA278.D343 2002
519.5'35—dc21 2001054913

ISBN 978-1-4419-2976-1 Printed on acid-free paper.

Originally published by Springer-Verlag New York, Inc. in 2002
Softcover reprint of the hardcover 1st edition 2002

9 8 7 6 5 4 3

www.springer-ny.com

Preface

I have endeavored to provide a comprehensive introduction to a wide variety of statistical methods for the analysis of repeated measurements. I envision this book primarily as a textbook, because the notes on which it is based have been used in a semester-length graduate course I have taught since 1991. This course is primarily taken by graduate students in biostatistics and statistics, although students and faculty from other departments have audited the course. I also anticipate that the book will be a useful reference for practicing statisticians. This assessment is based on the positive responses I have received to numerous short courses I have taught on this topic to academic and industry groups.

Although my intent is to provide a reasonably comprehensive overview of methods for the analysis of repeated measurements, I do not view this book as a definitive "state of the art" compendium of research in this area. Some general approaches are extremely active areas of current research, and it is not feasible, given the goals of this book, to include a comprehensive summary and list of references. Instead, my focus is primarily on methods that are implemented in standard statistical software packages. As a result, the level of detail on some topics is less than in other books, and some more recent methods of analysis are not included. One particular example is the topic of nonlinear mixed models for the analysis of repeated measurements (Davidian and Giltinan, 1995; Vonesh and Chinchilli, 1996). With respect to some of the more recent methods of analysis, I do attempt to mention some of the areas of current research.

The prerequisites for a course based on this book include knowledge of mathematical statistics at the level of Hogg and Craig (1995) and a course in linear regression and ANOVA at the level of Neter et al. (1985). Individuals without these prerequisites who have audited the graduate course or attended short courses have also been able to benefit from much of the material.

Because a wide variety of methods are covered, knowledge of topics such as multivariate normal distribution theory, categorical data analysis, and generalized linear models would also be useful. However, my philosophy is not to assume any particular knowledge of these areas and to present the necessary background material in the book.

When I began to develop my graduate course on the analysis of repeated measurements, no suitable text was available for the course as I envisioned it, and I made the decision to prepare my own notes. Since then, multiple books on the analysis of repeated measurements have been published. I regularly refer to the following books (listed chronologically): Hand and Taylor (1987), Crowder and Hand (1990) [updated as Hand and Crowder (1996)], Diggle (1990), Jones (1993), Diggle et al. (1994), Kshirsagar and Smith (1995), Vonesh and Chinchilli (1996), and Lindsey (1999), among others. Although some of the existing books are reasonably comprehensive in their coverage, others are more narrowly focused on specialized topics. This book is more comprehensive than many and is targeted at a lower mathematical level and focused more on applications than most. In summary, it is more oriented toward statistical practitioners than to statistical researchers.

Two obvious distinctions of this book are the extensive use of real data sets and the inclusion of numerous homework problems. Eighty real data sets are used in the examples and homework problems. These data sets are available from the website www.springer-ny.com (click on "author websites"). Because many of the data sets can be used to demonstrate multiple methods of analysis, instructors can easily develop additional homework problems and exam questions based on the data sets provided.

The inclusion of homework problems makes this book especially well-suited as a course text. Approximately 85% of the homework problems involve data analysis. The focus of these problems is not on providing a definitive analysis of the data but rather on providing the reader with experience in knowing when, and learning how, to select and apply appropriate methods of analysis. Although many of the examples and homework problems have a biomedical focus, the principles and methods apply to other subject areas as well.

My graduate course and short course notes include numerous examples of the use of, and output from, statistical software packages, primarily SAS (SAS Institute, 1999). I have purposely chosen not to include programming statements or computer output in the book. I do provide the raw data for nearly all examples as well as the key results of all analyses. In this way, readers will be able to carry out and verify the results of their own analyses using their choice of software.

The notes on which this book is based are in the form of overhead transparencies produced using TeX (Knuth, 1986). This format is well-suited for instructors. The course notes also include programming statements and computer output for the examples, prepared primarily using SAS. Course instructors interested in obtaining this supplemental material, as well as solutions to homework problems, should contact Springer-Verlag.

I would like to thank John Kimmel of Springer-Verlag for initially encouraging me to write this book and for his support and advice during its preparation. I am also grateful to the graduate students who have participated in my course since 1991 and to the attendees at external short courses; both groups have motivated me to develop and expand the notes on which this book is based. I also thank Michelle Larson for her assistance in the preparation of solutions to the homework problems and Kathy Clark for her careful review of the manuscript. Finally, I thank my wife, Ruth, and our children, Michael, Carrie, and Nathan, for their understanding and support during this endeavor.

San Diego, California — Charles S. Davis
November 2001

Contents

List of Tables

List of Figures

1
Introduction

1.1 Repeated Measurements

This book describes, discusses, and demonstrates a variety of statistical methods for the analysis of repeated measurements. The term "repeated measurements" refers broadly to data in which the response of each experimental unit or subject is observed on multiple occasions or under multiple conditions. Although the response variable could itself be either univariate or multivariate, we restrict consideration to univariate response variables measured at multiple occasions for each subject. The term "multiple" will usually mean "more than two," since the topic of paired measurements is addressed in many other books.

The term "longitudinal data" is also often used to describe repeated measurements data. Some authors use this term when referring to data in which the repeated measurements factor is time. In this usage, longitudinal data could be viewed as a special case of repeated measurements data. Other authors make an alternative distinction and use the term "longitudinal data" to refer to data collected over an extended period of time, often under uncontrolled conditions. The term "repeated measurements" is then used to describe data collected over a relatively short time period, frequently under experimental conditions. Using this definition, repeated measurements data can be regarded as a special case of longitudinal data. In this book, we will use the term "repeated measurements" in the broad sense to refer to the situation in which multiple measurements of the response variable are obtained from each experimental unit.

Research in many areas of application frequently involves study designs in which repeated measurements are obtained. Studies in which the response variable is measured at multiple points in time from each subject are one important and commonly used application. In other applications, the response from each experimental unit is measured under multiple conditions rather than at multiple time points.

In some settings in which repeated measurements data are obtained, the independent experimental units are not individual subjects. For example, in a toxicological study, the experimental units might be litters; responses are then obtained from the multiple newborns in each litter. In a genetic study, experimental units might be defined by families; responses are then obtained from the members of each family.

1.2 Advantages and Disadvantages of Repeated Measurements Designs

A key strength of studies in which repeated measurements are obtained from each subject is that this is the only type of design in which it is possible to obtain information concerning individual patterns of change. This type of design also economizes on subjects. For example, when studying the effects of a treatment over time, it is usually desirable to observe the same subjects repeatedly rather than to observe different subjects at each specified time point. Another advantage is that subjects can serve as their own controls in that the outcome variable can be measured under both control and experimental conditions for each subject. Because between-subjects sources of variability can be excluded from the experimental error, repeated measurements designs often provide more efficient estimators of relevant parameters than cross-sectional designs with the same number and pattern of measurements. A final consideration is that data can often be collected more reliably in a study in which the same subjects are followed repeatedly than in a cross-sectional study.

There are two main difficulties in the analysis of data from repeated measures studies. First, the analysis is complicated by the dependence among repeated observations made on the same experimental unit. Second, the investigator often cannot control the circumstances for obtaining measurements, so that the data may be unbalanced or partially incomplete. For example, in a longitudinal study, the response from a subject may be missing at one or more of the time points due to factors that are unrelated to the outcome of interest. In toxicology or genetic studies, litter or family sizes are variable rather than fixed; hence, the number of repeated measures is not constant across experimental units.

Although many approaches to the analysis of repeated measures data have been studied, most are restricted to the setting in which the response

TABLE 1.1. General layout for repeated measurements

Subject	Time Point	Missing Indicator	Response	Covariates		
1	1	δ_{11}	y_{11}	x_{111}	$\cdots$	x_{11p}
	$\vdots$	$\vdots$	$\vdots$	$\vdots$	$\ddots$	$\vdots$
	j	δ_{1j}	y_{1j}	x_{1j1}	$\cdots$	x_{1jp}
	$\vdots$	$\vdots$	$\vdots$	$\vdots$	$\ddots$	$\vdots$
	t_1	δ_{1t_1}	y_{1t_1}	x_{1t_11}	$\cdots$	x_{1t_1p}
$\cdots$	$\cdots$	$\cdots$	$\cdots$	$\cdots$	$\cdots$	$\cdots$
i	1	δ_{i1}	y_{i1}	x_{i11}	$\cdots$	x_{i1p}
	$\vdots$	$\vdots$	$\vdots$	$\vdots$	$\ddots$	$\vdots$
	j	δ_{ij}	y_{ij}	x_{ij1}	$\cdots$	x_{ijp}
	$\vdots$	$\vdots$	$\vdots$	$\vdots$	$\ddots$	$\vdots$
	t_i	δ_{it_i}	y_{it_i}	x_{it_i1}	$\cdots$	x_{it_ip}
$\cdots$	$\cdots$	$\cdots$	$\cdots$	$\cdots$	$\cdots$	$\cdots$
n	1	δ_{n1}	y_{n1}	x_{n11}	$\cdots$	x_{n1p}
	$\vdots$	$\vdots$	$\vdots$	$\vdots$	$\ddots$	$\vdots$
	j	δ_{nj}	y_{nj}	x_{nj1}	$\cdots$	x_{njp}
	$\vdots$	$\vdots$	$\vdots$	$\vdots$	$\ddots$	$\vdots$
	t_n	δ_{nt_n}	y_{nt_n}	x_{nt_n1}	$\cdots$	x_{nt_np}

variable is normally distributed and the data are balanced and complete. Although the development of methods for the analysis of repeated measures categorical data has received substantially less attention in the past, this has more recently become an important and active area of research. Still, the methodology is not nearly as well-developed as for continuous, normally distributed outcomes. The practical application of methods for repeated categorical outcomes also lags behind that for normal-theory methods due to the lack of readily accessible software.

1.3 Notation for Repeated Measurements

The notation used to describe methods for the analysis of repeated measurements varies considerably in the statistical literature. Table 1.1 shows the general layout for repeated measurements that will be used in this book. Let n denote the number of independent experimental units (subjects) from which repeated measurements are obtained, let t_i denote the number of measurements from subject i, and let y_{ij} be the response from subject i at time point (or occasion) j for $j = 1, \ldots, t_i$ and $i = 1, \ldots, n$. In addition, let p denote the number of covariates, and let $\boldsymbol{x}_{ij} = (x_{ij1}, \ldots, x_{ijp})'$ denote the vector of covariates associated with y_{ij}. In general, the values of the covariates may vary across the repeated measurements from a subject; such occasion-specific variables are called time-dependent or within-subject covariates. Because there may be missing values of y_{ij} and/or missing components in the vector $\boldsymbol{x}_{ij}$, it is convenient to define indicator variables

$$\delta_{ij} = \begin{cases} 1 & \text{if } y_{ij} \text{ and } \boldsymbol{x}_{ij} \text{ are observed,} \\ 0 & \text{otherwise.} \end{cases}$$

One special case of the general layout shown in Table 1.1 is when repeated measurements are obtained (or scheduled to be obtained) at a common set of t measurement occasions for all subjects. In this case, $t_1 = \cdots = t_n = t$.

An important and commonly occurring situation is when repeated measurements are obtained from s subpopulations (groups) of subjects at a common set of t time points (or measurement occasions). In this case, let n_h be the number of subjects in group h for $h = 1, \ldots, s$. In terms of the general notation, $n = \sum_{h=1}^{s} n_h$. The s groups may be defined by the s levels of a single covariate. In other situations, the groups may be defined by the cross-classification of the levels of several categorical covariates. In terms of the general layout shown in Table 1.1, the s groups can be described in terms of $p = s - 1$ time-independent (or between-subject) categorical covariates. Although data of this type can be displayed using the general layout of Table 1.1, it may be more convenient to present the data as shown in Table 1.2. In this case, instead of letting y_{ij} denote the response at time j from subject i, we let y_{hij} denote the response at time j from subject i in group h for $j = 1, \ldots, t$, $i = 1, \ldots, n_h$, and $h = 1, \ldots, s$.

The final special case we will consider is the situation where repeated measurements are obtained (or scheduled to be obtained) at t time points from n subjects from a single population. In this case, the data can be displayed in an $n \times t$ matrix, as shown in Table 1.3. Here, y_{ij} denotes the jth measurement from the ith subject for $j = 1, \ldots, t$, $i = 1, \ldots, n$. The corresponding missing value indicators are defined by

$$\delta_{ij} = \begin{cases} 1 & \text{if } y_{ij} \text{ is observed,} \\ 0 & \text{otherwise.} \end{cases}$$

1.4 Missing Data

As was mentioned in Section 1.2, the occurrence of missing data is common in studies where repeated measurements are obtained. Although this book does not focus specifically on the analysis of incomplete repeated measurements, many of the methods described in subsequent chapters can

TABLE 1.2. Layout for the special case of multiple samples

Group	Subject	Time Point 1	…	j	…	t
1	1	y_{111}	…	y_{11j}	…	y_{11t}
	⋮	⋮	⋱	⋮	⋱	⋮
	i	y_{1i1}	…	y_{1ij}	…	y_{1it}
	⋮	⋮	⋱	⋮	⋱	⋮
	n_1	y_{1n_11}	…	y_{1n_1j}	…	y_{1n_1t}
⋯	⋯	⋯	⋯	⋯	⋯	⋯
h	1	y_{h11}	…	y_{h1j}	…	y_{h1t}
	⋮	⋮	⋱	⋮	⋱	⋮
	i	y_{hi1}	…	y_{hij}	…	y_{hit}
	⋮	⋮	⋱	⋮	⋱	⋮
	n_h	y_{hn_h1}	…	y_{hn_hj}	…	y_{hn_ht}
⋯	⋯	⋯	⋯	⋯	⋯	⋯
s	1	y_{s11}	…	y_{s1j}	…	y_{s1t}
	⋮	⋮	⋱	⋮	⋱	⋮
	i	y_{si1}	…	y_{sij}	…	y_{sit}
	⋮	⋮	⋱	⋮	⋱	⋮
	n_s	y_{sn_s1}	…	y_{sn_sj}	…	y_{sn_st}

TABLE 1.3. Layout for the one-sample case

Subject	Time Point 1	…	j	…	t
1	y_{11}	…	y_{1j}	…	y_{1t}
⋮	⋮	⋱	⋮	⋱	⋮
i	y_{i1}	…	y_{ij}	…	y_{it}
⋮	⋮	⋱	⋮	⋱	⋮
n	y_{n1}	…	y_{nj}	…	y_{nt}

be used when the data are incomplete. The mechanism that results in missing data must, however, be considered when selecting an appropriate method of analysis. Little and Rubin (1987) and Schafer (1997) provide comprehensive treatments of the analysis of incomplete data. Laird (1988), Gornbein et al. (1992), Heyting et al. (1992), Little (1995), and Kenward and Molenberghs (1999) provide reviews focused specifically on repeated measurements.

In particular, Little and Rubin (1987) have described missing-data mechanisms as follows:

1. Missing completely at random (MCAR): if the probability of observing the response is independent of both the observed and unobserved outcome values;

2. Missing at random (MAR): if the probability of observing the response depends on the observed outcome values but is independent of the unobserved outcome values;

3. Nonignorable: if the probability of observing the response depends on the unobserved outcome values.

The nonignorable missing-data mechanism is also called informative or nonrandom.

With specific reference to repeated measurements, consider a study in which the outcome variable of interest is scheduled to be measured at a fixed number of occasions (visits) for each subject. The missing-data mechanism is MCAR if subjects miss their visits totally at random. A MAR missing-data mechanism would result if the probability of missing a visit is directly related to prior observed responses. An example of a nonrandom (nonignorable) missing-data mechanism would be if, in addition to prior observed responses affecting whether the response at a specific subsequent visit is missing, subjects would be more or less likely to miss a visit based on the unobserved value of their response at that specific visit.

In their discussion of missing data in repeated measurements, Diggle and Kenward (1994) refer to MCAR as the completely random dropout (CRD) mechanism. They propose the term "random dropout" (RD) for the MAR mechanism. The situation in which the missing-data mechanism is nonignorable is called the informative dropout (ID) mechanism.

The preceding characterizations of missing-data mechanisms refer only to the response variable and do not address the effect of covariates on the missing-data mechanism. For example, it may be important to consider the influence of a fully observed covariate on the probability of response. Little and Rubin (1987) have classified the mechanisms that govern missing data when the influence of a covariate is taken into account. If the probability of response is independent of the covariate and of the observed and unobserved responses, then the missing-data mechanism is said to be MCAR. If the probability of response depends on the covariate but is independent of the unobserved responses, then the missing-data mechanism is said to be MAR provided that we have conditioned on the value of the covariate. If the probability of response depends on the unobserved responses with a possible (but not necessary) dependence on the covariate, then the missing-data mechanism is said to be nonignorable.

Suppose that the probability of observing a response depends on the value of the covariate but not on the observed and unobserved responses. For example, suppose that the probability of dropping out of a study varies according to the value of a covariate. Little and Rubin (1987) classify this mechanism as MAR due to the dependence on the covariate. There are, however, differing opinions on the classification of the missing-data mechanism in this situation. Diggle and Kenward (1994), among others, have classified this mechanism as MCAR provided that one conditions on the covariate in the analysis. Little (1995) suggests using the term covariate dependent dropout to describe this situation (provided that one conditions on all of the necessary covariates) and reserves the term MCAR only for a dropout that is independent of the covariate and observed and unobserved responses.

If the missing-data mechanism is MCAR, most standard approaches to analysis will be valid, and the issue of interest is simply the difficulty in implementing an analysis when the data are incomplete. In particular, analyses that omit experimental units with missing data ("complete case" analyses) are valid, although they may be inefficient. If the missing-data mechanism is MAR, then the nonresponse mechanism is said to be ignorable. In this case, likelihood-based inferences are still valid. Moment-based analysis methods, however, are biased when the missing-data mechanism is MAR. Although MAR is a weaker assumption than MCAR, nonignorable missing-data mechanisms are certainly much more common than either MCAR or MAR mechanisms.

If the missing-data mechanism is nonignorable, both likelihood-based and moment-based methods of analysis are biased. The development of methods for the analysis of repeated measurements that are valid in the case of nonignorable missingness is a difficult task.

Wu and Carroll (1988) discuss a special type of nonignorable missingness that they call "informative dropout;" this special case has been studied by several authors. In particular, Wu and Carroll (1988), Wu and Bailey (1989), and Mori et al. (1992, 1994) propose methodology for estimating the rate of change of a continuous repeated outcome when the dropout mechanism is informative. This approach has been extended to generalized linear mixed models (Follmann and Wu, 1995) and to repeated count data (Albert and Follmann, 2000).

Other authors have considered other types of models that adjust for nonignorable missingness. These include the approaches of Stasny (1987), Conaway (1992, 1993, 1994), Dawson and Lagakos (1993), Diggle and Kenward (1994), Follmann et al. (1994), Cook and Lawless (1997), Molenberghs et al. (1997), and Albert (2000). Such methods for the analysis of repeated measurements when the missing-data mechanism is nonignorable are not yet available in standard statistical software packages.

As an alternative to parametrically modeling the dropout process, Verbeke et al. (2001) recommend the use of a sensitivity analysis based on local influence (Cook, 1986) to examine the potential effects of nonrandom dropout. Rotnitzky et al. (1998) also propose a procedure for carrying out a sensitivity analysis that examines how inferences concerning regression parameters change depending on assumptions about the nonresponse mechanism. Kenward (1998) provides an example illustrating the use of sensitivity analyses for repeated measurements. For normally distributed endpoints, Brown (1990) proposes a "protective" estimator that also does not require one to address the missingness model explicitly. Michiels and Molenberghs (1997) extend Brown's approach to repeated categorical outcomes with nonrandom dropout.

1.5 Sample Size Estimation

This book describes methods for the analysis of data when the response variable is measured repeatedly for each independent experimental unit. Although the design of repeated measurements studies is equally important, this is not, however, a focus of the following chapters.

One important issue in study design is estimating the sample size required to detect an effect of a given magnitude with specified power or to estimate the power with which an effect of a given magnitude can be detected using a specified sample size. When the outcome variable is measured once for each experimental unit, procedures for estimating sample size and power are well-known and widely applied. The corresponding situation for repeated measurements data, however, is less well-developed. The complexity is due both to the fact that repeated observations from the same experimental unit are correlated and also that the repeated measurements situation requires more assumptions and parameters to be specified.

Lefante (1990), Kirby et al. (1994), and Overall and Doyle (1994) consider sample size estimation when the focus is on hypotheses characterized in terms of a univariate summary statistic across the repeated measurements. These approaches are relevant to the methods of analysis presented in Chapter 2 of this book. Overall et al. (1998) compare the Kirby et al. (1994) and Overall and Doyle (1994) approaches, and Ahn et al. (2001) provide a computer program for sample size estimation.

Several sample size estimation methodologies are available when the response at each time point is normally distributed. These approaches are relevant to the methods of analysis discussed in Chapters 3–6 of this book.

Bloch (1986) and Lui and Cumberland (1992) describe methods for sample size estimation based on the univariate split-plot analysis-of-variance model. Vonesh and Schork (1986) and Rochon (1991) provide sample size estimation procedures based on Hotelling's T^2 statistic. Muller and Barton (1989) and Muller et al. (1992) consider sample size and power for the full multivariate analysis-of-variance model. Diggle et al. (1994, pp. 29–31) and Lindsey (2001) also discuss sample size estimation for normally distributed outcome variables.

Sample size estimation when the response variable at each time point is binary has also been studied; these approaches can be used in the situations discussed in Chapters 7–9 of this book. Lui (1991) and Shoukri and Martin (1992) extend the univariate split-plot model to the binary case. Lee and Dubin (1994) base their approach on the concept of the design effect from sample survey methodology. Rochon (1989) and Lipsitz and Fitzmaurice (1994) use weighted least squares procedures for sample size estimation with binary repeated measurements.

Approaches for estimation of sample size and power based on extensions of generalized linear model methodology to the repeated measurements situation are also available. These methods are useful in conjunction with the analysis approaches described in Chapter 9 of this book. Section 9.5.6 provides references and basic descriptions of the sample size estimation methods proposed by Liu and Liang (1997), Shih (1997), Rochon (1998), and Pan (2001b).

1.6 Outline of Topics

Many approaches to the analysis of repeated measurements have been proposed and studied. In addition, numerous books have been published dealing wholly or predominantly with the analysis of repeated measurements. Table 1.4 provides a listing of books that I am aware of that have their focus on statistical methodology for repeated measurements. Useful tutorials and articles reviewing methods for the analysis of repeated measurements include the papers by Everitt (1995), Cnaan et al. (1997), Albert (1999), and Omar et al. (1999). Diggle and Donnelly (1989) provide a selected bibliography on general methods for the analysis of repeated measurements.

Although I have found many of these other references to be quite useful, this book has a somewhat different purpose. Because it is often difficult to select, implement, and apply appropriate statistical methodology, I have sought to provide a broad survey of traditional and modern methods for the analysis of repeated measurements. Whereas some of the existing books are reasonably comprehensive in their coverage, others are more narrowly focused on specialized topics. This book is more comprehensive than many, and is targeted at a lower mathematical level and focused more on ap-

TABLE 1.4. Books focusing on methodology for repeated measurements

Crowder, M.J. and Hand, D.J. (1990). *Analysis of Repeated Measures.* Chapman and Hall, London.
Davidian, M. and Giltinan, D.M. (1995). *Nonlinear Models for Repeated Measurement Data.* Chapman and Hall, London.
Diggle, P.J. (1990). *Time Series: A Biostatistical Introduction.* Oxford University Press, New York.
Diggle, P.J. et al. (1994, 2002). *Analysis of Longitudinal Data.* Oxford University Press, Oxford.
Dwyer, J.H. et al. (1992). *Statistical Models for Longitudinal Studies of Health.* Oxford University Press, New York.
Fahrmeir, L. and Tutz, G. (2001). *Multivariate Statistical Modelling Based on Generalized Linear Models.* Springer-Verlag, New York.
Girden, E.R. (1992). *ANOVA: Repeated Measures.* Sage Publications, Newbury Park, CA.
Goldstein, H. (1979). *The Design and Analysis of Longitudinal Studies: Their Role in the Measurement of Change.* Academic Press, New York.
Hagenaars, J.A. (1990). *Categorical Longitudinal Data: Log-linear Panel, Trend, and Cohort Analysis.* Sage Publications, Newbury Park, CA.
Hand, D.J. and Crowder, M.J. (1996). *Practical Longitudinal Data Analysis.* Chapman and Hall, London.
Hand, D.J. and Taylor, C.C. (1987). *Multivariate Analysis of Variance and Repeated Measures.* Chapman and Hall, London.
Jones, R.H. (1993). *Longitudinal Data with Serial Correlation: A State-Space Approach.* Chapman and Hall, London.
Kshirsagar, A.M. and Smith, W.B. (1995). *Growth Curves.* Marcel Dekker, New York.
Lindsey, J.K. (1999). *Models for Repeated Measurements.* Oxford University Press, New York.
McCulloch, C.E. and Searle, S.R. (2000). *Generalized, Linear, and Mixed Models.* John Wiley and Sons, New York.
Müller, H.G. (1988). *Nonparametric Regression Analysis of Longitudinal Data.* Springer-Verlag, Berlin.
Nesselroade, J.R. and Baltes, P.B. (1980). *Longitudinal Methodology in the Study of Behavior and Development.* Academic Press, New York.
Pan, J.X. and Fang, K.T. (2001). *Growth Curve Models with Statistical Diagnostics.* Springer-Verlag, New York.
Pickles, A. (1990). *Longitudinal Data and the Analysis of Change.* Oxford University Press, New York.
Plewis, I. (1985). *Analysing Change: Measurement and Explanation Using Longitudinal Data.* John Wiley and Sons, New York.
Verbeke, G. and Molenberghs, G. (1997). *Linear Mixed Models in Practice.* Springer-Verlag, New York.
Verbeke, G. and Molenberghs, G. (2000). *Linear Mixed Models for Longitudinal Data.* Springer-Verlag, New York.
Vonesh, E.F. and Chinchilli, V.M. (1996). *Linear and Nonlinear Models for the Analysis of Repeated Measurements.* Marcel Dekker, New York.
von Eye, A. (1990). *Statistical Methods in Longitudinal Research. Volumes I and II.* Academic Press, New York.

plications than most. It is designed to be used both as a textbook in a semester-length course and also as a useful reference for statisticians and data analysts.

I have attempted to provide sufficient background material on the methods that are presented to ensure that students and readers will have a good understanding of the methodology. At the same time, the focus is on applying the approaches discussed to real data. Because of this, there are numerous examples in each chapter as well as homework problems at the end of each chapter.

The remaining chapters discuss methods for the analysis of repeated measurements when the response variable is

- continuous and normally distributed;
- categorical;
- continuous and nonnormal.

Note that categorical outcome variables include dichotomous responses, polytomous variables (more than two possible values, not necessarily ordered), ordered categorical responses, and count variables. For each type of outcome variable, methods that can be used in the following settings are discussed:

- one sample ($p = 0$);
- multiple samples (one categorical covariate);
- multiple samples (p categorical covariates);
- regression (quantitative covariates).

Chapter 2 first discusses some simple univariate approaches to the analysis of repeated measurements. These methods involve reducing the multiple measurements obtained from each subject to a single "derived variable" or "summary statistic." Chapters 3–6 discuss methods for normally distributed response variables. These chapters cover both traditional and modern approaches to the analysis of repeated measurements.

Chapter 7 then describes the weighted least squares approach for the analysis of categorical response variables. Chapter 8 presents the randomization model approach for the analysis of one-sample repeated measurements; this method can be applied both to categorical and continuous outcome variables. Chapter 9 describes extensions of generalized linear model methodology for the analysis of repeated measurements; these methods also can be used for categorical and continuous outcome variables. Finally, Chapter 10 discusses nonparametric methods for the analysis of repeated measurements.

1.7 Choosing the "Best" Method of Analysis

This book describes several methods for the analysis of repeated measurements. Although some are old and others are more recent, I have found all (with one exception to be mentioned later in this section) to be useful. Here are some guidelines for selecting an appropriate statistical method for a given application. Additional comments on the advantages and disadvantages of the various methods are provided in each chapter.

Chapter 2 discusses methods that reduce the vector of multiple measurements from each experimental unit to a single measurement. This approach avoids the issue of correlation among the repeated measurements from a subject and is often a useful preliminary or exploratory method of analysis. In situations where the distribution of the outcome variable is unusual, or where the sample size is too small or the number and pattern of repeated measurements are too irregular to permit the use of other methods, the univariate approach to the analysis of repeated measurements may be the only feasible one.

When the outcome variable at each time point is continuous and approximately normally distributed, the methods described in Chapters 3, 4, and 6 should be considered. Although Chapter 5 describes the use of classical repeated measures analysis of variance (ANOVA) for the analysis of continuous, normally distributed repeated measurements, I do not recommend the use of this methodology. I have included a short chapter on repeated measures ANOVA only because this approach is still widely used in some areas of application. Therefore, it is important to describe the restrictive assumptions and shortcomings of this methodology.

Chapter 6 discusses the linear mixed model, the most recent approach to the analysis of normally distributed repeated measurements. A natural question is whether the older multivariate analysis methods described in Chapters 3 and 4 are still necessary. First, the unstructured multivariate analysis approaches based on Hotelling's T^2 statistic, multivariate analysis of variance, and growth curve analysis are valid methods of analysis when repeated measurements are obtained at a fixed set of time points and there are no missing data. Second, the classical methods described in Chapters 3 and 4 are often based on fewer assumptions than are considered in practical applications of linear mixed model methodology. Third, because the unstructured multivariate analysis approaches are commonly used in some areas of application, familiarity with them is desirable. A final comment is that the simulation studies described in Section 6.5.3 indicate that the unstructured multivariate test statistics may perform better in small and moderate samples than the linear mixed model statistics. Thus, although the methods of Chapter 6 are important, the unstructured multivariate analysis approaches based on Hotelling's T^2 statistic, multivariate analysis of variance, and growth curve analysis are still often worthy of consideration.

When the outcome variable is categorical, the methods of Chapters 7–9 can be considered. Of these, the weighted least squares (WLS) methodology of Chapter 7 and the methods based on extensions of generalized linear model methodology (Chapter 9) are the most general approaches to the analysis of repeated categorical outcomes. Although some might argue that the methods of Chapter 9 are always to be preferred over the older WLS approach, the methods of Chapter 7 are quite useful when the number of repeated measurements is relatively small and all covariates are categorical. In particular, the WLS approach can be used for analyzing a wide variety of types of linear and nonlinear response functions and also provides a lack-of-fit statistic for assessing the appropriateness of the chosen model.

The methods described in Chapter 9 can also be used to analyze continuous repeated measurements when the marginal distribution at each time point is a member of the exponential family of distributions, such as the normal, gamma, and inverse Gaussian distributions. In particular, when the response is approximately normally distributed, the methods in Chapter 9 provide alternatives to the methods of Chapters 3–6 that may be more robust to departures from assumptions. Wu et al. (2001) discuss the relationships between the methods of Chapters 6 and 9 when the data are normally distributed.

Section 9.8 describes methods appropriate for the analysis of ordered categorical outcomes. These offer the advantage of being able to accommodate continuous covariates but require the restrictive proportional-odds assumption. The WLS approach (Chapter 7) can fit more flexible models to ordered categorical responses and also provides an overall goodness-of-fit test. The disadvantages are that covariates must be categorical and that the sample size must be quite large if any of (a) the number of levels of the response variable, (b) the number of time points, or (c) the number of levels of the cross-classification of the covariates is large.

Chapter 8 discusses the randomization model approach using Cochran–Mantel–Haenszel (CMH) statistics. This methodology requires minimal assumptions concerning the distribution of the response and can be used for both continuous and categorical outcomes. In addition, CMH statistics are applicable in situations where the sample size is too small to justify the use of alternative approaches. The major shortcoming of this method is that it is appropriate only for one-sample problems (i.e., when there are no covariates). In addition, the randomization model approach provides procedures for hypothesis testing only; it is not possible to estimate the parameters of a model.

When the response variable is continuous but nonnormal, nonparametric approaches (Chapter 10) may be the only reasonable option other than the summary-statistic approach. In this case, the Chapter 10 approaches allow one to consider the multivariate nature of the data rather than reducing the multiple responses to a summary measure. The shortcomings include the lack of estimation procedures and the fact that the repeated measurements nature of the data is not fully taken into account.

2
Univariate Methods

2.1 Introduction

The simplest approach to the analysis of repeated measurements is to reduce the vector of multiple measurements from each experimental unit to a single measurement. Thus, a multivariate response is reduced to a univariate response. This avoids the issue of correlation among the repeated measurements from a subject. In the special case of two measurements per subject, well-known methods of this type include the paired t test for continuous responses and McNemar's test for dichotomous responses.

Wishart (1938) appears to have been the first researcher to document the use of this approach. Pocock (1983), Matthews et al. (1990), Dawson and Lagakos (1991, 1993) , Frison and Pocock (1992), and Dawson (1994) refer to these types of methods as the "summary-statistic approach." Crowder and Hand (1990) and Diggle et al. (1994) call such methods "response feature analysis" and "derived variable analysis," respectively. When the univariate summary statistic is the least squares regression slope, this approach has been referred to as the "NIH method," because the use of this particular summary statistic appears to have been popularized at the U.S. National Institutes of Health.

The univariate approach to the analysis of repeated measurements is most applicable when complete data at a common set of measurement times are obtained from each subject. This approach is most straightforward when the data come from a single sample (as displayed in Table 1.3) or

TABLE 2.1. Ventilation volumes from eight subjects

	Temperature (°C)					
Subject	−10	25	37	50	65	80
1	74.5	81.5	83.6	68.6	73.1	79.4
2	75.5	84.6	70.6	87.3	73.0	75.0
3	68.9	71.6	55.9	61.9	60.5	61.8
4	57.0	61.3	54.1	59.2	56.6	58.8
5	78.3	84.9	64.0	62.2	60.1	78.7
6	54.0	62.8	63.0	58.0	56.0	51.5
7	72.5	68.3	67.8	71.5	65.0	67.7
8	80.8	89.9	83.2	83.0	85.7	79.6

from multiple samples defined by the levels of one or more categorical covariates (as displayed in Table 1.2).

2.2 One Sample

We first consider the situation in which repeated measurements are obtained (or scheduled to be obtained) at t time points from each of n subjects, as displayed in Table 1.3. The goal of the analysis is to determine whether the distribution of the response is changing over time.

One approach to this problem would be to carry out separate comparisons between pairs of time points. For example, if the response variable is continuous and normally distributed, multiple paired t tests could be performed. For nonnormal responses, the Wilcoxon signed rank test or the sign test could be used instead. With t time points, $t(t-1)/2$ tests are required. These test statistics are correlated due to the dependence between repeated measurements for each subject and the fact that the data from each time point are used in multiple tests. Thus, this method is not recommended.

If instead the summary-statistic approach is used, the goal is to reduce each subject's data to a single meaningful measure of association between the response variable and time. For example, the summary statistic could be the slope of the regression line for each subject or a parametric or nonparametric correlation coefficient. Appropriate statistical methods can then be used to test whether the mean (or median) of the derived measure differs from zero. This approach is often useful even when the repeated measurements are irregularly spaced. One must realize, however, that the results of the summary-statistic approach may be misleading if the selected summary measure does not adequately describe each subject's data.

As an example, Table 2.1 displays data from Deal et al. (1979). In this study, ventilation volumes (l/min) were measured in eight subjects under six different temperatures of inspired dry air. The goal of the analysis is to

TABLE 2.2. Estimated slopes for ventilation volume data

Subject	Slope	Signed Rank
1	−0.00916	−2
2	−0.02009	−4
3	−0.10439	−7
4	0.00443	1
5	−0.12029	−8
6	−0.03838	−5
7	−0.05672	−6
8	−0.01336	−3

determine whether ventilation volume is affected by temperature.

One approach would be to assume that the relationship between temperature and ventilation volume for each subject can be adequately summarized by the slope of the least squares regression line. Let x_{ij} and y_{ij} denote the temperature and ventilation volume, respectively, on the jth occasion for the ith subject, for $j = 1, \ldots, 6$ and $i = 1, \ldots, 8$. The estimated slope for subject i is

$$\widehat{\beta}_i = \frac{\sum_{j=1}^{6}(x_{ij} - \overline{x}_i)(y_{ij} - \overline{y}_i)}{\sum_{j=1}^{6}(x_{ij} - \overline{x}_i)^2} = \frac{\sum_{j=1}^{6}(x_{ij} - \overline{x}_i)y_{ij}}{\sum_{j=1}^{6}(x_{ij} - \overline{x}_i)^2},$$

where $\overline{x}_i$ and $\overline{y}_i$ are the sample means of temperature and ventilation volume, respectively, for subject i. For each subject, $\overline{x}_i = 41.167$ and

$$\sum_{j=1}^{6}(x_{ij} - \overline{x}_i)^2 = 5050.83.$$

Therefore, $\widehat{\beta}_i = \sum_{j=1}^{6} w_i y_{ij}$, where $w_1 = -0.010130$, $w_2 = -0.003201$, $w_3 = -0.000825$, $w_4 = 0.001749$, $w_5 = 0.004719$, and $w_6 = 0.007688$. Thus, the summary statistic $\widehat{\beta}_i$ is seen to be a weighted sum of the responses y_{ij}.

Table 2.2 displays the estimated slopes for each of the eight subjects as well as the signed ranks of these slopes. The sample mean and standard deviation of the slopes are −0.04475 and 0.04586, respectively. Assuming that the estimated slopes are approximately normally distributed, the one-sample t test yields

$$t = \frac{\sqrt{8}(-0.04475 - 0)}{0.04586} = -2.76$$

with seven degrees of freedom (df). The two-sided p-value is 0.028, indicating that the population mean slope is significantly different from zero. Alternatively, the Wilcoxon signed rank test gives an exact two-sided p-value of 0.032.

TABLE 2.3. Estimated Spearman correlation coefficients for ventilation volume data

	Temperature (°C)						
Subject	−10	25	37	50	65	80	r_s
1	3	5	6	1	2	4	−0.257
2	4	5	1	6	2	3	−0.257
3	5	6	1	4	2	3	−0.543
4	3	6	1	5	2	4	−0.086
5	4	6	3	2	1	5	−0.314
6	2	5	6	4	3	1	−0.371
7	6	4	3	5	1	2	−0.771
8	2	6	4	3	5	1	−0.257

As an alternative to using the least square regression slope as the summary statistic, one could make the weaker assumption that the relationship between temperature and ventilation volume is monotonic. Table 2.3 displays the within-subject ranks of ventilation volume as well as the values of Spearman's rank correlation coefficient r_s for each subject. The values of r_s are negative for all eight subjects. The exact two-sided p-value from the Wilcoxon signed rank statistic is 0.008, and the two-sided exact sign test yields $p = 0.0078$. All of these analyses indicate that ventilation volume tends to decrease as temperature increases.

Another example of the usefulness of the summary-statistic approach uses data from a study at the University of Iowa Mental Health Clinical Research Center in which 44 schizophrenic patients participated in a four-week antipsychotic medication washout. The severity of extrapyramidal side effects was assessed just prior to discontinuation of antipsychotic medication and at weeks 1, 2, 3, and 4 during the washout period. Because these types of side effects frequently accompany the use of antipsychotic medications, the investigators were interested in determining whether such symptoms improve during washout. Arndt et al. (1993) further describe the study.

Table 2.4 displays the resulting ratings on the Simpson–Angus (SA) scale (Simpson and Angus, 1970). The SA scale rates ten aspects (e.g., elbow rigidity, arm dropping) from 0 to 4 (normal to extremely symptomatic) and yields a total score ranging from 0 to 40. High scores indicate greater symptom severity. The character '.' is used to denote a few missing values in Table 2.4.

Figure 2.1 displays modified box plots (Moore and McCabe, 1993, pp. 42–43) of the weekly SA ratings. At each time point, the first quartile (25th percentile), median, third quartile (75th percentile), and sample mean (denoted by $\times$) are displayed. Data points more than 1.5 times the interquartile range beyond the quartiles are displayed individually ($*$); otherwise,

TABLE 2.4. Weekly Simpson–Angus ratings from 44 schizophrenic patients

Patient	Week 0	Week 1	Week 2	Week 3	Week 4
1	1	4	0	0	0
2	4	5	8	9	3
3	1	2	2	1	1
4	8	7	0	5	5
5	1	1	0	1	1
6	3	2	0	0	0
7	4	4	4	.	2
8	.	.	1	9	6
9	6	6	0	0	0
10	3	3	0	0	0
11	6	4	1	0	0
12	0	0	0	0	.
13	3	0	17	5	22
14	8	1	2	2	0
15	0	0	0	0	0
16	0	0	5	1	2
17	1	5	4	5	2
18	2	1	.	.	.
19	0	0	0	0	0
20	0	0	6	8	5
21	0	0	0	0	.
22	11	12	0	0	0
23	10	6	0	0	1
24	3	0	2	1	1
25	1	0	1	1	0
26	0	5	0	2	4
27	0	0	0	.	.
28	3	0	0	0	.
29	7	7	3	4	5
30	12	22	15	24	5
31	3	0	0	0	0
32	0	0	0	0	0
33	1	0	0	0	0
34	0	0	0	0	0
35	7	1	10	7	5
36	2	0	0	1	0
37	10	5	5	8	2
38	2	0	4	0	1
39	5	2	1	3	2
40	0	0	0	.	.
41	1	1	0	1	3
42	0	0	0	0	.
43	0	0	0	0	0
44	1	0	2	1	1

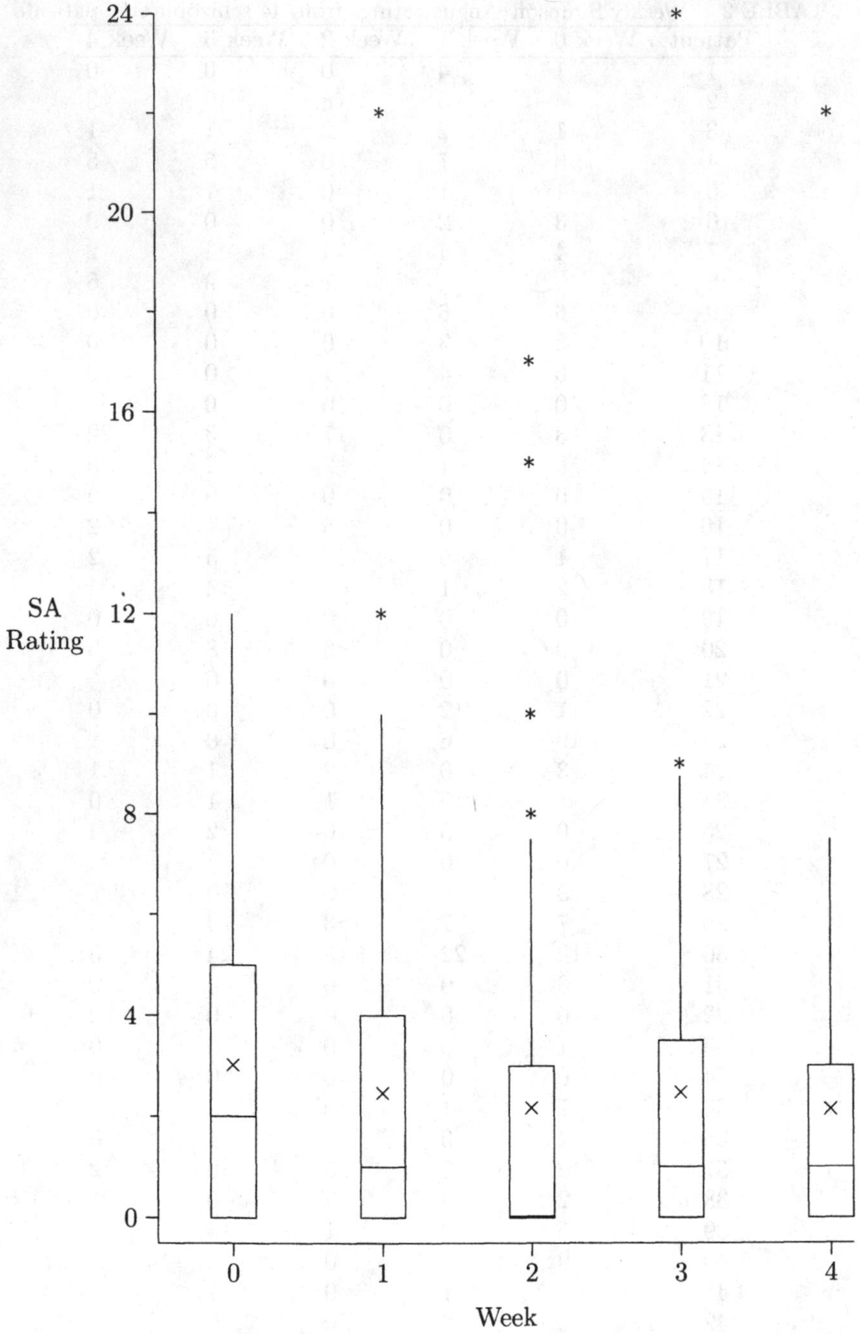

FIGURE 2.1. Modified box plots of weekly Simpson–Angus ratings for 44 schizophrenic patients

the upper and lower limits of each plot extend to the largest and smallest observations.

The marginal distributions of the SA ratings are clearly nonnormal. At each time point, both the minimum value and the 25th percentile are equal to zero, as is the median at week 2. The median SA ratings at weeks 0–4 are 2, 1, 0, 1, and 1, respectively. The mean ratings of 3.0, 2.5, 2.2, 2.5, and 2.1 also indicate a tendency for SA ratings to decrease following the withdrawal of antipsychotic medications.

The summary-statistic approach is one possible method of assessing whether there is an association between SA ratings and measurement week. In this example, the least squares slope is not likely to be a useful summary statistic. When the Spearman rank correlation coefficient between SA rating and week is computed for each subject, the correlation coefficients range from -1 to 0.8. Of the 32 nonzero correlations, eight are positive and 24 are negative. Based on the sign test, the exact two-sided p-value is 0.007. Using the Wilcoxon signed rank test, the sum of the ranks corresponding to positive correlations is 103 and the sum of the ranks of negative correlations is 425. The normal approximation to the distribution of the Wilcoxon statistic yields $p = 0.003$. Both tests indicate the tendency of SA ratings to decrease over time.

Although most of the subjects in Table 2.4 have observations at all five measurement times, there are eight subjects with missing data. Four subjects have four of the five measurements, three subjects have three of the five measurements, and one subject has only two measurements. As an alternative to weighting the individual Spearman correlation coefficients equally, one could consider giving lower weight to those from subjects with missing data.

2.3 Multiple Samples

Table 1.2 displays the general layout for the case of repeated measurements from multiple samples. In this setting, y_{hij} is the response at time point j for subject i in group h for $h = 1, \ldots, s$, $i = 1, \ldots, n_h$, and $j = 1, \ldots, t$. Within-group comparisons among time points might be of interest. In this case, the methods of Section 2.2 can be used. A more common goal of the analysis in this setting, however, is to determine whether the pattern of change over time is the same across the s groups.

One approach to this problem would be to carry out separate comparisons among groups at each of the t time points. For example, if the response variable was continuous and normally distributed, one-way analysis of variance (ANOVA) could be used to compare the groups at each measurement occasion. For nonnormal responses, the Kruskal–Wallis test could be used. If the response at each time point is categorical, Pearson's chi-square test

TABLE 2.5. Body weights of 16 rats

	Day										
ID	1	8	15	22	29	36	43	44	50	57	64
Group 1:											
1	240	250	255	260	262	258	266	266	265	272	278
2	225	230	230	232	240	240	243	244	238	247	245
3	245	250	250	255	262	265	267	267	264	268	269
4	260	255	255	265	265	268	270	272	274	273	275
5	255	260	255	270	270	273	274	273	276	278	280
6	260	265	270	275	275	277	278	278	284	279	281
7	275	275	260	270	273	274	276	271	282	281	284
8	245	255	260	268	270	265	265	267	273	274	278
Group 2:											
9	410	415	425	428	438	443	442	446	456	468	478
10	405	420	430	440	448	460	458	464	475	484	496
11	445	445	450	452	455	455	451	450	462	466	472
12	555	560	565	580	590	597	595	595	612	618	628
Group 3:											
13	470	465	475	485	487	493	493	504	507	518	525
14	535	525	530	533	535	540	525	530	543	544	559
15	520	525	530	540	543	546	538	544	553	555	548
16	510	510	520	515	530	538	535	542	550	553	569

of homogeneity would be appropriate. The primary disadvantage of this type of univariate analysis approach is that t separate tests are required.

If instead the summary-statistic approach is used, the goal is to first reduce each subject's data to a single, meaningful measure of association between the response variable and time, as in Section 2.2. In the multiple-sample case, parametric or nonparametric methods can then be used to test for differences among the s groups.

For example, Table 2.5 displays data from a nutrition study conducted in three groups of rats (Crowder and Hand, 1990, p. 19). The three groups were put on different diets, and each animal's body weight (grams) was recorded repeatedly (approximately weekly) over a nine-week period. The goal of the analysis is to determine whether the growth profiles of the three groups differ.

One approach would be to assume that the relationship between body weight and measurement time can be adequately summarized by the slope of the least squares regression line. Let x_{ij} and y_{ij} denote the measurement day and body weight, respectively, on the jth occasion for the ith animal, for $j = 1, \ldots, 11$ and $i = 1, \ldots, 16$. The estimated slope for the ith animal

TABLE 2.6. Estimated slopes for rat body weight data

Group	ID	Slope	Group	ID	Slope
1	1	0.484	2	9	1.011
	2	0.330		10	1.341
	3	0.398		11	0.363
	4	0.330		12	1.148
	5	0.406	3	13	0.919
	6	0.318		14	0.315
	7	0.202		15	0.493
	8	0.409		16	0.905

is

$$\widehat{\beta}_i = \frac{\sum_{j=1}^{11}(x_{ij} - \overline{x}_i)(y_{ij} - \overline{y}_i)}{\sum_{j=1}^{11}(x_{ij} - \overline{x}_i)^2} = \frac{\sum_{j=1}^{11}(x_{ij} - \overline{x}_i)y_{ij}}{\sum_{j=1}^{11}(x_{ij} - \overline{x}_i)^2},$$

where $\overline{x}_i$ and $\overline{y}_i$ are the sample means of x and y for animal i. Note that $\overline{x}_i = 33.545$ and

$$\sum_{j=1}^{11}(x_{ij} - \overline{x}_i)^2 = 4162.73$$

for $i = 1, \ldots, 16$. Therefore, $\widehat{\beta}_i = \sum_{j=1}^{11} w_i y_{ij}$, where

$$\begin{aligned}
w_1 &= -0.007818, & w_7 &= 0.002271,\\
w_2 &= -0.006137, & w_8 &= 0.002511,\\
w_3 &= -0.004455, & w_9 &= 0.003953,\\
w_4 &= -0.002774, & w_{10} &= 0.005634,\\
w_5 &= -0.001092, & w_{11} &= 0.007316.\\
w_6 &= 0.000590, & &
\end{aligned}$$

Table 2.6 displays the estimated slopes for each animal; these slopes are positive for all animals in each of the three groups. The sample means of the slopes in groups 1, 2, and 3 are 0.3596, 0.9655, and 0.6580, respectively, indicating that the rate of weight gain is, on average, greatest in group 2 and least in group 1. The corresponding sample standard deviations are 0.0845, 0.4242, and 0.3022.

One possible method of analysis is to compare the three groups using one-way ANOVA. The resulting F statistic with 2 and 13 df is 7.57 ($p = 0.007$). Because the assumptions of the one-way ANOVA model may not be satisfied, the Kruskal–Wallis test could also be used to compare the distributions of the estimated slopes in the three groups. This test gives a chi-square statistic of 5.80 with 2 df ($p = 0.055$). The parametric analysis indicates that the mean slopes in the three groups differ significantly; the nonparametric test gives a nearly significant result.

TABLE 2.7. Successive two-week seizure counts: first ten subjects in each of the two treatment groups

Treatment	ID	Week 2	Week 4	Week 6	Week 8
Progabide	101	11	14	9	8
	102	8	7	9	4
	103	0	4	3	0
	108	3	6	1	3
	110	2	6	7	4
	111	4	3	1	3
	112	22	17	19	16
	113	5	4	7	4
	117	2	4	0	4
	121	3	7	7	7
Placebo	104	5	3	3	3
	106	3	5	3	3
	107	2	4	0	5
	114	4	4	1	4
	116	7	18	9	21
	118	5	2	8	7
	123	6	4	0	2
	126	40	20	23	12
	130	5	6	6	5
	135	14	13	6	0

As a second example, Leppik et al. (1987) conducted a clinical trial in 59 epileptic subjects. In this study, individuals suffering from simple or complex partial seizures were randomized to receive either the antiepileptic drug progabide (31 subjects) or a placebo (28 subjects). At each of four successive postrandomization visits, the number of seizures occurring during the previous two weeks was reported. The medical question of interest is whether progabide reduces the frequency of epileptic seizures.

Table 2.7 displays the seizure counts during the successive two-week periods from the first ten subjects in each of the two groups. These data were obtained from Thall and Vail (1990). Figure 2.2 displays side-by-side modified box plots (Moore and McCabe, 1993, pp. 42–43) for the two treatments at each assessment time. The sample means in the progabide and placebo groups are denoted by filled and open circles, respectively. During each two-week period, there appears to be a slight tendency for seizure counts to be lower in progabide-treated patients than in placebo-treated patients. The median number of seizures in the progabide group at weeks 2, 4, 6, and 8 is 4, 5, 4, and 4, respectively. The corresponding medians in the placebo group are 5, 4.5, 5, and 5, respectively.

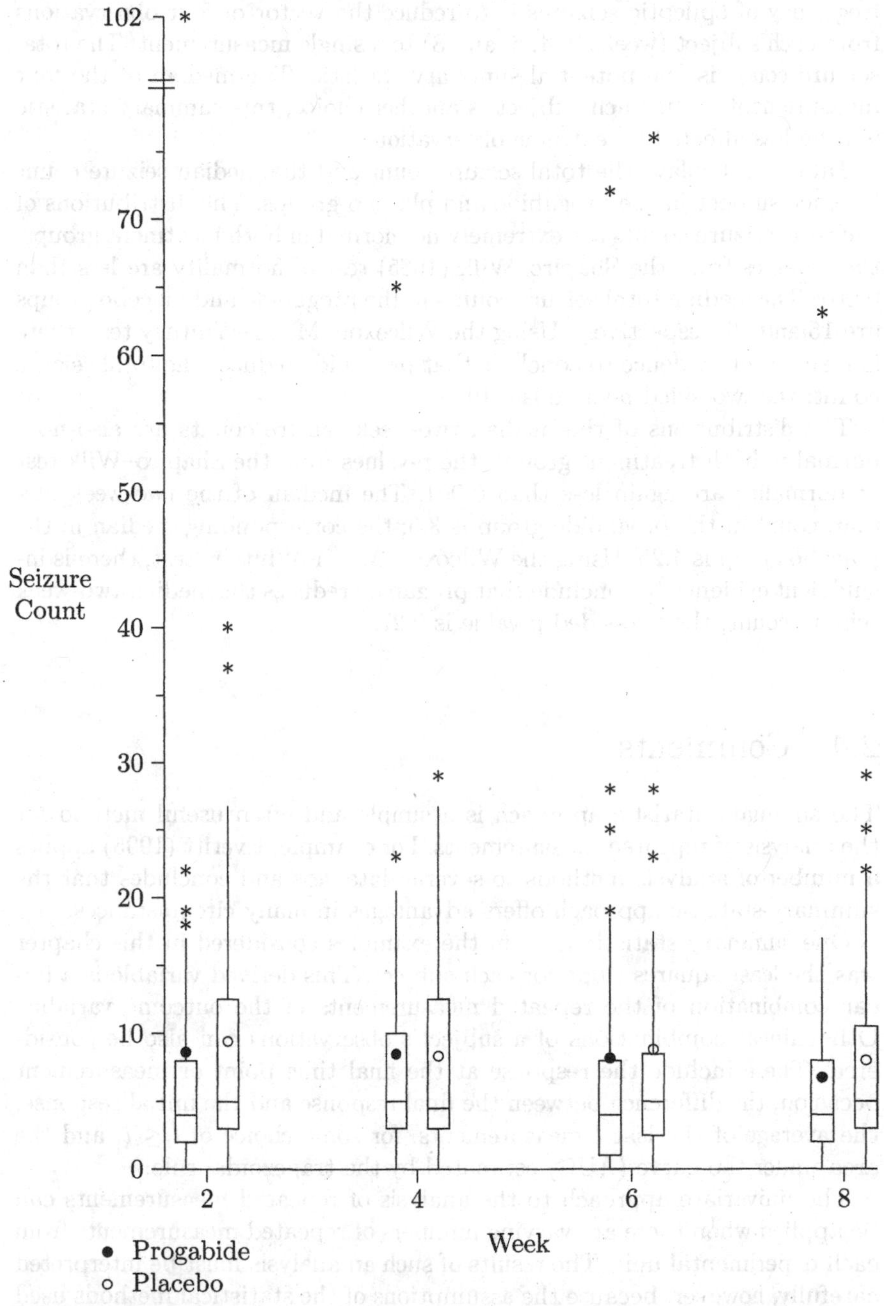

FIGURE 2.2. Modified box plots of successive two-week seizure counts for 59 subjects with epilepsy

One possible approach to determining whether progabide reduces the frequency of epileptic seizures is to reduce the vector of four observations from each subject (weeks 2, 4, 6, and 8) to a single measurement. The total seizure count is one potential summary statistic. The median of the four measurements from each subject is another choice; this summary statistic will be less affected by extreme observations.

Table 2.8 displays the total seizure count and the median seizure count for each subject in the progabide and placebo groups. The distributions of the total seizure counts are extremely nonnormal in both treatment groups; the p-values from the Shapiro–Wilk (1965) test of normality are less than 0.001. The median total seizure counts in the progabide and placebo groups are 15 and 16, respectively. Using the Wilcoxon–Mann–Whitney test, there is insufficient evidence to conclude that progabide reduces the total seizure count; the two-sided p-value is 0.19.

The distributions of the median two-week seizure counts are also nonnormal in both treatment groups; the p-values from the Shapiro–Wilk test of normality are again less than 0.001. The median of the two-week median count in the progabide group is 3.5; the corresponding median in the placebo group is 4.25. Using the Wilcoxon–Mann–Whitney test, there is insufficient evidence to conclude that progabide reduces the median two-week seizure count; the two-sided p-value is 0.27.

2.4 Comments

The summary-statistic approach is a simple and often useful method for the analysis of repeated measurements. For example, Everitt (1995) applies a number of analysis methods to several data sets and concludes that the summary-statistic approach offers advantages in many circumstances.

One summary statistic used in the examples considered in this chapter was the least squares slope for each subject. This derived variable is a linear combination of the repeated measurements of the outcome variable. Other linear combinations of a subject's observations can also be considered. These include the response at the final time point or measurement occasion, the difference between the final response and the initial response, the average of the last l measurements, for some choice of $l \leq t$, and the area under the curve (AUC) estimated by the trapezoidal rule.

The univariate approach to the analysis of repeated measurements can be applied when there are varying numbers of repeated measurements from each experimental unit. The results of such an analysis must be interpreted carefully, however, because the assumptions of the statistical methods used in making comparisons among groups may not be satisfied when each experimental unit does not contribute the same number and pattern of measurements. In this case, one approach that can be considered is to carry out

TABLE 2.8. Total and median seizure counts from 31 subjects in the progabide group and 28 subjects in the placebo group

Group	ID	Total	Median	ID	Total	Median
Progabide	101	42	10.0	143	39	7.0
	102	28	7.5	147	7	1.5
	103	7	1.5	203	32	8.0
	108	13	3.0	204	3	0.5
	110	19	5.0	207	302	68.5
	111	11	3.0	208	13	3.5
	112	74	18.0	209	26	6.5
	113	20	4.5	211	10	2.0
	117	10	3.0	214	70	15.5
	121	24	7.0	218	13	3.5
	122	29	4.5	221	15	3.5
	124	4	1.0	225	51	13.5
	128	6	1.0	228	6	1.5
	129	12	3.5	232	0	0.0
	137	65	14.5	236	10	2.5
	139	26	6.5			
Placebo	104	14	3.0	205	59	13.0
	106	14	3.0	206	16	2.5
	107	11	3.0	210	6	1.5
	114	13	4.0	213	123	29.0
	116	55	13.5	215	15	4.0
	118	22	6.0	217	16	4.5
	123	12	3.0	219	14	3.5
	126	95	21.5	220	14	3.5
	130	22	5.5	222	13	3.0
	135	33	9.5	226	30	8.0
	141	66	17.0	227	143	24.5
	145	30	7.0	230	6	1.5
	201	16	4.0	234	10	2.5
	202	42	10.5	238	53	13.0

a weighted analysis of the summary statistics. Matthews (1993) studies the use of a weighted summary-statistic approach in the context of an example in which the number of repeated measurements per subject ranges from 4 to 36.

Although the univariate approach can be useful in certain situations, a shortcoming is that the results may be misleading if the selected univariate summary measure does not adequately describe each subject's data. Ghosh et al. (1973) describe multivariate methods based on the use of two or more summary statistics for each subject. This extension of the univariate summary-statistic approach may be useful when multiple univariate statistics are necessary to adequately summarize each subject's data. Carr et al. (1989) describe a different type of multivariate approach based on summary statistics. They consider the situation in which an ordered categorical or interval response variable is measured at multiple time points for each subject in two or more ordered groups. Rank measures of association between group and response are constructed at each time point; the estimated covariance matrix of these summary measures is then used to test hypotheses concerning the rank measures of association.

2.5 Problems

In each of the following problems: (a) describe and justify your choice of statistical methodology; (b) present your results, along with documentation of how they were obtained; (c) state your conclusions and provide any necessary comments on their limitations and significance.

2.1 Table 2.9 displays data from a study to test whether pH alters action potential characteristics following administration of a drug. The response variable of interest (V_{max}) was measured at up to four pH levels for each of 25 subjects. Test the null hypothesis that there is no relationship between pH and V_{max}.

2.2 Forty male subjects were randomly assigned to one of two treatment groups. Each patient had his BPRS factor measured before treatment (week 0) and at weekly intervals for eight weeks. Table 2.10 displays the resulting data. Test whether the BPRS response profiles are the same for the two treatments using an appropriate summary statistic.

2.3 Kenward (1987) describes an experiment to compare two treatments for controlling intestinal parasites in calves. There were 30 calves in each of the two groups, and the weight of each calf was determined at 11 measurement times. Table 2.11 displays the data from the first ten calves in each group. Use an appropriate summary statistic to compare the two treatments.

TABLE 2.9. Effect of pH on action potential characteristics in 25 subjects

	pH Level			
Subject	6.5	6.9	7.4	7.9
1		284	310	326
2			261	292
3		213	224	240
4		222	235	247
5			270	286
6			210	218
7		216	234	237
8		236	273	283
9	220	249	270	281
10	166	218	244	
11	227	258	282	286
12	216		284	
13			257	284
14	204	234	268	
15			258	267
16		193	224	235
17	185	222	252	263
18		238	301	300
19		198	240	
20		235	255	
21		216	238	
22		197	212	219
23		234	238	
24			295	281
25			261	272

TABLE 2.10. BPRS measurements from 40 subjects

		Week								
Treatment	Subject	0	1	2	3	4	5	6	7	8
1	1	42	39	36	43	41	40	38	47	41
	2	58	68	61	55	43	34	28	28	28
	3	54	55	41	38	43	28	29	25	24
	4	55	77	49	54	56	50	47	42	46
	5	72	75	72	65	50	39	32	38	32
	6	48	43	41	38	36	29	33	27	25
	7	71	61	47	30	27	40	30	31	31
	8	30	36	38	38	31	26	26	25	24
	9	41	43	39	35	28	22	20	23	21
	10	57	51	51	55	53	43	43	39	32
	11	30	34	34	41	36	36	38	36	36
	12	55	52	49	54	48	43	37	36	31
	13	36	32	36	31	25	25	21	19	22
	14	38	35	36	34	25	27	25	26	26
	15	66	68	65	49	36	32	27	30	37
	16	41	35	45	42	31	31	29	26	30
	17	45	38	46	38	40	33	27	31	27
	18	39	35	27	25	29	28	21	25	20
	19	24	28	31	28	29	21	22	23	22
	20	38	34	27	25	25	27	21	19	21
2	1	52	73	42	41	39	38	43	62	50
	2	30	23	32	24	20	20	19	18	20
	3	65	31	33	28	22	25	24	31	32
	4	37	31	27	31	31	26	24	26	23
	5	59	67	58	61	49	38	37	36	35
	6	30	33	37	33	28	26	27	23	21
	7	69	52	41	33	34	37	37	38	35
	8	62	54	49	39	55	51	55	59	66
	9	38	40	38	27	31	24	22	21	21
	10	65	44	31	34	39	34	41	42	39
	11	78	95	75	76	66	64	64	60	75
	12	38	41	36	27	29	27	21	22	23
	13	63	65	60	53	52	32	37	52	28
	14	40	37	31	38	35	30	33	30	27
	15	40	36	55	55	42	30	26	30	37
	16	54	45	35	27	25	22	22	22	22
	17	33	41	30	32	46	43	43	43	43
	18	28	30	29	33	30	26	36	33	30
	19	52	43	26	27	24	32	21	21	21
	20	47	36	32	29	25	23	23	23	23

TABLE 2.11. Weights of 60 calves at 11 measurement times: first ten animals in each group

		Week										
Trt.	ID	0	2	4	6	8	10	12	14	16	18	19
1	1	233	224	245	258	271	287	287	287	290	293	297
	2	231	238	260	273	290	300	311	313	317	321	326
	3	232	237	245	265	285	298	304	319	317	334	329
	4	239	246	268	288	308	309	327	324	327	336	341
	5	215	216	239	264	282	299	307	321	328	332	337
	6	236	226	242	255	263	277	290	299	300	308	310
	7	219	229	246	265	279	292	299	299	298	300	290
	8	231	245	270	292	302	321	322	334	323	337	337
	9	230	228	243	255	272	276	277	289	289	300	303
	10	232	240	247	263	275	286	294	302	308	319	326
2	1	210	215	230	244	259	266	277	292	292	290	264
	2	230	240	258	277	277	293	300	323	327	340	343
	3	226	233	248	277	297	313	322	340	354	365	362
	4	233	239	253	277	292	310	318	333	336	353	338
	5	238	241	262	282	300	314	319	331	338	348	338
	6	225	228	237	261	271	288	300	316	319	333	330
	7	224	225	239	257	268	290	304	313	310	318	318
	8	237	241	255	276	293	307	312	336	336	344	328
	9	237	224	234	239	256	266	276	300	302	293	269
	10	233	239	259	283	294	313	320	347	348	362	352

TABLE 2.12. Body weights of 27 rats

Group	Rat	Week 0	1	2	3	4
Control	1	57	86	114	139	172
	2	60	93	123	146	177
	3	52	77	111	144	185
	4	49	67	100	129	164
	5	56	81	104	121	151
	6	46	70	102	131	153
	7	51	71	94	110	141
	8	63	91	112	130	154
	9	49	67	90	112	140
	10	57	82	110	139	169
Thyroxin	1	59	85	121	146	181
	2	54	71	90	110	138
	3	56	75	108	151	189
	4	59	85	116	148	177
	5	57	72	97	120	144
	6	52	73	97	116	140
	7	52	70	105	138	171
Thiouracil	1	61	86	109	120	129
	2	59	80	101	111	122
	3	53	79	100	106	133
	4	59	88	100	111	122
	5	51	75	101	123	140
	6	51	75	92	100	119
	7	56	78	95	103	108
	8	58	69	93	116	140
	9	46	61	78	90	107
	10	53	72	89	104	122

2.4 Box (1950) describes an experiment in which 30 rats were randomly assigned to three treatment groups. Group 1 was a control group, group 2 had thyroxin added to their drinking water, and group 3 had thiouracil added to their drinking water. Whereas there were ten rats in each of groups 1 and 3, group 2 consisted of only seven rats (due to an unspecified accident at the beginning of the experiment). The body weights of each of the 27 rats were recorded at the beginning of the experiment and at weekly intervals for four weeks, as shown in Table 2.12. Test for differences among the three groups using an appropriate summary statistic.

2.5 Table 2.13 displays data from 27 patients involved in a pilot study for a new treatment for AIDS (Thompson, 1991). Three variables (TMHR scores, Karnofsky scores, and T-4 cell counts) were measured at baseline and at 90 and 180 days after the beginning of treatment. For each variable, test whether the treatment has an effect over time.

2.6 In an investigation of the effects of various dosages of radiation therapy on psychomotor skills (Danford et al., 1960), 45 cancer patients were trained to operate a psychomotor testing device. Six patients were not given radiation and served as controls, whereas the remainder were treated with dosages of 25–50 R, 75–100 R, or 125–250 R. Table 2.14 displays the psychomotor test scores on the three days following radiation treatment. Test for differences among the four groups using an appropriate summary statistic.

2.7 In a study of the association of hyperglycemia and relative hyperinsulinemia, standard glucose tolerance tests were administered to three groups of subjects: 13 controls, 12 nonhyperinsulinemic obese patients, and 8 hyperinsulinemic obese patients (Zerbe, 1979b; Zerbe and Murphy, 1986). Table 2.15 displays plasma inorganic phosphate measurements obtained from blood samples drawn 0, 0.5, 1, 1.5, 2, 3, 4, and 5 hours after a standard-dose oral glucose challenge. Test for differences among the three groups using an appropriate summary statistic.

2.8 Sixty female rats were randomly assigned to one of four dosages of a drug (control, low dose, medium dose, or high dose). The body weight of each animal, in grams, was recorded at week 0 (just prior to initiation of treatment) and at weekly intervals for 9 weeks. Table 2.16 displays the data from the first five animals in each group. Test for differences among the four dosage groups using an appropriate summary statistic.

2.9 In the Iowa Cochlear Implant Project, the effectiveness of two types of cochlear implants was studied in profoundly and bilaterally deaf patients. In one group of 23 subjects, the "type A" implant was used. A second group of 21 subjects received the "type B" implant. In both groups, the electrode array was surgically implanted five to six weeks prior to electrical connection to the external speech processor. A sentence test was then administered at 1, 9, 18, and 30 months after connection. The outcome variable of interest at each time point was the percentage of correct scores. Table 2.17 displays the resulting data, which were originally analyzed by Núñez Antón (1993). Test for a difference between the two implant types using an appropriate summary statistic.

2.10 Davis (1991) discusses a clinical trial comparing two treatments for maternal pain relief during labor. In this study, 83 women in labor were randomized to receive an experimental pain medication (43 subjects) or placebo (40 subjects). Treatment was initiated when the cervical dilation was 8 cm. At 30-minute intervals, the amount of pain was self-reported by placing a mark on a 100-mm line (0 = no pain, 100 = very much pain). Table 2.18 displays the data from the first 20 subjects in each group. Test

TABLE 2.13. Measurements at days 0, 90, and 180 from a pilot study of a new treatment for AIDS

	TMHR Scores			Karnofsky Scores			T-4 Cell Counts		
ID	0	90	180	0	90	180	0	90	180
1	7.25	1.5	2.50	70	90	100	285	406	199
2	7.50	1.0	1.00	70	90	100	234	227	384
3	2.00	0.0	0.00	90	100	100	629	724	731
4	7.00	2.5	3.50	50	90	90	39	43	64
5	3.00	1.5	2.50	90	100	100	266	323	367
6	4.50	2.5	2.50	80	90	100	84	70	53
7	6.00	1.5	1.00	60	90	100	178	211	157
8	1.75	1.5	2.00	100	100	100	1076	1184	678
9	7.00	5.0	5.00	90	90	80	17	4	2
10	6.25	3.5	4.75	80	80	90	33	9	1
11	11.00	4.5	4.00	50	80	80	41	24	33
12	9.50	4.5	4.00	60	80	80	138	186	61
13	3.25	0.5	0.00	80	100	100	677	687	561
14	2.00	0.5	0.00	80	100	100	554	696	653
15	2.00	0.5	0.50	80	90	100	375	215	308
16	7.50	1.5	1.50	90	100	100	206	191	243
17	6.50	2.0	2.00	80	90	100	35	53	38
18	6.50	3.0	4.50	50	70	80	53	17	11
19	4.75	1.0	0.50	90	100	100	500	578	462
20	2.25	0.5	1.75	100	100	100	464	384	214
21	1.50	0.5	1.00	90	100	100	460	651	410
22	6.50	5.0	3.00	90	90	100	138	80	221
23	7.50	3.0	2.50	90	100	100	213	89	114
24	5.50	1.0	2.50	80	90	100	480	239	170
25	6.50	0.5	1.50	90	100	100	580	890	1024
26	2.50	1.0	1.00	90	90	100	411	256	447
27	4.00	0.5	0.50	80	100	100	585	595	327

TABLE 2.14. Psychomotor test scores from 45 cancer patients

Group	ID	Day 1	Day 2	Day 3	Group	ID	Day 1	Day 2	Day 3
Control	1	223	242	248	75–100 R	4	119	149	196
	2	72	81	66		5	144	169	164
	3	172	214	239		6	170	202	181
	4	171	191	203		7	93	122	145
	5	138	204	213		8	237	243	281
	6	22	24	24		9	208	235	249
25–50 R	1	53	102	104		10	187	199	205
	2	45	50	54		11	95	102	96
	3	47	45	34		12	46	67	28
	4	167	188	209		13	95	137	99
	5	193	206	210		14	59	76	101
	6	91	154	152		15	186	198	201
	7	115	133	136	125–250 R	1	202	229	232
	8	32	97	86		2	126	159	157
	9	38	37	40		3	54	75	75
	10	66	131	148		4	158	168	175
	11	210	221	251		5	175	217	235
	12	167	172	212		6	147	183	181
	13	23	18	30		7	105	107	92
	14	234	260	269		8	213	263	260
75–100 R	1	206	199	237		9	258	248	257
	2	208	222	237		10	257	269	270
	3	224	224	261					

TABLE 2.15. Plasma inorganic phosphate levels from 33 subjects

Group	ID	Hours after Glucose Challenge 0	0.5	1	1.5	2	3	4	5
Control	1	4.3	3.3	3.0	2.6	2.2	2.5	3.4	4.4
	2	3.7	2.6	2.6	1.9	2.9	3.2	3.1	3.9
	3	4.0	4.1	3.1	2.3	2.9	3.1	3.9	4.0
	4	3.6	3.0	2.2	2.8	2.9	3.9	3.8	4.0
	5	4.1	3.8	2.1	3.0	3.6	3.4	3.6	3.7
	6	3.8	2.2	2.0	2.6	3.8	3.6	3.0	3.5
	7	3.8	3.0	2.4	2.5	3.1	3.4	3.5	3.7
	8	4.4	3.9	2.8	2.1	3.6	3.8	4.0	3.9
	9	5.0	4.0	3.4	3.4	3.3	3.6	4.0	4.3
	10	3.7	3.1	2.9	2.2	1.5	2.3	2.7	2.8
	11	3.7	2.6	2.6	2.3	2.9	2.2	3.1	3.9
	12	4.4	3.7	3.1	3.2	3.7	4.3	3.9	4.8
	13	4.7	3.1	3.2	3.3	3.2	4.2	3.7	4.3
Nonhyper-insulinemic obese	1	4.3	3.3	3.0	2.6	2.2	2.5	2.4	3.4
	2	5.0	4.9	4.1	3.7	3.7	4.1	4.7	4.9
	3	4.6	4.4	3.9	3.9	3.7	4.2	4.8	5.0
	4	4.3	3.9	3.1	3.1	3.1	3.1	3.6	4.0
	5	3.1	3.1	3.3	2.6	2.6	1.9	2.3	2.7
	6	4.8	5.0	2.9	2.8	2.2	3.1	3.5	3.6
	7	3.7	3.1	3.3	2.8	2.9	3.6	4.3	4.4
	8	5.4	4.7	3.9	4.1	2.8	3.7	3.5	3.7
	9	3.0	2.5	2.3	2.2	2.1	2.6	3.2	3.5
	10	4.9	5.0	4.1	3.7	3.7	4.1	4.7	4.9
	11	4.8	4.3	4.7	4.6	4.7	3.7	3.6	3.9
	12	4.4	4.2	4.2	3.4	3.5	3.4	3.9	4.0
Hyperinsulinemic obese	1	4.9	4.3	4.0	4.0	3.3	4.1	4.2	4.3
	2	5.1	4.1	4.6	4.1	3.4	4.2	4.4	4.9
	3	4.8	4.6	4.6	4.4	4.1	4.0	3.8	3.8
	4	4.2	3.5	3.8	3.6	3.3	3.1	3.5	3.9
	5	6.6	6.1	5.2	4.1	4.3	3.8	4.2	4.8
	6	3.6	3.4	3.1	2.8	2.1	2.4	2.5	3.5
	7	4.5	4.0	3.7	3.3	2.4	2.3	3.1	3.3
	8	4.6	4.4	3.8	3.8	3.8	3.6	3.8	3.8

TABLE 2.16. Body weights of 60 female rats: First five animals in each group

		Week									
Group	ID	0	1	2	3	4	5	6	7	8	9
Control	1	152	178	198	200	214	237	240	246	524	255
	2	135	152	165	173	184	200	209	208	224	235
	3	142	162	184	200	220	230	239	244	259	262
	4	159	183	214	233	251	269	280	283	292	295
	5	159	180	196	210	216	230	237	247	255	258
Low	1	155	178	194	217	224	230	251	268	279	293
	2	158	181	213	254	254	271	280	276	312	318
	3	158	185	212	229	250	263	299	290	290	305
	4	163	187	214	233	252	259	275	282	295	368
	5	159	184	188	229	244	255	270	276	279	285
Medium	1	196	183	208	231	237	261	252	281	282	285
	2	159	200	230	265	281	314	330	339	333	353
	3	158	185	224	239	254	275	283	292	298	303
	4	154	216	234	268	300	338	339	367	373	368
	5	142	173	186	214	226	241	256	255	260	272
High	1	167	204	225	258	248	282	284	304	306	333
	2	165	193	197	231	229	242	267	268	279	265
	3	163	186	212	244	255	264	270	293	290	308
	4	175	200	223	247	253	274	282	288	300	290
	5	144	177	218	252	269	278	305	308	324	326

TABLE 2.17. Sentence test results in 44 deaf patients

Type A Implant					Type B Implant				
	Month					Month			
ID	1	9	18	30	ID	1	9	18	30
1	28.57	53.00	57.83	59.22	1		0.00	0.90	1.61
2		13.00	21.00	26.50	2	0.00	0.00	0.00	
3	60.37	86.41			3	0.00	0.00		
4	33.87	55.50	61.06		4	8.76	24.42		
5	1.61	0.69			5	0.00	20.79	27.42	31.80
6	26.04	61.98	67.28		6	2.30	12.67	28.80	24.42
7		59.00	66.80	83.20	7	12.90	28.34		
8	11.29	38.02			8		45.50	43.32	36.80
9	0.00	0.00	0.00	2.76	9	68.00	96.08	97.47	99.00
10		35.10	37.79	54.80	10	20.28	41.01	51.15	61.98
11	16.00	33.00	45.39	40.09	11	65.90	81.30	71.20	70.00
12	40.55	50.69	41.70	52.07	12	0.00	8.76	16.59	14.75
13	3.90	11.06	4.15	14.90	13	0.00	0.00	0.00	0.00
14	1.80	2.30	2.53	2.53	14	9.22	14.98	9.68	
15	0.00	17.74	44.70	48.85	15	11.29	44.47	62.90	68.20
16	64.75	84.50	92.40		16	30.88	29.72		
17	38.25	81.57	89.63		17	29.72	41.40	64.00	
18	67.50	91.47	92.86		18	0.00	43.55	48.16	
19	45.62	58.00			19	0.00	0.00		
20	0.00	0.00	37.00		20	8.76	60.00		
21	51.15	66.13			21	8.00	25.00	30.88	55.53
22	0.00	48.16							
23	0.00	0.92							

for a difference between the groups using an appropriate summary statistic.

2.11 The National Cooperative Gallstone Study evaluated the safety of the drug chenodiol for the treatment of cholesterol gallstones. This drug dissolves gallstones by altering the metabolic pathway of cholesterol to reduce cholesterol secretion into gallbladder bile. One potential side effect, however, was that it might also increase serum cholesterol, a known risk factor for atherosclerotic disease. In a group of 113 patients with floating gallstones, 65 patients received 750 mg/day of chenodiol and 48 patients received a placebo. Serum cholesterol was measured in these patients prior to treatment and at 6, 12, 20, and 24 months of follow-up. Many cholesterol measurements were missing because patient follow-up was terminated, visits were missed, or laboratory specimens were lost or inadequate. The two groups have rather different missing value patterns, mainly because of the termination of follow-up for different reasons.

Tables 2.19 and 2.20 display the data from 103 patients, 41 from the placebo group and 62 from the high-dose chenodiol group (Wei and Lachin, 1984). Note that a few patients from each group who had only one cholesterol measurement are excluded. Using an appropriate summary statistic, test whether the two treatments differ with respect to their effects on serum cholesterol levels.

2.12 Everitt (1994a, 1994b) reports the results from a 100 kilometer (km) road race held in 1984 in the United Kingdom. The data consist of the "split" times for 80 runners in each 10-km section of the race as well as the age of each runner. Table 2.21 displays the data from the first 15 runners.

(a) Using an appropriate summary statistic, assess whether the "split" times tend to increase, decrease, or remain the same across the 10-km sections of the race.

(b) Repeat part (a) separately for the first 80 km and the last 20 km of the race.

(c) Use an appropriate summary statistic to assess whether the association between "split" time and section of the race changes with the age of the runner.

2.13 In an arthritis clinical trial, 227 subjects were randomized to one of two treatments (labeled as A and B). The outcome variable of interest was the time (seconds) required to walk 50 feet; this was measured at baseline (prior to the initiation of treatment) and at four-week intervals during a 40-week treatment period. Table 2.22 displays the data from the first 10 subjects.

(a) Suggest and defend an appropriate summary statistic for comparing the two treatments.

TABLE 2.18. Pain scores from 83 women in labor: First 20 subjects in each group

		Self-Reported Pain Scores at 30-Minute Intervals						
Group	Patient	0	30	60	90	120	150	180
1	1	0.0	0.0	0.0	0.0			
	2	0.0	0.0	0.0	0.0	2.5	2.3	14.0
	3	38.0	5.0	1.0	1.0	0.0	5.0	
	4	6.0	48.0	85.0	0.0	0.0		
	5	19.0	5.0					
	6	7.0	0.0	0.0	0.0			
	7	44.0	42.0	42.0	45.0			
	8	1.0	0.0	0.0	0.0	0.0	6.0	24.0
	9	24.5	35.0	13.0				
	10	1.0	30.5	81.5	67.5	98.5	97.0	
	11	35.5	44.5	55.0	69.0	72.5	39.5	26.0
	12	0.0	0.0	0.0	0.0	0.0	0.0	0.0
	13	8.0	30.5	26.0	24.0	29.0	45.0	91.0
	14	7.0	6.5	7.0	4.0	10.0		
	15	6.0	8.5	19.5	16.5	42.5	45.5	48.5
	16	32.5	9.5	7.5	5.5	4.5	0.0	7.0
	17	10.5	10.0	18.0	32.5	0.0	0.0	0.0
	18	11.5	20.5	32.5	37.0	39.0		
	19	72.0	91.5	4.5	32.0	10.5	10.5	10.5
	20	0.0	0.0	0.0	0.0	13.5	7.0	
2	1	4.0	9.0	30.0	75.0	49.0	97.0	
	2	0.0	0.0	1.0	27.5	95.0	100.0	
	3	9.0	6.0	25.0				
	4	52.5	18.0	12.5				
	5	90.5	99.0	100.0	100.0	100.0	100.0	100.0
	6	74.0	70.0	81.5	94.5	97.0		
	7	0.0	0.0	0.0	1.5	0.0	18.0	71.0
	8	0.0	51.5	56.0				
	9	6.5	7.0	7.0	9.0	25.0	36.0	20.0
	10	19.0	31.0	41.0	58.0			
	11	6.0	23.0	45.0	67.0	90.5		
	12	42.0	64.0	6.0				
	13	86.5	53.0	88.0	100.0	100.0		
	14	50.0	100.0	100.0	100.0	100.0		
	15	27.5	36.5	74.0	97.0	100.0	100.0	95.0
	16	0.0	0.0	6.0	6.0			
	17	62.0	79.0	80.5	85.0	90.0	97.5	97.0
	18	17.5	27.5	21.0	60.0	80.0	97.0	
	19	6.5	5.5	18.5	20.0	36.5	63.5	81.5
	20	8.0	9.0	35.5	39.0	70.0	92.0	98.0

TABLE 2.19. Serum cholesterol measurements from 103 patients in the National Cooperative Gallstone Study: Placebo group

Patient	Baseline	Month 6	Month 12	Month 20	Month 24
1	251	262	239	234	248
2	233	218	230	251	273
3	250	258	258	286	240
4	141	143	157	162	169
5	418	371	363	384	387
6	229	218	228	244	179
7	271	289	270	296	346
8	312	323	318	383	310
9	194	220	214	256	204
10	211	232	189	230	231
11	205	299	278	259	266
12	191	248	283	268	233
13	249	217	236	266	235
14	301	270	282	287	268
15	201	214	247	274	224
16	251	257	237	266	
17	277	242	249	293	306
18	294	313	295	295	271
19	212	236	235	272	287
20	230	315	300	305	341
21	206	242	236	239	
22	246	205	249	225	236
23	245	192	215	214	242
24	179	202	194	239	234
25	165	142	188	192	200
26	262	274	245	275	278
27	212	216	228	221	223
28	285	292	300	319	277
29	166	171	166	186	220
30	179	206	214	189	250
31	298	280	280	328	318
32	238	267	269	268	280
33	172	180	216	183	
34	191	208	162	218	206
37	282	282			
38	213	249	219	209	
44	171	188			
45	242	268			
46	197	224	214		
47	230	228	266		
48	373	309	332		

TABLE 2.20. Serum cholesterol measurements from 103 patients in the National Cooperative Gallstone Study: High-dose chenodiol group

Patient	Baseline	Month 6	Month 12	Month 20	Month 24
1	178	246	295	228	274
2	254	260	278	245	340
3	185	232	215	220	292
4	219	268	241	260	320
5	205	232	265	242	230
6	182	213	173	200	193
7	310	334	290	286	248
8	191	204	227	228	196
9	245	270	209	255	213
10	229	200	238	259	221
11	245	293	261	297	231
12	240	313	251	307	291
13	234	281	277	235	210
14	210	252	275	235	237
15	275	231	285	238	251
16	269	332	300	320	335
17	148	180	184	231	184
18	181	194	212	217	205
19	165	242	250	249	312
20	293	276	276	278	306
21	195	190	205	217	238
22	210	230	249	240	194
23	212	224	246	271	256
24	243	271	304	273	318
25	259	279	296	262	283
26	202	214	192	239	172
27	184	192	205	253	217
28	238	272	297	282	251
29	263	283	248	334	271
30	144	226	261	227	283
31	220	272	222	246	253
32	225	260	253	202	265
33	224	273	242	274	
34	307	252	316	258	283
35	313	300	313	317	397
36	231	252	267	299	
37	206	177	194	194	212
38	285	291	291	268	260
41	250	269			
42	175	214			
43	201	219	220		
44	268	296	314	330	
45	202	186	253		
46	260	268			
48	209	207	167		
49	197	218			
50	248	262			
51	212	253	225		
52	276	326	304		
53	163	179	199		
54	239	243	265		
55	204	203	198		
56	247	211	225		
57	195	250	272		
58	228	228	279		
59	290	264	260		
60	284	288	268	261	
61	217	231	276	257	
62	209	200	269	233	
63	200	261	264	300	
64	227	247			220
65	193	189		232	211

TABLE 2.21. Ten-kilometer "split" times for 80 runners in a 100-kilometer road race: Runners 1–15

		10-Kilometer Section									
ID	Age	1	2	3	4	5	6	7	8	9	10
1	39	37.0	37.8	36.6	39.6	41.0	41.0	41.3	45.7	45.1	43.1
2	39	39.5	42.2	40.0	42.3	40.6	40.8	42.0	43.7	41.0	43.9
3	36	37.0	37.8	36.6	39.6	41.0	44.8	44.5	49.4	44.6	47.7
4	.	37.1	38.0	37.7	42.4	41.6	43.5	48.7	49.7	44.8	47.0
5	34	42.2	44.5	41.9	43.4	43.0	47.2	49.1	49.9	46.8	52.3
6	46	43.0	44.6	41.2	42.1	42.5	46.8	47.5	55.8	56.6	58.6
7	35	43.2	44.4	41.0	43.4	43.0	47.2	52.4	57.3	54.4	53.5
8	47	43.2	46.7	44.8	47.5	47.4	47.7	49.9	52.1	50.7	50.0
9	30	38.5	41.4	40.1	43.2	43.2	51.5	56.7	71.5	56.2	48.2
10	.	42.5	43.1	40.6	44.5	45.4	52.3	59.7	59.3	55.0	49.6
11	48	38.0	40.1	39.1	43.8	46.6	51.9	59.2	63.5	57.6	58.4
12	39	46.0	50.4	46.8	47.4	44.1	43.4	46.3	55.0	64.9	56.2
13	32	44.8	46.0	43.1	46.5	46.3	49.0	52.5	58.4	60.9	55.2
14	43	44.8	46.0	43.1	46.5	46.3	49.0	52.5	58.4	60.9	55.2
15	35	47.0	49.4	46.8	48.6	47.8	50.8	50.3	54.0	54.4	53.6

(b) Test whether the profiles over time differ between the two treatments.

(c) Repeat part (b) for males and females separately.

(d) Summarize your conclusions from this study.

TABLE 2.22. Measurements of time (seconds) to walk 50 feet from 227 subjects in an arthritis clinical trial: First ten subjects

			Week										
ID	Sex	Trt.	0	4	8	12	16	20	24	28	32	36	40
1	F	A	20.0	18.0	18.0	16.0	18.0	18.0	20.0	16.0	20.0	20.0	16.0
2	M	B	16.0	14.0	.	.	.	.	.	.	.	.	.
3	M	A	12.0	12.0	12.0	12.0	12.0	14.0	12.0	14.0	.	16.0	16.0
4	F	A	18.0	14.0	18.0	18.0	18.0	16.0	18.0	20.0	.	.	.
5	F	A	20.0	20.0	.	.	.	.	.	.	.	.	.
6	F	A	18.0	18.0	12.0	16.0	16.0	16.0	12.0	14.0	14.0	12.0	14.0
7	F	B	20.0	16.0	20.0	16.0	12.0	18.0	18.0	28.0	20.0	.	.
8	M	B	16.0	14.0	12.0	12.0	18.0	.	.	.	.	.	.
9	F	A	16.0	18.0	16.0	16.0	14.0	16.0	16.0	16.0	16.0	18.0	14.0
10	F	B	20.0	16.0	16.0	20.0	16.0	18.0	18.0	16.0	16.0	16.0	18.0

3

Normal-Theory Methods: Unstructured Multivariate Approach

3.1 Introduction

The univariate methods described in Chapter 2 reduce the vector of repeated measurements from each experimental unit to a single number. Although this permits the use of simple analysis methods, the resulting loss of information may not be desirable.

Chapters 3–6 consider alternative methods that are useful when the response y_{ij} from subject i at time point j is normally distributed. These approaches use the multivariate nature of a subject's observations. Thus, rather than reduce the vector of repeated measurements from each subject to a single summary measurement, all of the data are used.

Chapter 3 covers the use of the unstructured multivariate approach for one-sample and two-sample problems. In both of these settings, hypotheses of interest can be tested using Hotelling's T^2 statistic (Hotelling, 1931). This statistic is a generalization of the usual one-sample and two-sample t statistics for univariate outcomes. Section 3.2 reviews multivariate normal distribution theory, Section 3.3 discusses the analysis of repeated measurements from a single sample, and Section 3.4 covers the two-sample setting. Sections 3.3 and 3.4 also include examples illustrating the use of Hotelling's T^2 statistic for the analysis of repeated measurements.

3.2 Multivariate Normal Distribution Theory

3.2.1 The Multivariate Normal Distribution

Let $\boldsymbol{x} = (x_1, \ldots, x_p)'$ be a p-component random vector having a multivariate normal distribution with mean vector $\boldsymbol{\mu} = (\mu_1, \ldots, \mu_p)'$ and $p \times p$ covariance matrix

$$\boldsymbol{\Sigma} = \begin{pmatrix} \sigma_{11} & \cdots & \sigma_{1p} \\ \vdots & \ddots & \vdots \\ \sigma_{p1} & \cdots & \sigma_{pp} \end{pmatrix}.$$

The probability density function of $\boldsymbol{x}$ is

$$f(x_1, \ldots, x_p) = (2\pi)^{-p/2} |\boldsymbol{\Sigma}|^{-1/2} \exp(-0.5(\boldsymbol{x} - \boldsymbol{\mu})' \boldsymbol{\Sigma}^{-1} (\boldsymbol{x} - \boldsymbol{\mu}))$$

for $-\infty < x_i < \infty$, $i = 1, \ldots, p$. We write this distribution as $\boldsymbol{x} \sim N_p(\boldsymbol{\mu}, \boldsymbol{\Sigma})$.

Now, consider a sample of n such vectors:

$$\boldsymbol{x}_1 = (x_{11}, \ldots, x_{1p})', \ldots, \boldsymbol{x}_n = (x_{n1}, \ldots, x_{np})'.$$

These data can be summarized in the $n \times p$ data matrix

$$\boldsymbol{X} = \begin{pmatrix} x_{11} & \cdots & x_{1p} \\ \vdots & \ddots & \vdots \\ x_{n1} & \cdots & x_{np} \end{pmatrix} = \begin{pmatrix} \boldsymbol{x}_1' \\ \vdots \\ \boldsymbol{x}_n' \end{pmatrix}.$$

The maximum likelihood estimator of $\boldsymbol{\mu}$ is $\widehat{\boldsymbol{\mu}} = \overline{\boldsymbol{x}} = (\overline{x}_1, \ldots, \overline{x}_p)'$, where $\overline{x}_j = \sum_{i=1}^n x_{ij}/n$. The maximum likelihood estimator of Σ is

$$\widehat{\boldsymbol{\Sigma}} = \frac{1}{n} \boldsymbol{A},$$

where $\boldsymbol{A}$ is a $p \times p$ matrix with elements $a_{jk} = \sum_{i=1}^n (x_{ij} - \overline{x}_j)(x_{ik} - \overline{x}_k)$. In matrix notation,

$$\boldsymbol{A} = \sum_{i=1}^n (\boldsymbol{x}_i - \overline{\boldsymbol{x}})(\boldsymbol{x}_i - \overline{\boldsymbol{x}})' = \sum_{i=1}^n \boldsymbol{x}_i \boldsymbol{x}_i' - n \overline{\boldsymbol{x}}\, \overline{\boldsymbol{x}}'.$$

An unbiased estimator of $\boldsymbol{\Sigma}$ is given by

$$\boldsymbol{S} = \frac{1}{n-1} \boldsymbol{A}.$$

3.2.2 The Wishart Distribution

Let $\boldsymbol{z}_1, \ldots, \boldsymbol{z}_n$ be independent random vectors with $\boldsymbol{z}_i \sim N_p(\boldsymbol{0}_p, \boldsymbol{\Sigma})$, where $\boldsymbol{0}_p$ is the p-component vector $(0, \ldots, 0)'$. Let $\boldsymbol{A} = \sum_{i=1}^n \boldsymbol{z}_i \boldsymbol{z}_i'$. The $p \times p$

matrix $\boldsymbol{A}$ has the (central) Wishart distribution with parameters n and $\boldsymbol{\Sigma}$. We write $\boldsymbol{A} \sim W_p(n, \boldsymbol{\Sigma})$.

The probability density function of $\boldsymbol{A}$ is given by

$$\frac{|\boldsymbol{A}|^{(n-p-1)/2} \exp\left(-\frac{1}{2}\mathrm{tr}(\boldsymbol{\Sigma}^{-1}\boldsymbol{A})\right)}{2^{np/2}\, \pi^{p(p-1)/4}\, |\boldsymbol{\Sigma}|^{n/2} \prod_{i=1}^{p} \Gamma\left((n+1-i)/2\right)}$$

for $\boldsymbol{A}$ positive-definite and 0 otherwise, where $\Gamma(x) = \int_0^\infty u^{x-1}e^{-u}du$. In the case where $p = 1$ and $\boldsymbol{\Sigma} = 1$, this reduces to the density of the chi-square distribution with n degrees of freedom (χ^2_n). Note that $\boldsymbol{A}$ does not have a density if $n < p$, although the distribution is nevertheless defined.

3.2.3 Wishart Matrices

Let $\boldsymbol{x}_1, \ldots, \boldsymbol{x}_n$ be independent $N_p(\boldsymbol{\mu}, \boldsymbol{\Sigma})$ random vectors. The sample covariance matrix (from Section 3.2.1) is given by

$$\boldsymbol{S} = \frac{1}{n-1}\sum_{i=1}^{n}(\boldsymbol{x}_i - \overline{\boldsymbol{x}})(\boldsymbol{x}_i - \overline{\boldsymbol{x}})'.$$

Let $\boldsymbol{A} = (n-1)\boldsymbol{S}$ denote the matrix of corrected sums of squares and products of multivariate normal variates. The matrix $\boldsymbol{A}$ is called a Wishart matrix and is said to have the Wishart distribution with parameters $n-1$ and $\boldsymbol{\Sigma}$; we write $\boldsymbol{A} \sim W_p(n-1, \boldsymbol{\Sigma})$.

One important property of a Wishart matrix is that the sample mean vector $\overline{\boldsymbol{x}}$ and the Wishart matrix $\boldsymbol{A}$ computed from the same sample are independent. Another useful property is that if $\boldsymbol{A}_1, \ldots, \boldsymbol{A}_s$ are independent Wishart matrices with $\boldsymbol{A}_h \sim W_p(n_h, \boldsymbol{\Sigma})$, then $\sum_{h=1}^{s} \boldsymbol{A}_h \sim W_p(n, \boldsymbol{\Sigma})$, where $n = \sum_{h=1}^{s} n_h$.

3.2.4 Hotelling's T^2 Statistic

Let $\boldsymbol{x} \sim N_p(\boldsymbol{\mu}, \boldsymbol{\Sigma})$. Let $n\boldsymbol{W}$ be a $p \times p$ matrix, independent of $\boldsymbol{x}$, such that $n\boldsymbol{W} \sim W_p(n, \boldsymbol{\Sigma})$. The statistic

$$T^2 = \boldsymbol{x}'\boldsymbol{W}^{-1}\boldsymbol{x}$$

has the T^2 distribution with noncentrality parameter

$$\delta = \boldsymbol{\mu}'\boldsymbol{\Sigma}^{-1}\boldsymbol{\mu}$$

and degrees of freedom (df) p and n. We write $T^2 \sim T^2_{p,n,\delta}$. Hotelling (1931) proposed this statistic and derived its distribution.

The distribution of T^2 is related to that of the ratio of independent χ^2 random variables in that

$$F = \frac{n-p+1}{np}T^2$$

has the noncentral F distribution with parameters p, $n-p+1$ and noncentrality parameter δ (written as $F_{p,n-p+1,\delta}$). If $\boldsymbol{\mu} = \mathbf{0}_p$, the random variable F has the central F distribution ($F_{p,n-p+1}$).

3.2.5 Hypothesis Tests

Let $\boldsymbol{x}_1, \ldots, \boldsymbol{x}_n$ be a random sample from $N_p(\boldsymbol{\mu}, \boldsymbol{\Sigma})$. Suppose that we wish to test $H_0\colon \boldsymbol{\mu} = \boldsymbol{\mu}_0$ for some specified vector $\boldsymbol{\mu}_0 = (\mu_{01}, \ldots, \mu_{0p})'$. The test is constructed using the following results:

1. $\sqrt{n}(\overline{\boldsymbol{x}} - \boldsymbol{\mu}_0) \sim N_p(\sqrt{n}(\boldsymbol{\mu} - \boldsymbol{\mu}_0), \boldsymbol{\Sigma})$.

2. The sample covariance matrix $\boldsymbol{S}$ is independent of $\overline{\boldsymbol{x}}$.

3. $(n-1)\boldsymbol{S} \sim W_p(n-1, \boldsymbol{\Sigma})$.

In this case, Hotelling's T^2 statistic is

$$T^2 = \left(\sqrt{n}(\overline{\boldsymbol{x}} - \boldsymbol{\mu}_0)\right)' \boldsymbol{S}^{-1} \left(\sqrt{n}(\overline{\boldsymbol{x}} - \boldsymbol{\mu}_0)\right) = n(\overline{\boldsymbol{x}} - \boldsymbol{\mu}_0)' \boldsymbol{S}^{-1} (\overline{\boldsymbol{x}} - \boldsymbol{\mu}_0).$$

The statistic

$$F = \frac{(n-1) - p + 1}{(n-1)p} T^2 = \frac{n-p}{(n-1)p} T^2$$

has the $F_{p,n-p,\delta}$ distribution, where

$$\delta = n(\boldsymbol{\mu} - \boldsymbol{\mu}_0)' \boldsymbol{\Sigma}^{-1} (\boldsymbol{\mu} - \boldsymbol{\mu}_0).$$

If H_0 is true, $F \sim F_{p,n-p}$.

This test can only be used when $n > p$. The test based on T^2 can also be derived as the likelihood ratio test of H_0. The null distribution of T^2 is approximately valid even if the distribution of $\boldsymbol{x}_1, \ldots, \boldsymbol{x}_n$ is not normal (Anderson, 1984, p. 163).

Another general type of hypothesis of interest is $H_0\colon \boldsymbol{C}\boldsymbol{\mu} = \mathbf{0}_c$, where $\boldsymbol{C}$ is a $c \times p$ matrix of rank c with $c \le p$. Let $\boldsymbol{z}_i = \boldsymbol{C}\boldsymbol{x}_i$ for $i = 1, \ldots, n$; $\boldsymbol{z}_1, \ldots, \boldsymbol{z}_n$ are independent random vectors from the $N_c(\boldsymbol{C}\boldsymbol{\mu}, \boldsymbol{C}\boldsymbol{\Sigma}\boldsymbol{C}')$ distribution. Let

$$\overline{\boldsymbol{z}} = \frac{1}{n}\sum_{i=1}^{n} \boldsymbol{z}_i = \frac{1}{n}\sum_{i=1}^{n} \boldsymbol{C}\boldsymbol{x}_i = \boldsymbol{C}\overline{\boldsymbol{x}}.$$

The distribution of $\overline{\boldsymbol{z}}$ is

$$N_c(\boldsymbol{C}\boldsymbol{\mu}, n^{-1}\boldsymbol{C}\boldsymbol{\Sigma}\boldsymbol{C}'),$$

and so $\sqrt{n}\overline{\boldsymbol{z}} \sim N_c(\sqrt{n}\boldsymbol{C}\boldsymbol{\mu}, \boldsymbol{C}\boldsymbol{\Sigma}\boldsymbol{C}')$.

The sample covariance matrix of $\boldsymbol{z}_1, \ldots, \boldsymbol{z}_n$ is given by

$$\begin{aligned}
\boldsymbol{S_z} &= \frac{1}{n-1}\sum_{i=1}^{n}(\boldsymbol{z}_i - \overline{\boldsymbol{z}})(\boldsymbol{z}_i - \overline{\boldsymbol{z}})' \\
&= \frac{1}{n-1}\sum_{i=1}^{n}(\boldsymbol{C}\boldsymbol{x}_i - \boldsymbol{C}\overline{\boldsymbol{x}})(\boldsymbol{C}\boldsymbol{x}_i - \boldsymbol{C}\overline{\boldsymbol{x}})' \\
&= \frac{1}{n-1}\sum_{i=1}^{n}\boldsymbol{C}(\boldsymbol{x}_i - \overline{\boldsymbol{x}})[\boldsymbol{C}(\boldsymbol{x}_i - \overline{\boldsymbol{x}})]' \\
&= \frac{1}{n-1}\sum_{i=1}^{n}\boldsymbol{C}(\boldsymbol{x}_i - \overline{\boldsymbol{x}})(\boldsymbol{x}_i - \overline{\boldsymbol{x}})'\boldsymbol{C}' \\
&= \boldsymbol{CSC}'.
\end{aligned}$$

Because $(n-1)\boldsymbol{S_z} = (n-1)\boldsymbol{CSC}' \sim W_c(n-1, \boldsymbol{C\Sigma C}')$ and $\boldsymbol{S_z} = \boldsymbol{CSC}'$ is independent of $\overline{\boldsymbol{z}}$, the statistic

$$T^2 = (\sqrt{n}\overline{\boldsymbol{z}})'\boldsymbol{S_z}^{-1}(\sqrt{n}\overline{\boldsymbol{z}}) = n(\boldsymbol{C}\overline{\boldsymbol{x}})'(\boldsymbol{CSC}')^{-1}(\boldsymbol{C}\overline{\boldsymbol{x}})$$

has the $T^2_{c,n-1,\delta}$ distribution with noncentrality parameter

$$\delta = n(\boldsymbol{C\mu})'(\boldsymbol{C\Sigma C}')^{-1}(\boldsymbol{C\mu}).$$

The statistic

$$F = \frac{(n-1)-c+1}{(n-1)c}T^2 = \frac{n-c}{(n-1)c}T^2 \tag{3.1}$$

has the $F_{c,n-c,\delta}$ distribution. If H_0 is true, $F \sim F_{c,n-c}$. This test can be used if $n > c$.

3.3 One-Sample Repeated Measurements

3.3.1 Methodology

Consider the one-sample layout of Table 1.3. Let y_{ij} denote the response from subject i at time j, for $i = 1, \ldots, n$, $j = 1, \ldots, t$. The vectors

$$\boldsymbol{y}_i = (y_{i1}, \ldots, y_{it})', \qquad i = 1, \ldots, n,$$

are a random sample from $N_t(\boldsymbol{\mu}, \boldsymbol{\Sigma})$, where $\boldsymbol{\mu} = (\mu_1, \ldots, \mu_t)'$.

Suppose that we wish to test $H_0\colon \mu_1 = \cdots = \mu_t$. Let $y^*_{ij} = y_{ij} - y_{i,j+1}$ for $j = 1, \ldots, t-1$. The $\boldsymbol{y}^*_i = (y^*_{i1}, \ldots, y^*_{i,t-1})'$ vectors are a random sample from $N_{t-1}(\boldsymbol{\mu}^*, \boldsymbol{\Sigma}^*)$, where

$$\boldsymbol{\mu}^* = (\mu_1 - \mu_2, \mu_2 - \mu_3, \ldots, \mu_{t-1} - \mu_t)'.$$

The hypothesis $H_0\colon \mu_1 = \cdots = \mu_t$ is then equivalent to

$$H_0^*\colon \boldsymbol{\mu}^* = (0, \ldots, 0)'.$$

The test of H_0^* can be carried out using the T^2 statistic computed from the sample mean vector and covariance matrix of the y_{ij}^* values. Because $\sqrt{n}\overline{\boldsymbol{y}}^* \sim N_{t-1}(\sqrt{n}\boldsymbol{\mu}^*, \boldsymbol{\Sigma}^*)$ and $(n-1)\boldsymbol{S}^* \sim W_{t-1}(n-1, \boldsymbol{\Sigma}^*)$, the statistic T^2 is given by

$$T^2 = n\overline{\boldsymbol{y}}^{*'}\boldsymbol{S}^{*-1}\overline{\boldsymbol{y}}^* \sim T^2_{t-1,n-1,\delta^*},$$

where $\delta^* = n\boldsymbol{\mu}^{*'}\boldsymbol{\Sigma}^{*-1}\boldsymbol{\mu}^*$. The statistic

$$F = \frac{(n-1)-(t-1)+1}{(n-1)(t-1)}T^2 = \frac{n-t+1}{(n-1)(t-1)}T^2$$

has the $F_{t-1,n-t+1}$ distribution if H_0^* is true.

Using vector and matrix notation, $\boldsymbol{y}_i^* = \boldsymbol{C}\boldsymbol{y}_i$, where $\boldsymbol{C}$ is the $(t-1) \times t$ matrix

$$\begin{pmatrix} 1 & -1 & 0 & \ldots & 0 & 0 \\ 0 & 1 & -1 & \ldots & 0 & 0 \\ \ldots & \ldots & \ldots & \ldots & \ldots & \ldots \\ 0 & 0 & 0 & \ldots & 1 & -1 \end{pmatrix}.$$

Thus, $\boldsymbol{y}_i^* \sim N_{t-1}(\boldsymbol{C}\boldsymbol{\mu}, \boldsymbol{C}\boldsymbol{\Sigma}\boldsymbol{C}')$ and

$$T^2 = n(\boldsymbol{C}\overline{\boldsymbol{y}})'(\boldsymbol{C}\boldsymbol{S}\boldsymbol{C}')^{-1}(\boldsymbol{C}\overline{\boldsymbol{y}}).$$

The value of T^2 is invariant with respect to the specific choice of $\boldsymbol{C}$. For example, another choice is

$$\boldsymbol{C} = \begin{pmatrix} -1 & 1 & 0 & \ldots & 0 & 0 \\ -1 & 0 & 1 & \ldots & 0 & 0 \\ \ldots & \ldots & \ldots & \ldots & \ldots & \ldots \\ -1 & 0 & 0 & \ldots & 0 & 1 \end{pmatrix}.$$

Other types of hypotheses of the general form $H_0\colon \boldsymbol{C}\boldsymbol{\mu} = 0$ can also be tested.

3.3.2 Examples

Table 2.1 displays data from a study in which ventilation volumes (l/min) were measured in eight subjects under six different temperatures of inspired dry air (Deal et al., 1979). In Section 2.2, these data were analyzed using the summary-statistic approach. Figure 3.1 displays the response profiles for each of the eight subjects as well as the mean profile.

Because the individual profiles display no clear pattern, this plot might lead one to conclude that the summary-statistic approach may not be the

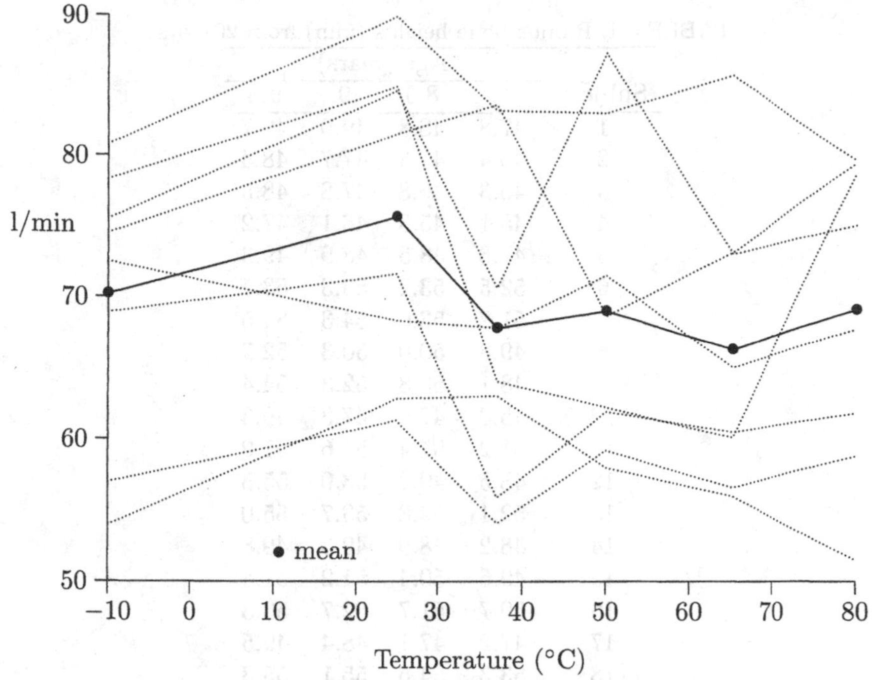

FIGURE 3.1. Ventilation volumes (l/min) from eight subjects

most appropriate method to use in testing whether ventilation volume is affected by temperature.

Let $\mu_1, \ldots, \mu_6$ denote the mean ventilation volumes at temperatures −10, 25, 37, 50, 65, and 80°C, respectively. Under the assumption that ventilation volumes are normally distributed, Hotelling's T^2 can be used to test $H_0\colon \mu_1 = \cdots = \mu_6$. In this example, $T^2 = 34.155$ and

$$F = \frac{n-t+1}{(n-1)(t-1)} T^2 = \frac{8-6+1}{7 \times 5} T^2 = \frac{3}{35} T^2 = 2.9276.$$

With reference to the $F_{5,3}$ distribution, $p = 0.20$. At the 5% level of significance, there is insufficient evidence to conclude that the mean ventilation volumes at the six temperatures differ significantly.

As a second example, Table 3.1 lists the data from a dental study in which the height of the ramus bone (mm) was measured in 20 boys at ages 8, 8.5, 9, and 9.5 years (Elston and Grizzle, 1962). Figure 3.2 displays the response profiles for each of the 20 boys as well as the mean profile.

One question of interest is to determine whether bone height changes with age. Let $\boldsymbol{\mu} = (\mu_1, \ldots, \mu_4)'$ denote the vector of mean ramus bone heights at ages 8, 8.5, 9, and 9.5 years of age, respectively. Under the assumption that ramus bone heights are normally distributed, Hotelling's T^2 can be used to test $H_0\colon \mu_1 = \cdots = \mu_4$. The T^2 statistic is equal to 73.16

TABLE 3.1. Ramus bone heights (mm) from 20 boys

	Age (years)			
Subject	8	8.5	9	9.5
1	47.8	48.8	49.0	49.7
2	46.4	47.3	47.7	48.4
3	46.3	46.8	47.8	48.5
4	45.1	45.3	46.1	47.2
5	47.6	48.5	48.9	49.3
6	52.5	53.2	53.3	53.7
7	51.2	53.0	54.3	54.5
8	49.8	50.0	50.3	52.7
9	48.1	50.8	52.3	54.4
10	45.0	47.0	47.3	49.3
11	51.2	51.4	51.6	51.9
12	48.5	49.2	53.0	55.5
13	52.1	52.8	53.7	55.0
14	48.2	48.9	49.3	49.8
15	49.6	50.4	51.2	51.8
16	50.7	51.7	52.7	53.3
17	47.2	47.7	48.4	49.5
18	53.3	54.6	55.1	55.3
19	46.2	47.5	48.1	48.4
20	46.3	47.6	51.3	51.8

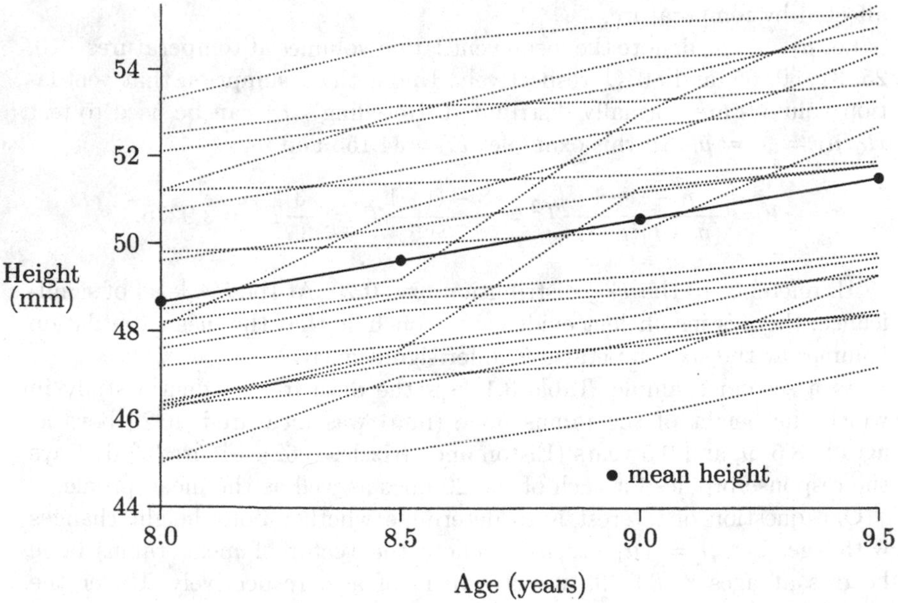

FIGURE 3.2. Ramus bone heights (mm) from 20 boys

TABLE 3.2. Orthogonal polynomial coefficients for four equally spaced time points

Number of Points	Order				
4	Linear	−3	−1	1	3
	Quadratic	1	−1	−1	1
	Cubic	−1	3	−3	1

and

$$F = \frac{n-t+1}{(n-1)(t-1)} T^2 = \frac{20-4+1}{19 \times 3} T^2 = \frac{17}{57} T^2 = 21.82.$$

With reference to the $F_{3,17}$ distribution, this result is highly significant ($p < 0.001$).

In this example, the result that bone height changes with age in young boys is perhaps too obvious to be of great interest. Another question of interest is to assess whether the relationship between bone height and age is linear. Because the four measurements are equally spaced, the test of nonlinearity can be carried out using orthogonal polynomial coefficients (Pearson and Hartley, 1966, Table 47).

Table 3.2 displays orthogonal polynomial coefficients for the case of four equally spaced time points. The hypothesis that the nonlinear (quadratic and cubic) effects of age on ramus bone height are jointly equal to zero is assessed by testing $H_0\colon \boldsymbol{C\mu} = \mathbf{0}_2$, where

$$\boldsymbol{C} = \begin{pmatrix} 1 & -1 & -1 & 1 \\ -1 & 3 & -3 & 1 \end{pmatrix}.$$

In this case, the F statistic is given by Equation (3.1) with $c = 2$. The T^2 statistic is 0.038 and

$$F = \frac{(n-1)-c+1}{(n-1)c} T^2 = \frac{n-c}{(n-1)c} T^2 = \frac{18}{38} T^2 = 0.018.$$

With reference to the $F_{2,18}$ distribution, the p-value is 0.98. Thus, the relationship between ramus bone height and age appears to be linear.

In this example, published tables of orthogonal polynomial coefficients for equally spaced data were used. Although orthogonal polynomial coefficients for unequally spaced time points are not tabulated, these can be generated using computer programs. Another (equivalent) approach is the method of divided differences (Hills, 1968).

Suppose that measurements are obtained at time points $x_1, \ldots, x_t$. Let

$$d_j = \frac{1}{x_{j+1} - x_j}$$

for $j = 1, \ldots, t-1$. The test of nonlinearity is $H_0: \boldsymbol{C\mu} = \boldsymbol{0}_{t-2}$, where $\boldsymbol{C}$ is the $(t-2) \times t$ matrix

$$\begin{pmatrix} -d_1 & d_1+d_2 & -d_2 & 0 & \cdots & 0 & 0 & 0 \\ 0 & -d_2 & d_2+d_3 & -d_3 & \cdots & 0 & 0 & 0 \\ \cdots & \cdots & \cdots & \cdots & \cdots & \cdots & \cdots & \cdots \\ 0 & 0 & 0 & 0 & \cdots & -d_{t-2} & d_{t-2}+d_{t-1} & -d_{t-1} \end{pmatrix}.$$

For example, if the measurements in this example had instead been obtained at ages 8, 8.5, 9, and 10,

$$d_1 = \frac{1}{8.5-8} = 2, \qquad d_2 = \frac{1}{9-8.5} = 2, \qquad d_3 = \frac{1}{10-9} = 1,$$

and

$$\boldsymbol{C} = \begin{pmatrix} -2 & 4 & -2 & 0 \\ 0 & -2 & 3 & -1 \end{pmatrix}.$$

Note that if the time points $x_1, \ldots, x_t$ are equally spaced, then

$$d_1 = \cdots = d_{t-1} = 1$$

and

$$\boldsymbol{C} = \begin{pmatrix} -1 & 2 & -1 & 0 & \cdots & 0 & 0 & 0 \\ 0 & -1 & 2 & -1 & \cdots & 0 & 0 & 0 \\ \cdots & \cdots & \cdots & \cdots & \cdots & \cdots & \cdots & \cdots \\ 0 & 0 & 0 & 0 & \cdots & -1 & 2 & -1 \end{pmatrix}.$$

3.3.3 Comments

The unstructured multivariate approach to the analysis of repeated measurements from one sample assumes multivariate normality but does not require any assumptions concerning the covariance matrix of the multivariate normal distribution. This approach is analogous to the univariate paired t test.

One disadvantage of this approach is that it is necessary to estimate the $t \times t$ covariance matrix $\boldsymbol{\Sigma}$. If t is large, many degrees of freedom are used in estimating covariance parameters. As a consequence, hypothesis tests using this approach will have low power when the denominator df of the F statistic is small. In addition, this method can only be used when the number of linearly independent components of the hypothesis is less than the number of subjects. For example, to test $H_0: \mu_1 = \cdots = \mu_t$, the number of subjects n must be greater than t. Finally, this approach can not be easily adapted for situations in which there are missing data.

3.4 Two-Sample Repeated Measurements

3.4.1 Methodology

The extension of the unstructured multivariate approach to the situation when repeated measurements at t time points are obtained from two independent groups of subjects is straightforward. Consider the data layout of Table 1.2 for the special case where $s = 2$. Let $\boldsymbol{y}_{hi} = (y_{hi1}, \ldots, y_{hit})'$ denote the vector of observations from the ith subject in group h for $i = 1, \ldots, n_h$, $h = 1, 2$. We assume that the vectors $\boldsymbol{y}_{11}, \ldots, \boldsymbol{y}_{1n_1}$ are an independent random sample from the $N_t(\boldsymbol{\mu}_1, \boldsymbol{\Sigma})$ distribution, where $\boldsymbol{\mu}_1 = (\mu_{11}, \ldots, \mu_{1t})'$. We similarly assume that the vectors $\boldsymbol{y}_{21}, \ldots, \boldsymbol{y}_{2n_2}$ are an independent random sample from the $N_t(\boldsymbol{\mu}_2, \boldsymbol{\Sigma})$ distribution, where $\boldsymbol{\mu}_2 = (\mu_{21}, \ldots, \mu_{2t})'$. Note that the covariance matrices of the two distributions are assumed equal.

One hypothesis of general interest is $H_0\colon \boldsymbol{\mu}_1 = \boldsymbol{\mu}_2$. Based on the properties of linear combinations of multivariate normal random vectors, we have the following results:

$$\overline{\boldsymbol{y}}_h \sim N_t\left(\boldsymbol{\mu}_h, \frac{1}{n_h}\boldsymbol{\Sigma}\right), \quad h = 1, 2,$$

$$\overline{\boldsymbol{y}}_1 - \overline{\boldsymbol{y}}_2 \sim N_t\left(\boldsymbol{\mu}_1 - \boldsymbol{\mu}_2, \left(\frac{1}{n_1} + \frac{1}{n_2}\right)\boldsymbol{\Sigma}\right),$$

$$\sqrt{\frac{n_1 n_2}{n_1 + n_2}}\left(\overline{\boldsymbol{y}}_1 - \overline{\boldsymbol{y}}_2\right) \sim N_t\left(\sqrt{\frac{n_1 n_2}{n_1 + n_2}}\left(\boldsymbol{\mu}_1 - \boldsymbol{\mu}_2\right), \boldsymbol{\Sigma}\right).$$

The pooled estimator of the covariance matrix $\boldsymbol{\Sigma}$ is given by

$$\boldsymbol{S} = \frac{(n_1 - 1)\boldsymbol{S}_1 + (n_2 - 1)\boldsymbol{S}_2}{n_1 + n_2 - 2},$$

where

$$\boldsymbol{S}_h = \frac{1}{n_h - 1}\sum_{i=1}^{n_h}(\boldsymbol{y}_{hi} - \overline{\boldsymbol{y}}_h)(\boldsymbol{y}_{hi} - \overline{\boldsymbol{y}}_h)'$$

is the sample covariance matrix in group h for $h = 1, 2$. Because

$$(n_h - 1)\boldsymbol{S}_h \sim W_t(n_h - 1, \Sigma),$$

it follows that

$$(n_1 - 1)\boldsymbol{S}_1 + (n_2 - 1)\boldsymbol{S}_2 \sim W_t(n_1 + n_2 - 2, \boldsymbol{\Sigma})$$

and that

$$(n_1 + n_2 - 2)\boldsymbol{S} \sim W_t(n_1 + n_2 - 2, \boldsymbol{\Sigma}).$$

Therefore, the statistic

$$T^2 = \frac{n_1 n_2}{n_1 + n_2}(\overline{\boldsymbol{y}}_1 - \overline{\boldsymbol{y}}_2)'\boldsymbol{S}^{-1}(\overline{\boldsymbol{y}}_1 - \overline{\boldsymbol{y}}_2) \qquad (3.2)$$

has the $T^2_{t,n_1+n_2-2,\delta}$ distribution with noncentrality parameter

$$\delta = \frac{n_1 n_2}{n_1 + n_2}(\boldsymbol{\mu}_1 - \boldsymbol{\mu}_2)'\boldsymbol{\Sigma}^{-1}(\boldsymbol{\mu}_1 - \boldsymbol{\mu}_2).$$

Consequently, the statistic

$$F = \frac{(n_1 + n_2 - 2) - t + 1}{(n_1 + n_2 - 2)t} T^2 = \frac{n_1 + n_2 - t - 1}{(n_1 + n_2 - 2)t} T^2$$

has the $F_{t,n_1+n_2-t-1,\delta}$ distribution. If $H_0\colon \boldsymbol{\mu}_1 = \boldsymbol{\mu}_2$ is true, then $\delta = 0$ and $F \sim F_{t,n_1+n_2-t-1}$.

Tests of other hypotheses can be similarly constructed. For example, suppose that we wish to test $H_0\colon \boldsymbol{C}(\boldsymbol{\mu}_1 - \boldsymbol{\mu}_2) = \boldsymbol{0}_c$, where $\boldsymbol{C}$ is a $c \times t$ matrix of rank c ($c \le t$). Let $\boldsymbol{z}_{hi} = \boldsymbol{C}\boldsymbol{y}_{hi}$ for $h = 1, 2$. Because

$$\overline{\boldsymbol{y}}_1 - \overline{\boldsymbol{y}}_2 \sim N_t\left(\boldsymbol{\mu}_1 - \boldsymbol{\mu}_2, \left(\frac{1}{n_1} + \frac{1}{n_2}\right)\boldsymbol{\Sigma}\right),$$

it follows that

$$\overline{\boldsymbol{z}}_1 - \overline{\boldsymbol{z}}_2 \sim N_c\left(\boldsymbol{C}(\boldsymbol{\mu}_1 - \boldsymbol{\mu}_2), \left(\frac{n_1 + n_2}{n_1 n_2}\right)\boldsymbol{C}\boldsymbol{\Sigma}\boldsymbol{C}'\right).$$

Let $\boldsymbol{S}_{zh} = \boldsymbol{C}\boldsymbol{S}_h\boldsymbol{C}'$ denote the sample covariance matrix of the transformed observations $\boldsymbol{z}_{hi}$ from group h, and let

$$\boldsymbol{S}_z = \frac{(n_1 - 1)\boldsymbol{S}_{z1} + (n_2 - 1)\boldsymbol{S}_{z2}}{n_1 + n_2 - 2}$$

denote the pooled covariance matrix. Because

$$(n_1 + n_2 - 2)\boldsymbol{S}_z \sim W_c(n_1 + n_2 - 2, \boldsymbol{C}\boldsymbol{\Sigma}\boldsymbol{C}'),$$

the statistic

$$T^2 = \frac{n_1 n_2}{n_1 + n_2}(\overline{\boldsymbol{y}}_1 - \overline{\boldsymbol{y}}_2)'\boldsymbol{C}'\left(\boldsymbol{C}\boldsymbol{S}\boldsymbol{C}'\right)^{-1}\boldsymbol{C}(\overline{\boldsymbol{y}}_1 - \overline{\boldsymbol{y}}_2)$$

has the $T^2_{c,n_1+n_2-2,\delta}$ distribution with noncentrality parameter

$$\delta = \frac{n_1 n_2}{n_1 + n_2}(\boldsymbol{\mu}_1 - \boldsymbol{\mu}_2)'\boldsymbol{C}'(\boldsymbol{C}\boldsymbol{\Sigma}\boldsymbol{C}')^{-1}\boldsymbol{C}(\boldsymbol{\mu}_1 - \boldsymbol{\mu}_2).$$

The statistic

$$F = \frac{(n_1 + n_2 - 2) - c + 1}{(n_1 + n_2 - 2)c} T^2 = \frac{n_1 + n_2 - c - 1}{(n_1 + n_2 - 2)c} T^2$$

then has the $F_{c,n_1+n_2-c-1,\delta}$ distribution. If $H_0\colon \boldsymbol{C}\boldsymbol{\mu}_1 = \boldsymbol{C}\boldsymbol{\mu}_2$ is true, F has the central F distribution F_{c,n_1+n_2-c-1}.

For example, if $H_0\colon \boldsymbol{\mu}_1 = \boldsymbol{\mu}_2$ is rejected, a weaker, and often more realistic, hypothesis is that the mean profiles in the two groups are parallel; that is, that the $\boldsymbol{\mu}_1$ and $\boldsymbol{\mu}_2$ profiles differ only by a constant vertical shift. This hypothesis of parallelism can be expressed as

$$\begin{aligned} H_0\colon \mu_{12} - \mu_{11} &= \mu_{22} - \mu_{21}, \\ \mu_{13} - \mu_{12} &= \mu_{23} - \mu_{22}, \\ &\ \vdots \\ \mu_{1t} - \mu_{1,t-1} &= \mu_{2t} - \mu_{2,t-1}. \end{aligned}$$

In matrix notation, this is $H_0\colon \boldsymbol{C}(\boldsymbol{\mu}_1 - \boldsymbol{\mu}_2) = \boldsymbol{0}_{t-1}$, where $\boldsymbol{C}$ is the $(t-1)\times t$ matrix

$$\begin{pmatrix} -1 & 1 & 0 & 0 & \cdots & 0 & 0 \\ 0 & -1 & 1 & 0 & \cdots & 0 & 0 \\ \cdots & \cdots & \cdots & \cdots & \cdots & \cdots & \cdots \\ 0 & 0 & 0 & 0 & \cdots & -1 & 1 \end{pmatrix}.$$

3.4.2 *Example*

Potthoff and Roy (1964) describe a study conducted at the University of North Carolina Dental School in two groups of children (16 boys and 11 girls). At ages 8, 10, 12, and 14, the distance (mm) from the center of the pituitary gland to the pterygomaxillary fissure was measured. Table 3.3 lists the individual measurements as well as the sample means and standard deviations in both groups. Figure 3.3 displays the individual profiles for the 16 boys, and Figure 3.4 displays the corresponding profiles for the 11 girls. Figure 3.5 shows the mean profiles in boys and girls.

Let $\boldsymbol{\mu}_b = (\mu_{b,8}, \mu_{b,10}, \mu_{b,12}, \mu_{b,14})'$ and $\boldsymbol{\mu}_g = (\mu_{g,8}, \mu_{g,10}, \mu_{g,12}, \mu_{g,14})'$ denote the mean profiles for boys and girls, respectively. One question of interest is to assess whether the profiles for boys and girls are the same (i.e., to test $H_0\colon \boldsymbol{\mu}_b = \boldsymbol{\mu}_g$). Hotelling's T^2 statistic is 16.51 and

$$F = \frac{n_1 + n_2 - t - 1}{(n_1 + n_2 - 2)t} T^2 = \frac{16 + 11 - 4 - 1}{25 \times 4} T^2 = \frac{22}{100} T^2 = 3.63,$$

with $t = 4$ and $n_1 + n_2 - t - 1 = 22$ df. With reference to the $F_{4,22}$ distribution, $p = 0.02$. At the 5% level of significance, one would conclude that the profiles for boys and girls are not the same.

The weaker hypothesis of parallelism is given by

$$\begin{aligned} H_0\colon \mu_{b,10} - \mu_{b,8} &= \mu_{g,10} - \mu_{g,8}, \\ \mu_{b,12} - \mu_{b,10} &= \mu_{g,12} - \mu_{g,10}, \\ \mu_{b,14} - \mu_{b,12} &= \mu_{g,14} - \mu_{g,12}. \end{aligned}$$

TABLE 3.3. Dental measurements from 16 boys and 11 girls

Group	ID	Age 8	Age 10	Age 12	Age 14
Boys	1	26.0	25.0	29.0	31.0
	2	21.5	22.5	23.0	26.5
	3	23.0	22.5	24.0	27.5
	4	25.5	27.5	26.5	27.0
	5	20.0	23.5	22.5	26.0
	6	24.5	25.5	27.0	28.5
	7	22.0	22.0	24.5	26.5
	8	24.0	21.5	24.5	25.5
	9	23.0	20.5	31.0	26.0
	10	27.5	28.0	31.0	31.5
	11	23.0	23.0	23.5	25.0
	12	21.5	23.5	24.0	28.0
	13	17.0	24.5	26.0	29.5
	14	22.5	25.5	25.5	26.0
	15	23.0	24.5	26.0	30.0
	16	22.0	21.5	23.5	25.0
	Mean	22.88	23.81	25.72	27.47
	S.D.	2.45	2.14	2.65	2.09
Girls	1	21.0	20.0	21.5	23.0
	2	21.0	21.5	24.0	25.5
	3	20.5	24.0	24.5	26.0
	4	23.5	24.5	25.0	26.5
	5	21.5	23.0	22.5	23.5
	6	20.0	21.0	21.0	22.5
	7	21.5	22.5	23.0	25.0
	8	23.0	23.0	23.5	24.0
	9	20.0	21.0	22.0	21.5
	10	16.5	19.0	19.0	19.5
	11	24.5	25.0	28.0	28.0
	Mean	21.18	22.23	23.09	24.09
	S.D.	2.12	1.90	2.36	2.44

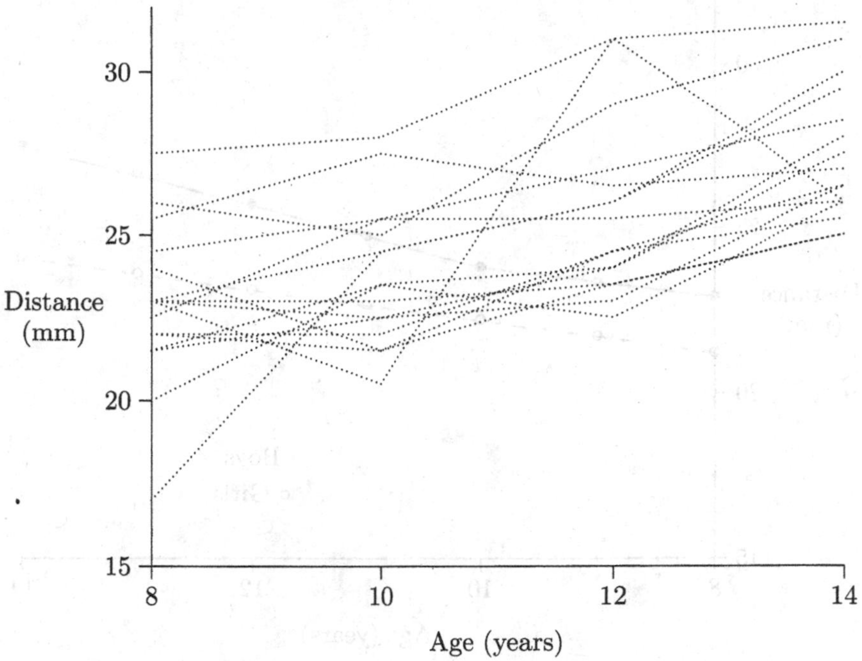

FIGURE 3.3. Dental measurements from 16 boys

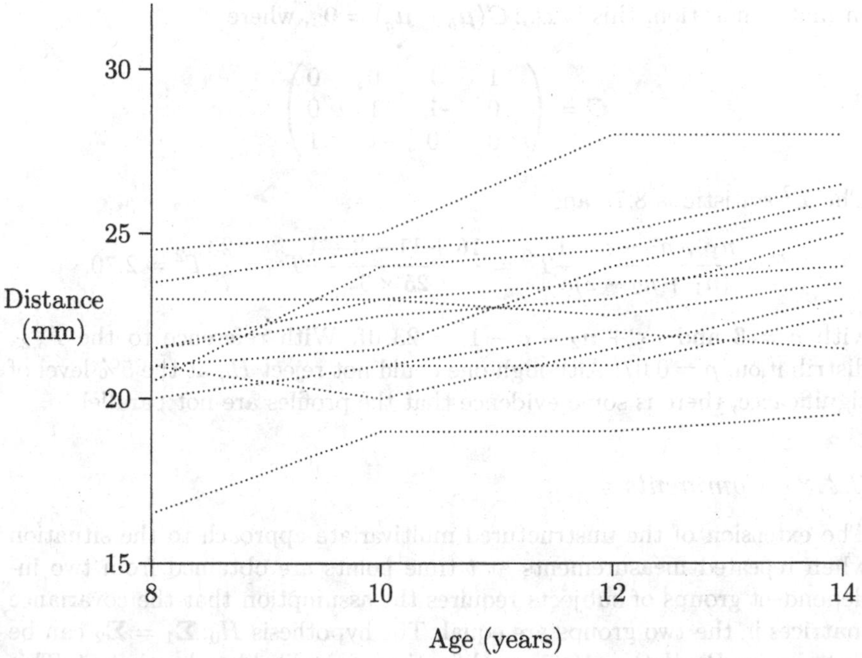

FIGURE 3.4. Dental measurements from 11 girls

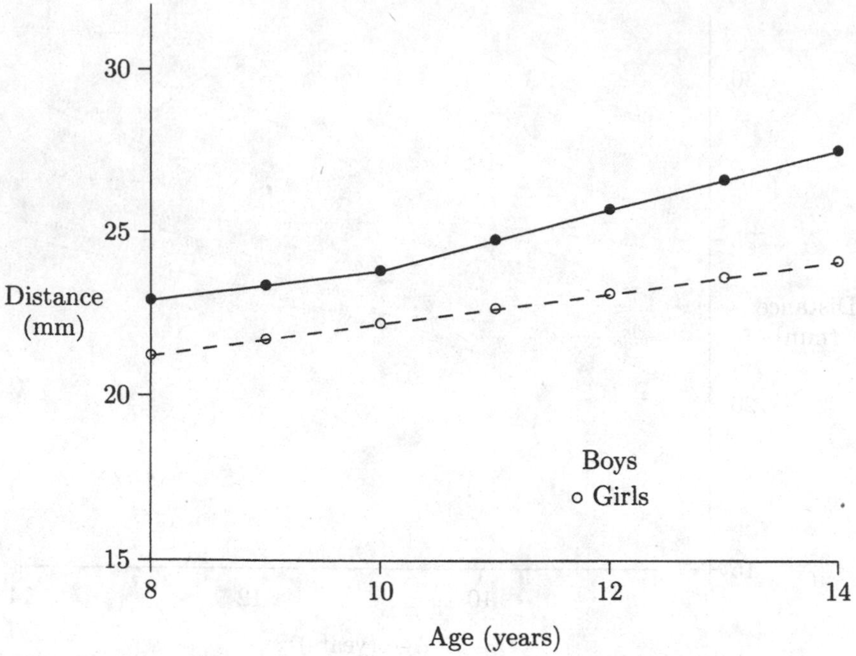

FIGURE 3.5. Sample means of dental measurements from 16 boys and 11 girls

In matrix notation, this is $H_0\colon \boldsymbol{C}(\boldsymbol{\mu}_b - \boldsymbol{\mu}_g) = \mathbf{0}_3$, where

$$\boldsymbol{C} = \begin{pmatrix} -1 & 1 & 0 & 0 \\ 0 & -1 & 1 & 0 \\ 0 & 0 & -1 & 1 \end{pmatrix}.$$

The T^2 statistic is 8.79 and

$$F = \frac{n_1 + n_2 - c - 1}{(n_1 + n_2 - 2)c} T^2 = \frac{16 + 11 - 3 - 1}{25 \times 3} T^2 = \frac{23}{75} T^2 = 2.70,$$

with $c = 3$ and $n_1 + n_2 - c - 1 = 23$ df. With reference to the $F_{3,23}$ distribution, $p = 0.07$. Although one could not reject H_0 at the 5% level of significance, there is some evidence that the profiles are not parallel.

3.4.3 Comments

The extension of the unstructured multivariate approach to the situation when repeated measurements at t time points are obtained from two independent groups of subjects requires the assumption that the covariance matrices in the two groups are equal. The hypothesis $H_0\colon \boldsymbol{\Sigma}_1 = \boldsymbol{\Sigma}_2$ can be tested using Bartlett's (1937) modification of the likelihood ratio test. This test is implemented in standard statistical software, such as the DISCRIM procedure of SAS (SAS Institute, 1999). The asymptotic distribution of the test criteria used in PROC DISCRIM is $\chi^2_{(s-1)t(t+1)/2}$, where s is the number of groups and t is the number of time points. Note that this test can be used when $s > 2$. Although the likelihood ratio test is unbiased, it is not robust to departures from multivariate normality. Parhizgari and Prakash (1989) provide a FORTRAN subroutine implementing an improved approximation to the distribution of the likelihood ratio test.

Anderson (1984, pp. 175–181) discusses the consequences and remedies for the situation in which the covariance matrices are unequal. If $\boldsymbol{\Sigma}_1 \neq \boldsymbol{\Sigma}_2$, the significance level of the T^2 test of $H_0\colon \boldsymbol{\mu}_1 = \boldsymbol{\mu}_2$ depends on $\boldsymbol{\Sigma}_1$ and $\boldsymbol{\Sigma}_2$. If the difference between $\boldsymbol{\Sigma}_1$ and $\boldsymbol{\Sigma}_2$ is small, or if the sample sizes n_1 and n_2 are large, there is no practical effect. Otherwise, the nominal significance level of the test may be distorted.

Two tests of $H_0\colon \boldsymbol{\mu}_1 = \boldsymbol{\mu}_2$ are possible without the assumption that $\boldsymbol{\Sigma}_1 = \boldsymbol{\Sigma}_2$. First, if $n_1 = n_2 = n/2$, the null hypothesis $H_0\colon \boldsymbol{\mu}_1 = \boldsymbol{\mu}_2$ can be tested using a $T^2_{t,(n-2)/2}$ statistic or, equivalently, an $F_{t,n/2-t}$ statistic. In comparison, the degrees of freedom of the F statistic are t and $n-t-1$ if the assumption that $\boldsymbol{\Sigma}_1 = \boldsymbol{\Sigma}_2$ is made. Thus, although the numerator df of the tests are the same, the denominator df are substantially reduced. A much more serious shortcoming is that this test depends on the ordering of the values in the two samples.

If $n_1 < n_2$, the hypothesis $H_0\colon \boldsymbol{\mu}_1 = \boldsymbol{\mu}_2$ can be tested using a T^2_{t,n_1-1} statistic, leading to an F_{t,n_1-t} statistic. This test is based on the difference between the sample means (using all the data), but it sacrifices observations in estimating the covariance matrix. In addition, the test statistic is not unique, because it depends on the ordering of the values in the two samples.

3.5 Problems

3.1 Show that the $W_p(n, \boldsymbol{\Sigma})$ distribution simplifies to the χ^2_n distribution when $p = 1$ and $\boldsymbol{\Sigma} = 1$.

3.2 Consider the one-sample repeated measures problem with data matrix as shown in Table 1.3. Suppose that the $\boldsymbol{y}_i = (y_{i1}, \ldots, y_{it})'$ vectors are a random sample from the $N_t(\boldsymbol{\mu}, \boldsymbol{\Sigma})$ distribution, where $\boldsymbol{\mu} = (\mu_1, \ldots, \mu_t)'$. Let $\overline{\boldsymbol{y}}$ and $\boldsymbol{S}$ denote the sample mean vector and covariance matrix of the observations $\boldsymbol{y}_i$, and let $\boldsymbol{C}$ be a $(t-1) \times t$ matrix of rank $t-1$ satisfying $\boldsymbol{C}\mathbf{1}_{t-1} = \mathbf{0}_{t-1}$, where $\mathbf{1}_{t-1}$ is the $(t-1)$-component vector $(1, \ldots, 1)'$. For example, one choice for $\boldsymbol{C}$ is the matrix

$$\begin{pmatrix} 1 & -1 & 0 & \cdots & 0 & 0 \\ 0 & 1 & -1 & \cdots & 0 & 0 \\ \cdots & \cdots & \cdots & \cdots & \cdots & \cdots \\ 0 & 0 & 0 & \cdots & 1 & -1 \end{pmatrix}.$$

The null hypothesis $H_0: \mu_1 = \ldots = \mu_t$ can be tested using the statistic

$$T^2 = n(\boldsymbol{C}\overline{\boldsymbol{y}})'(\boldsymbol{CSC}')^{-1}(\boldsymbol{C}\overline{\boldsymbol{y}}).$$

Prove that the value of T^2 is invariant with respect to the specific choice of $\boldsymbol{C}$.

3.3 Table 3.4 displays data from a study of affective facial expressions conducted in 22 subjects (Vasey and Thayer, 1987). In this study, several pieces of music were played to each subject in an attempt to elicit selected affective states. Trial 1 was a baseline, relaxing music condition. Trial 2 was designed to produce positive effects, trial 3 was designed to produce agitation, and trial 4 was meant to create sadness. Each trial lasted 90 seconds, and the response variable at each trial was the mean electromyographic (EMG) amplitude (μV) from the left brow region.

(a) Use Hotelling's T^2 statistic to test whether the mean EMG amplitude is the same across the four trials.

(b) Use Hotelling's T^2 statistic to compare each of trials 2–4 to the baseline condition (trial 1).

3.4 Table 3.5 displays data from a study of the effects of the hydrobromides of L-hyoscyamine, L-hyoscine, and DL-hyoscine (scopolamine) on the duration of sleep of ten mental patients (Cushny and Peebles, 1905; Bock, 1975, p. 465). Each of the drugs was tested a number of nights in each subject, and the response variable is the average number of hours of sleep per night. Test the following hypotheses using Hotelling's T^2 statistic:

(a) None of the three hypnotic drugs has an effect different from the control.

(b) The average effect of the three hypnotic drugs is not different from the control.

(c) The effect of L-hyoscyamine is not different from the average effect of L-hyoscine and DL-hyoscine.

(d) The effects of L-hyoscine and DL-hyoscine are not different.

3.5 In a pilot study of a new treatment for AIDS, TMHR scores, Karnofsky scores, and T-4 cell counts were measured at baseline and at 90 and 180 days after the beginning of treatment (Thompson, 1991). These data were considered previously in Problem 2.5 and are displayed in Table 2.13. For each variable, use Hotelling's T^2 statistic to test whether the treatment has an effect over time and whether the effect is linear. Would you recommend the use of this methodology to analyze the data from this study?

TABLE 3.4. Left brow EMG amplitudes from 22 subjects

	EMG Amplitude (μV)			
Subject	Trial 1	Trial 2	Trial 3	Trial 4
1	143	368	345	772
2	142	155	161	178
3	109	167	356	956
4	123	135	137	187
5	276	216	232	307
6	235	386	398	425
7	208	175	207	293
8	267	358	698	771
9	183	193	631	403
10	245	268	572	1383
11	324	507	556	504
12	148	378	342	796
13	130	142	150	173
14	119	171	333	1062
15	102	94	93	69
16	279	204	229	299
17	244	365	392	406
18	196	168	199	287
19	279	358	822	671
20	167	183	731	203
21	345	238	572	1652
22	524	507	520	504

TABLE 3.5. Effects of hypnotic drugs on duration of sleep in ten subjects

	Average Hours of Sleep			
Subject	Control	L-hyoscyamine	L-hyoscine	DL-hyoscine
1	0.6	1.3	2.5	2.1
2	3.0	1.4	3.8	4.4
3	4.7	4.5	5.8	4.7
4	5.5	4.3	5.6	4.8
5	6.2	6.1	6.1	6.7
6	3.2	6.6	7.6	8.3
7	2.5	6.2	8.0	8.2
8	2.8	3.6	4.4	4.3
9	1.1	1.1	5.7	5.8
10	2.9	4.9	6.3	6.4

TABLE 3.6. Left and right eye response times in seven volunteers

	Left Eye				Right Eye			
Subject	6/6	6/18	6/36	6/60	6/6	6/18	6/36	6/60
1	116	119	116	124	120	117	114	122
2	110	110	114	115	106	112	110	110
3	117	118	120	120	120	120	120	124
4	112	116	115	113	115	116	116	119
5	113	114	114	118	114	117	116	112
6	119	115	94	116	100	99	94	97
7	110	110	105	118	105	105	115	115

3.6 Table 3.6 displays data from a study measuring response times of the eyes to a stimulus (Crowder and Hand, 1990, p. 30). The variable of interest was the time lag (milliseconds) between the stimulus (a light flash) and the electrical response at the back of the cortex. In seven student volunteers, recordings were made for left and right eyes through lenses of powers 6/6, 6/18, 6/36, and 6/60. In the following questions, let $\mu_{l1}, \ldots, \mu_{l4}$ and $\mu_{r1}, \ldots, \mu_{r4}$ denote the mean values for the four left and right eye measurements, respectively.

(a) Consider the hypothesis $H_0\colon \mu_{l1} = \mu_{l2} = \cdots = \mu_{r3} = \mu_{r4}$ that there are no differences among the means for the eight repeated measurements. Is it possible to test this hypothesis using Hotelling's T^2? If so, carry out the test.

(b) Repeat (a) for the hypothesis $H_0\colon \mu_{l1} = \mu_{r1}, \ldots, \mu_{l4} = \mu_{r4}$ that there are no differences between eyes.

(c) Repeat (a) for the hypothesis $H_0\colon \mu_{l1} = \mu_{l2} = \mu_{l3} = \mu_{l4}, \mu_{r1} = \mu_{r2} = \mu_{r3} = \mu_{r4}$ that there are no differences within eyes.

3.7 Table 3.7 displays data from a study examining the effectiveness of three methods of suctioning an endotracheal tube: standard suctioning, a new method using a special vacuum, and manual bagging of the patient while suctioning is taking place (Weissfeld and Kshirsagar, 1992). Each of the three methods was applied in a random order to 25 patients in an intensive care unit. The outcome of interest, oxygen saturation, was then measured at five time points: baseline, first suctioning pass, second suctioning pass, third suctioning pass, and 5 minutes postsuctioning.

(a) Test whether the mean responses differ across the 15 measurements using Hotelling's T^2.

(b) At each of the five time points, test whether the mean responses differ among the three methods using Hotelling's T^2.

TABLE 3.7. Oxygen saturation measurements from 25 intensive care unit patients

	Standard					New					Manual Bagging				
ID	1	2	3	4	5	1	2	3	4	5	1	2	3	4	5
1	95	96	94	97	95	94	95	95	95	94	92	97	98	97	91
2	94	94	92	93	95	96	96	95	95	94	96	99	97	99	99
3	94	93	92	91	93	92	94	93	94	92	94	96	96	98	96
4	96	98	97	98	95	98	98	99	98	97	97	95	95	92	96
5	94	93	94	95	95	94	90	93	93	95	93	96	96	96	93
6	97	99	100	99	99	98	97	98	94	98	99	99	98	99	100
7	97	90	93	91	97	95	95	96	92	97	92	91	89	92	92
8	94	95	95	95	95	93	96	96	94	95	96	92	95	94	96
10	95	96	95	94	94	97	99	100	100	99	91	92	92	93	94
11	96	96	96	96	96	100	100	100	100	100	96	96	96	96	96
12	98	96	99	97	98	99	99	98	98	99	99	99	99	99	99
13	94	89	88	79	93	97	98	98	98	96	96	94	94	92	95
14	93	93	94	94	95	93	94	95	95	94	95	96	97	97	97
15	97	100	97	98	96	100	100	99	99	100	97	96	97	97	100
16	96	97	99	100	97	96	95	95	96	97	96	94	93	94	96
17	92	93	94	93	93	92	90	91	90	93	96	100	100	100	98
18	100	99	98	99	99	96	95	97	97	96	96	96	99	99	95
19	97	96	96	96	96	98	100	100	100	99	98	98	97	99	98
20	94	97	98	98	96	98	97	96	93	100	98	95	95	96	97
21	94	97	97	95	95	96	96	96	96	97	95	83	92	93	95
22	96	96	94	94	96	97	95	95	92	96	96	98	98	98	98
23	97	98	97	96	98	99	95	93	90	99	98	99	99	98	97
24	97	98	98	99	98	100	100	100	100	100	97	97	97	96	96
25	98	100	100	100	96	95	96	97	96	94	95	94	97	98	97
26	91	90	92	92	92	94	93	94	94	94	95	93	92	93	95

(c) For each of the three methods, test whether the mean responses differ across the five time points using Hotelling's T^2.

(d) Summarize the results of this study.

3.8 Twelve hospitalized patients underwent a dietary treatment regimen during which plasma ascorbic acid levels were recorded on each of seven occasions during a 16-week period. There were two measurements prior to treatment (weeks 1 and 2), three during treatment (weeks 6, 10, and 14), and two after (weeks 15 and 16) the treatment regimen. The data, which were originally reported in Crowder and Hand (1990, p. 32), are displayed in Table 3.8.

TABLE 3.8. Plasma ascorbic acid levels in 12 hospitalized patients

Patient	Week 1	2	6	10	14	15	16
1	0.22	0.00	1.03	0.67	0.75	0.65	0.59
2	0.18	0.00	0.96	0.96	0.98	1.03	0.70
3	0.73	0.37	1.18	0.76	1.07	0.80	1.10
4	0.30	0.25	0.74	1.10	1.48	0.39	0.36
5	0.54	0.42	1.33	1.32	1.30	0.74	0.56
6	0.16	0.30	1.27	1.06	1.39	0.63	0.40
7	0.30	1.09	1.17	0.90	1.17	0.75	0.88
8	0.70	1.30	1.80	1.80	1.60	1.23	0.41
9	0.31	0.54	1.24	0.56	0.77	0.28	0.40
10	1.40	1.40	1.64	1.28	1.12	0.66	0.77
11	0.60	0.80	1.02	1.28	1.16	1.01	0.67
12	0.73	0.50	1.08	1.26	1.17	0.91	0.87

(a) Use Hotelling's T^2 to test the null hypothesis that there were no changes within phases; that is, $H_0: \mu_1 = \mu_2, \mu_6 = \mu_{10} = \mu_{14}, \mu_{15} = \mu_{16}$.

(b) Use Hotelling's T^2 to test the null hypothesis that the nonlinear components of the relationship between plasma ascorbic acid and time are equal to zero (ignoring the fact that measurements were obtained during three phases).

3.9 Two drug treatments, both in tablet form, were compared using five volunteer subjects in a pilot trial. There were two phases, with a washout period in between. In each phase, blood samples were taken at times 1, 2, 3, and 6 hours after medication. The resulting antibiotic serum levels were reported in Crowder and Hand (1990, p. 9) and are displayed in Table 3.9. In the following questions, let μ_{A1}, μ_{A2}, μ_{A3}, and μ_{A6} denote the mean values at times 1, 2, 3, and 6 during phase A, and let μ_{B1}, μ_{B2}, μ_{B3}, and μ_{B6} denote the corresponding means during phase B.

(a) Consider the hypothesis

$$H_0: \mu_{A1} = \mu_{B1}, \mu_{A2} = \mu_{B2}, \mu_{A3} = \mu_{B3}, \mu_{A6} = \mu_{B6}$$

that there is no difference between phases A and B. Is it possible to test this hypothesis using Hotelling's T^2? If so, carry out the test.

(b) Repeat (a) for the hypothesis

$$H_0: \mu_{A1} = \mu_{A2} = \mu_{A3} = \mu_{A6},\ \mu_{B1} = \mu_{B2} = \mu_{B3} = \mu_{B6}$$

that there are no differences among the four times for both drugs.

TABLE 3.9. Antibiotic serum levels in five volunteers

	Drug A				Drug B			
Subject	1	2	3	6	1	2	3	6
1	1.08	1.99	1.46	1.21	1.48	2.50	2.62	1.95
2	1.19	2.10	1.21	0.96	0.62	0.88	0.68	0.48
3	1.22	1.91	1.36	0.90	0.65	1.52	1.32	0.95
4	0.60	1.10	1.03	0.61	0.32	2.12	1.48	1.09
5	0.55	1.00	0.82	0.52	1.48	0.90	0.75	0.44

(c) Repeat (a) for the hypothesis $H_0\colon \mu_{A1} = \mu_{A2} = \mu_{A3} = \mu_{A6}$ that there are no differences among the four times for drug A.

(d) Repeat (a) for the hypothesis $H_0\colon \mu_{B1} = \mu_{B2} = \mu_{B3} = \mu_{B6}$ that there are no differences among the four times for drug B.

(e) Repeat (a) for the hypothesis that there is no nonlinear effect of time for either of the two drugs.

3.10 Table 3.10 displays plasma inorganic phosphate measurements obtained from 13 control and 20 obese patients 0, 0.5, 1, 1.5, 2, and 3 hours after an oral glucose challenge (Zerbe, 1979b). The sample means are plotted in Figure 3.6.

(a) At the 5% level of significance, test the null hypothesis that the covariance matrices in the control group and the obese group are equal.

(b) Use Hotelling's T^2 statistic to test the null hypothesis that the group means are the same at all six measurement times.

(c) Use Hotelling's T^2 statistic to test whether the profiles in the two groups are parallel.

(d) Repeat parts (a), (b), and (c) using only the first three time points (hours 0, 0.5, and 1).

3.11 Kenward (1987) describes an experiment to compare two treatments for controlling intestinal parasites in calves. There were 30 calves in each of the two groups, and the weight of each calf was determined at 11 measurement times. These data were previously considered in Problem 2.3 and are partially displayed in Table 2.11.

(a) At each of the 11 measurement times, test the null hypothesis that the mean weight for treatment 1 is equal to the mean weight for treatment 2.

TABLE 3.10. Plasma inorganic phosphate levels from 13 control and 20 obese patients

		Hours After Glucose Challenge					
Group	Patient	0	0.5	1	1.5	2	3
Control	1	4.3	3.3	3.0	2.6	2.2	2.5
	2	3.7	2.6	2.6	1.9	2.9	3.2
	3	4.0	4.1	3.1	2.3	2.9	3.1
	4	3.6	3.0	2.2	2.8	2.9	3.9
	5	4.1	3.8	2.1	3.0	3.6	3.4
	6	3.8	2.2	2.0	2.6	3.8	3.6
	7	3.8	3.0	2.4	2.5	3.1	3.4
	8	4.4	3.9	2.8	2.1	3.6	3.8
	9	5.0	4.0	3.4	3.4	3.3	3.6
	10	3.7	3.1	2.9	2.2	1.5	2.3
	11	3.7	2.6	2.6	2.3	2.9	2.2
	12	4.4	3.7	3.1	3.2	3.7	4.3
	13	4.7	3.1	3.2	3.3	3.2	4.2
Obese	1	4.3	3.3	3.0	2.6	2.2	2.5
	2	5.0	4.9	4.1	3.7	3.7	4.1
	3	4.6	4.4	3.9	3.9	3.7	4.2
	4	4.3	3.9	3.1	3.1	3.1	3.1
	5	3.1	3.1	3.3	2.6	2.6	1.9
	6	4.8	5.0	2.9	2.8	2.2	3.1
	7	3.7	3.1	3.3	2.8	2.9	3.6
	8	5.4	4.7	3.9	4.1	2.8	3.7
	9	3.0	2.5	2.3	2.2	2.1	2.6
	10	4.9	5.0	4.1	3.7	3.7	4.1
	11	4.8	4.3	4.7	4.6	4.7	3.7
	12	4.4	4.2	4.2	3.4	3.5	3.4
	13	4.9	4.3	4.0	4.0	3.3	4.1
	14	5.1	4.1	4.6	4.1	3.4	4.2
	15	4.8	4.6	4.6	4.4	4.1	4.0
	16	4.2	3.5	3.8	3.6	3.3	3.1
	17	6.6	6.1	5.2	4.1	4.3	3.8
	18	3.6	3.4	3.1	2.8	2.1	2.4
	19	4.5	4.0	3.7	3.3	2.4	2.3
	20	4.6	4.4	3.8	3.8	3.8	3.6

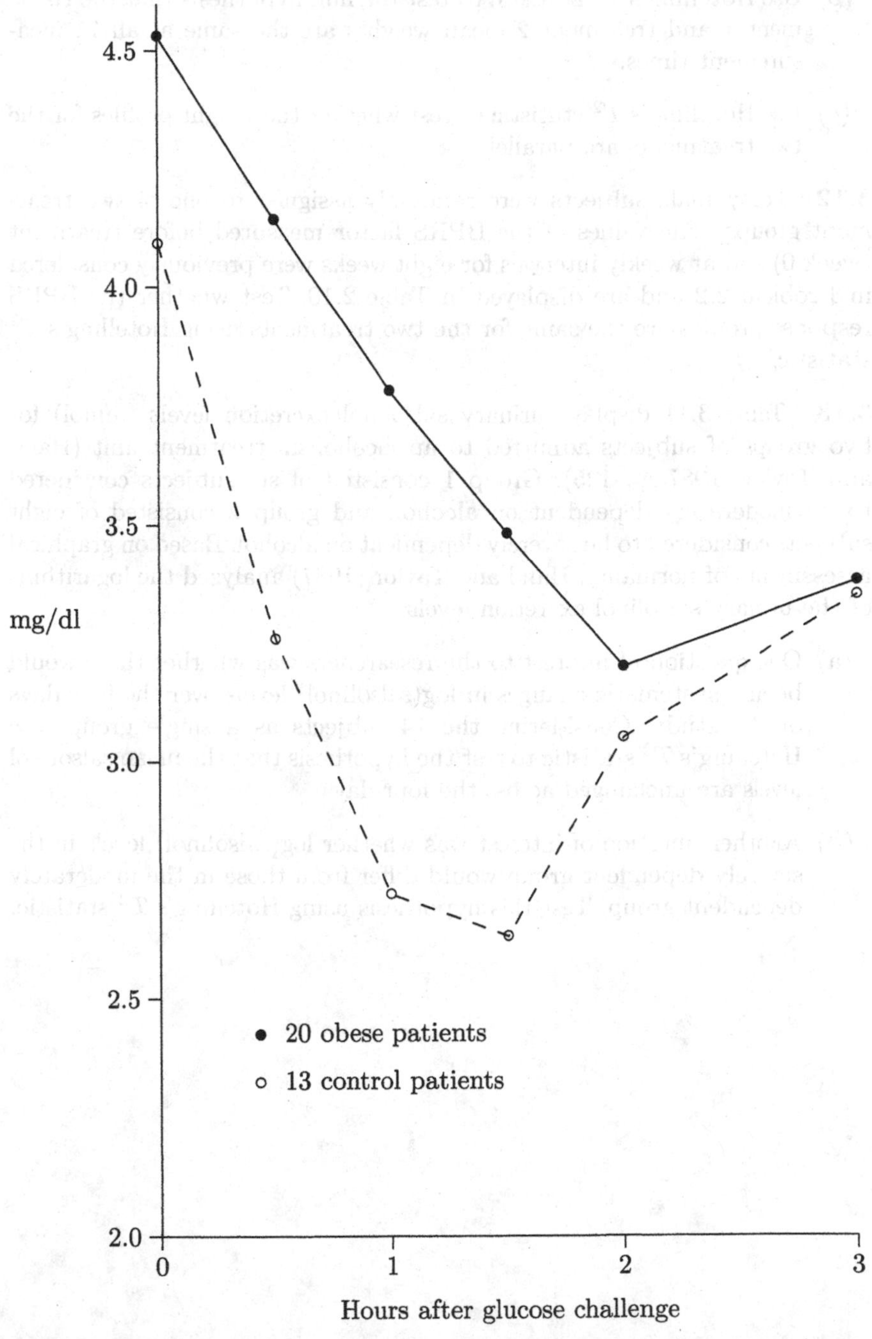

FIGURE 3.6. Mean plasma inorganic phosphate levels in 13 control subjects and 20 obese subjects

(b) Use Hotelling's T^2 statistic to test the null hypothesis that the treatment 1 and treatment 2 mean weights are the same at all 11 measurement times.

(c) Use Hotelling's T^2 statistic to test whether the weight profiles for the two treatments are parallel.

3.12 Forty male subjects were randomly assigned to one of two treatment groups. The values of the BPRS factor measured before treatment (week 0) and at weekly intervals for eight weeks were previously considered in Problem 2.2 and are displayed in Table 2.10. Test whether the BPRS response profiles are the same for the two treatments using Hotelling's T^2 statistic.

3.13 Table 3.11 displays urinary salsolinol excretion levels (mmol) for two groups of subjects admitted to an alcoholism treatment unit (Hand and Taylor, 1987, p. 125). Group 1 consisted of six subjects considered to be moderately dependent on alcohol, and group 2 consisted of eight subjects considered to be severely dependent on alcohol. Based on graphical assessments of normality, Hand and Taylor (1987) analyzed the logarithms of the urinary salsolinol excretion levels.

(a) One question of interest to the researchers was whether there would be any systematic changes in log(salsolinol) levels over the four days of the study. Considering the 14 subjects as a single group, use Hotelling's T^2 statistic to test the hypothesis that the mean salsolinol levels are unchanged across the four days.

(b) Another question of interest was whether log(salsolinol) levels in the severely dependent group would differ from those in the moderately dependent group. Test this hypothesis using Hotelling's T^2 statistic.

TABLE 3.11. Urinary salsolinol excretion levels (mmol) in 14 subjects admitted to an alcoholism treatment unit

Subject	Group	Day 1	Day 2	Day 3	Day 4
1	2	0.64	0.70	1.00	1.40
2	1	0.33	0.70	2.33	3.20
3	2	0.73	1.85	3.60	2.60
4	2	0.70	4.20	7.30	5.40
5	2	0.40	1.60	1.40	7.10
6	2	2.60	1.30	0.70	0.70
7	2	7.80	1.20	2.60	1.80
8	1	5.30	0.90	1.80	0.70
9	1	2.50	2.10	1.12	1.01
10	2	1.90	1.30	4.40	2.80
11	1	0.98	0.32	3.91	0.66
12	1	0.39	0.69	0.73	2.45
13	1	0.31	6.34	0.63	3.86
14	2	0.50	0.40	1.10	8.10

4

Normal-Theory Methods: Multivariate Analysis of Variance

4.1 Introduction

Chapter 3 described methods for the analysis of one-sample and two-sample problems based on Hotelling's T^2 statistic. This chapter extends this methodology to the situation in which there are more than two groups of experimental units.

Section 4.2 introduces the multivariate general linear model. This model extends the univariate linear model to the situation in which there is a vector of responses from each experimental unit. The algebra of the multivariate general linear model is essentially the same as the univariate case, with the differences that univariate variances are replaced by covariance matrices and univariate sums of squares are replaced by sums of squares and products (ssp) matrices. In addition, the distribution theory is analogous to that of the univariate case. In particular, the test criteria are analogs of F statistics. In univariate analysis of variance (ANOVA), the F tests are based on ratios of sums of squares. Because there is no such unique way of comparing matrices, multiple test criteria are available in the multivariate case. There is also more latitude in terms of the types of hypotheses that can be tested.

Section 4.3 discusses the use of profile analysis for the analysis of repeated measurements, and Section 4.4 discusses the growth curve model. Both of these sections also include examples illustrating the use of the corresponding methods for the analysis of repeated measurements.

4.2 The Multivariate General Linear Model

4.2.1 Notation and Assumptions

Consider the situation in which a t-component response vector is measured for each of n experimental units. Let y_{ij} denote the jth component of the response from subject i for $i = 1, \ldots, n$ and $j = 1, \ldots, t$. Also suppose that y_{ij} is generated from the linear model

$$y_{ij} = \boldsymbol{x}_i' \boldsymbol{\beta}_j + e_{ij},$$

where $\boldsymbol{x}_i = (x_{i1}, \ldots, x_{ip})'$ is a vector of p known coefficients specific to the ith subject (and common across the t components of the response) and $\boldsymbol{\beta}_j = (\beta_{1j}, \ldots, \beta_{pj})'$ is a vector of p unknown parameters (specific to the jth time point). To ensure that the covariance matrix of $\boldsymbol{y}_i = (y_{i1}, \ldots, y_{it})'$ is positive-definite, $p \leq n - t$.

Let $\boldsymbol{e}_i = (e_{i1}, \ldots, e_{it})'$ denote the vector of t residuals from the ith subject, and assume that $\boldsymbol{e}_i \sim N_t(\boldsymbol{0}_t, \boldsymbol{\Sigma})$. The $nt \times 1$ vector

$$\boldsymbol{e} = \begin{pmatrix} \boldsymbol{e}_1 \\ \vdots \\ \boldsymbol{e}_n \end{pmatrix}$$

has the $N_{nt}(\boldsymbol{0}_{nt}, \boldsymbol{I}_n \otimes \boldsymbol{\Sigma})$ distribution, where $\boldsymbol{I}_n$ denotes the $n \times n$ identity matrix and the operator $\otimes$ denotes the direct (Kronecker) product (Searle, 1982, p. 265). Thus, the $\boldsymbol{y}_i$ vectors are independent $N_t(\boldsymbol{\mu}_i, \boldsymbol{\Sigma})$ random vectors with

$$\boldsymbol{\mu}_i = \begin{pmatrix} \mu_{i1} \\ \vdots \\ \mu_{it} \end{pmatrix} = \begin{pmatrix} \boldsymbol{x}_i'\boldsymbol{\beta}_1 \\ \vdots \\ \boldsymbol{x}_i'\boldsymbol{\beta}_t \end{pmatrix}.$$

To express the model in terms of matrices, let $\boldsymbol{Y}$ denote the $n \times t$ data matrix

$$\boldsymbol{Y} = \begin{pmatrix} y_{11} & \cdots & y_{1t} \\ \cdots & \cdots & \cdots \\ y_{n1} & \cdots & y_{nt} \end{pmatrix} = \begin{pmatrix} \boldsymbol{y}_1' \\ \vdots \\ \boldsymbol{y}_n' \end{pmatrix}.$$

Let $\boldsymbol{X}$ denote the $n \times p$ known design matrix

$$\boldsymbol{X} = \begin{pmatrix} x_{11} & \cdots & x_{1p} \\ \cdots & \cdots & \cdots \\ x_{n1} & \cdots & x_{np} \end{pmatrix} = \begin{pmatrix} \boldsymbol{x}_1' \\ \vdots \\ \boldsymbol{x}_n' \end{pmatrix}$$

of rank $p \leq (n - t)$. Let $\boldsymbol{B}$ denote the $p \times t$ parameter matrix

$$\boldsymbol{B} = \begin{pmatrix} \beta_{11} & \cdots & \beta_{1t} \\ \cdots & \cdots & \cdots \\ \beta_{p1} & \cdots & \beta_{pt} \end{pmatrix} = (\boldsymbol{\beta}_1, \cdots, \boldsymbol{\beta}_t).$$

Let $\boldsymbol{E}$ denote the $n \times t$ matrix of random errors

$$\boldsymbol{E} = \begin{pmatrix} e_{11} & \cdots & e_{1t} \\ \cdots & \cdots & \cdots \\ e_{n1} & \cdots & e_{nt} \end{pmatrix} = \begin{pmatrix} \boldsymbol{e}'_1 \\ \vdots \\ \boldsymbol{e}'_n \end{pmatrix}.$$

The multivariate general linear model can now be written as

$$\boldsymbol{Y} = \boldsymbol{XB} + \boldsymbol{E},$$

where $\mathrm{E}(\boldsymbol{Y}) = \boldsymbol{XB}$ and

$$\mathrm{Var}\begin{pmatrix} \boldsymbol{y}_1 \\ \vdots \\ \boldsymbol{y}_n \end{pmatrix} = \boldsymbol{I}_n \otimes \boldsymbol{\Sigma}.$$

4.2.2 Parameter Estimation

The maximum likelihood estimator of $\boldsymbol{B}$ is

$$\widehat{\boldsymbol{B}} = (\boldsymbol{X}'\boldsymbol{X})^{-1}\boldsymbol{X}'\boldsymbol{Y}.$$

Note that $\widehat{\boldsymbol{B}}$ is also the least squares estimator of $\boldsymbol{B}$. Also note that if $\boldsymbol{U}_j$ denotes the jth column of $\boldsymbol{Y}$, then

$$\widehat{\boldsymbol{B}} = (\boldsymbol{X}'\boldsymbol{X})^{-1}\boldsymbol{X}'[\boldsymbol{U}_1, \ldots, \boldsymbol{U}_t] = (\widehat{\boldsymbol{\beta}}_1, \ldots, \widehat{\boldsymbol{\beta}}_t),$$

where $\widehat{\boldsymbol{\beta}}_j = (\boldsymbol{X}'\boldsymbol{X})^{-1}\boldsymbol{X}'\boldsymbol{U}_j$ is the usual univariate least squares estimator considering each column of $\boldsymbol{Y}$ as a separate variable.

The maximum likelihood estimator of $\boldsymbol{\Sigma}$ is

$$\widehat{\boldsymbol{\Sigma}} = \frac{1}{n}(\boldsymbol{Y} - \boldsymbol{X}\widehat{\boldsymbol{B}})'(\boldsymbol{Y} - \boldsymbol{X}\widehat{\boldsymbol{B}}).$$

An unbiased estimator of $\boldsymbol{\Sigma}$ is given by

$$\boldsymbol{S} = \frac{1}{n-p}(\boldsymbol{Y} - \boldsymbol{X}\widehat{\boldsymbol{B}})'(\boldsymbol{Y} - \boldsymbol{X}\widehat{\boldsymbol{B}}).$$

Estimation of linear functions of the elements of $\boldsymbol{B}$ is also often of interest. Let $\psi = \boldsymbol{a}'\boldsymbol{B}\boldsymbol{c}$, where $\boldsymbol{a}$ and $\boldsymbol{c}$ are $p \times 1$ and $t \times 1$ vectors of constants, respectively. Note that $\boldsymbol{a}'$ operates within time points and $\boldsymbol{c}$ operates between time points. The estimator $\widehat{\psi} = \boldsymbol{a}'\widehat{\boldsymbol{B}}\boldsymbol{c}$ has minimum variance among all linear unbiased estimates of ψ. The variance of $\widehat{\psi}$ is $\mathrm{Var}(\widehat{\psi}) = (\boldsymbol{c}'\boldsymbol{\Sigma}\boldsymbol{c})[\boldsymbol{a}'(\boldsymbol{X}'\boldsymbol{X})^{-1}\boldsymbol{a}]$.

4.2.3 Hypothesis Testing

Consider the general hypothesis H_0: $\boldsymbol{ABC} = \boldsymbol{D}$. The matrix $\boldsymbol{A}$ is an $a \times p$ matrix (of rank $a \leq p$) of coefficients permitting the testing of "within time" hypotheses (i.e., hypotheses on the elements within given columns of $\boldsymbol{B}$). The matrix $\boldsymbol{C}$ is a $t \times c$ matrix (with rank $c \leq t \leq n-p$) of coefficients permitting the testing of "between time" hypotheses (i.e., hypotheses on the elements within given rows of $\boldsymbol{B}$). Finally, $\boldsymbol{D}$ is an $a \times c$ matrix of constants. This framework for hypothesis tests is very general. In particular, special cases include $\boldsymbol{A} = \boldsymbol{I}_p$, $\boldsymbol{C} = \boldsymbol{I}_t$, and the elements of $\boldsymbol{D}$ all equal to zero.

Four test statistics are commonly used to test H_0: $\boldsymbol{ABC} = \boldsymbol{D}$. All of these statistics are computed using the hypothesis ssp matrix

$$\boldsymbol{Q}_h = (\boldsymbol{A}\widehat{\boldsymbol{B}}\boldsymbol{C} - \boldsymbol{D})'[\boldsymbol{A}(\boldsymbol{X}'\boldsymbol{X})^{-1}\boldsymbol{A}']^{-1}(\boldsymbol{A}\widehat{\boldsymbol{B}}\boldsymbol{C} - \boldsymbol{D})$$

and the residual ssp matrix

$$\boldsymbol{Q}_e = \boldsymbol{C}'\left[\boldsymbol{Y}'\boldsymbol{Y} - \widehat{\boldsymbol{B}}'(\boldsymbol{X}'\boldsymbol{X})\widehat{\boldsymbol{B}}\right]\boldsymbol{C}.$$

The matrix $\boldsymbol{Q}_h$ is analogous to the numerator of a univariate F test, and $\boldsymbol{Q}_e$ is analogous to the error sum of squares.

The likelihood ratio statistic is

$$\Lambda = \frac{|Q_e|}{|Q_h + Q_e|} = \prod \frac{1}{1+\lambda_i},$$

where λ_i are the solutions of the characteristic equation

$$|Q_h - \lambda Q_e| = 0. \tag{4.1}$$

This statistic is known as Wilks' Λ (Wilks, 1932). The Pillai trace statistic is

$$V = \text{trace}[Q_h(Q_h + Q_e)^{-1}] = \sum \theta_i,$$

where the θ_i values are the solutions of the characteristic equation

$$|Q_h - \theta(Q_h + Q_e)| = 0.$$

This statistic is also known as the Bartlett–Nanda–Pillai trace (Bartlett, 1939; Nanda, 1950; Pillai, 1955). The Hotelling–Lawley trace statistic is

$$U = \text{trace}[Q_h Q_e^{-1}] = \sum \lambda_i$$

(Lawley, 1938; Bartlett, 1939; Hotelling, 1947; Hotelling, 1951). This statistic is sometimes called the Lawley–Hotelling trace criterion. Roy's (1957) maximum root statistic is

$$\Theta = \frac{\lambda_1}{1+\lambda_1},$$

where λ_1 is the largest solution of Equation (4.1). Equivalently, Θ is the largest solution of the characteristic equation

$$|Q_h - \theta(Q_h + Q_e)| = 0.$$

In most cases, the exact null distributions of these four test criteria cannot be computed, and approximate tests are required. Approximate F statistics are often used in computer programs. In certain situations, the F approximation for the distribution of Wilks' Λ is exact (Rao, 1973, p. 556).

4.2.4 Comparisons of Test Statistics

The four test statistics have been compared theoretically as well as empirically. Anderson (1984, pp. 330–333) summarizes many of the theoretical and empirical comparisons among statistics. Morrison (1976, pp. 223–224) also summarizes empirical comparisons.

The statistics Λ, V, and U have been compared based on asymptotic expansions of their nonnull distributions in Mikhail (1965), Pillai and Jayachandran (1967), Lee (1971), and Rothenberg (1977). If the population characteristic roots are roughly equal, the ordering from most powerful to least powerful is $V > \Lambda > U$. If the roots are unequal, the ordering is $U > \Lambda > V$. Because the population characteristic roots are unknown in practice, these results support the general use of Λ.

With respect to empirical comparisons among statistics, Ito (1962) compared the large-sample power properties of Λ and U for a simple class of alternative hypotheses; he concluded that there was little difference between these two statistics. Pillai and Jayachandran (1967) compared all four statistics. When the population characteristic roots were very different, U tended to have the highest power. When the characteristic roots were equal, V was most powerful. In the situations they considered, Θ was least powerful.

Roy et al. (1971) also compared all four statistics. For equal population roots, V was most powerful, followed by Λ and U. For the case of a single large population root, Θ had the highest empirical power. In the simulation studies of Schatzoff (1966) and Olson (1974), Θ was most powerful if the alternative was one-dimensional. If, however, there were multiple nonzero characteristic roots, Θ was inferior.

Anderson (1984, p. 333) also discusses the robustness of the four test statistics. All four test procedures tend to be relatively robust to departures from normality. The limiting distributions of each criterion (suitably standardized) for nonnormal $\boldsymbol{y}_i$ are the same as when $\boldsymbol{y}_i$ is normal (as long as conditions such as bounded fourth moments are satisfied). Olson (1974) studied the robustness under departures from covariance homogeneity and departures from normality. Although Λ, U, and V were quite robust, Θ was least robust.

4.3 Profile Analysis

4.3.1 Methodology

Suppose that repeated measurements at t time points have been obtained from s groups of subjects. Let n_h denote the number of subjects in group h for $h = 1, \ldots, s$, and let $n = \sum_{h=1}^{s} n_h$ denote the total sample size. Let y_{hij} denote the response at time j from the ith subject in group h for $h = 1, \ldots, s$, $i = 1, \ldots, n_h$, and $j = 1, \ldots, t$. Note that this is the repeated measurements data layout displayed in Table 1.2.

We assume that the data vectors $\boldsymbol{y}_{hi} = (y_{hi1}, \ldots, y_{hit})'$ are independent and normally distributed with mean $\boldsymbol{\mu}_h = (\mu_{h1}, \ldots, \mu_{ht})'$ and common covariance matrix $\boldsymbol{\Sigma}$. Thus, $\boldsymbol{y}_{hi} \sim N_t(\boldsymbol{\mu}_h, \boldsymbol{\Sigma})$.

The profile analysis model is $y_{hij} = \mu_{hj} + e_{hij}$, where e_{hij} is the residual for subject i in group h at time j. The vector $\boldsymbol{e}_{hi} = (e_{hi1}, \ldots, e_{hit})'$ is the vector of residuals for the ith subject in group h. In terms of the multivariate general linear model,

$$\begin{pmatrix} \boldsymbol{y}'_{11} \\ \vdots \\ \boldsymbol{y}'_{1n_1} \\ \hline \boldsymbol{y}'_{21} \\ \vdots \\ \boldsymbol{y}'_{2n_2} \\ \hline \vdots \\ \hline \boldsymbol{y}'_{s1} \\ \vdots \\ \boldsymbol{y}'_{sn_s} \end{pmatrix} = \begin{pmatrix} 1 & 0 & \cdots & 0 \\ \vdots & \vdots & \cdots & \vdots \\ 1 & 0 & \cdots & 0 \\ \hline 0 & 1 & \cdots & 0 \\ \vdots & \vdots & \cdots & \vdots \\ 0 & 1 & \cdots & 0 \\ \hline & \vdots & & \\ \hline 0 & 0 & \cdots & 1 \\ \vdots & \vdots & \cdots & \vdots \\ 0 & 0 & \cdots & 1 \end{pmatrix} \begin{pmatrix} \mu_{11} & \cdots & \mu_{1t} \\ \mu_{21} & \cdots & \mu_{2t} \\ \vdots & \vdots & \vdots \\ \mu_{s1} & \cdots & \mu_{st} \end{pmatrix} + \begin{pmatrix} \boldsymbol{e}'_{11} \\ \vdots \\ \boldsymbol{e}'_{1n_1} \\ \hline \boldsymbol{e}'_{21} \\ \vdots \\ \boldsymbol{e}'_{2n_2} \\ \hline \vdots \\ \hline \boldsymbol{e}'_{s1} \\ \vdots \\ \boldsymbol{e}'_{sn_s} \end{pmatrix},$$

or $\boldsymbol{Y} = \boldsymbol{XB} + \boldsymbol{E}$, where $\boldsymbol{Y}$ and $\boldsymbol{E}$ are $n \times t$ matrices with rows $\boldsymbol{y}'_{11}, \ldots, \boldsymbol{y}'_{sn_s}$ and $\boldsymbol{e}'_{11}, \ldots, \boldsymbol{e}'_{sn_s}$, respectively, $\boldsymbol{X}$ is $n \times s$, and $\boldsymbol{B}$ is $s \times t$.

Three general hypotheses are of interest in profile analysis:

H_{01}: the profiles for the s groups are parallel (i.e., no group-by-time interaction);

H_{02}: no differences among groups;

H_{03}: no differences among time points.

Note that H_{01} should be tested first, because the acceptance or rejection of this hypothesis affects how the two other hypotheses can be tested. In addition, if H_{01} is rejected, we may wish to test hypotheses of the form:

H_{04}: no differences among groups within some subset of the total number of time points;

H_{05}: no differences among time points in a particular group (or subset of groups);

H_{06}: no differences within some subset of the total number of time points in a particular group (or subset of groups).

Test of Parallelism

The hypothesis of parallelism is

$$H_{01}: \begin{pmatrix} \mu_{11}-\mu_{12} \\ \mu_{12}-\mu_{13} \\ \vdots \\ \mu_{1,t-1}-\mu_{1t} \end{pmatrix} = \begin{pmatrix} \mu_{21}-\mu_{22} \\ \mu_{22}-\mu_{23} \\ \vdots \\ \mu_{2,t-1}-\mu_{2t} \end{pmatrix} \cdots = \begin{pmatrix} \mu_{s1}-\mu_{s2} \\ \mu_{s2}-\mu_{s3} \\ \vdots \\ \mu_{s,t-1}-\mu_{st} \end{pmatrix}.$$

In terms of the general hypothesis H_0: $\boldsymbol{ABC} = \boldsymbol{D}$,

$$\begin{aligned} \boldsymbol{A}_{(s-1)\times s} &= (\boldsymbol{I}_{s-1}, -\boldsymbol{1}_{s-1}), \\ \boldsymbol{C}_{t\times(t-1)} &= \begin{pmatrix} 1 & 0 & \cdots & 0 \\ -1 & 1 & \cdots & 0 \\ 0 & -1 & \cdots & 0 \\ \cdots & \cdots & \cdots & \cdots \\ 0 & 0 & \cdots & 1 \\ 0 & 0 & \cdots & -1 \end{pmatrix}, \\ \boldsymbol{D}_{(s-1)\times(t-1)} &= \begin{pmatrix} 0 & \cdots & 0 \\ \vdots & \ddots & \vdots \\ 0 & \cdots & 0 \end{pmatrix}. \end{aligned}$$

Testing this hypothesis is equivalent to carrying out a one-way multivariate analysis of variance (MANOVA) model on the $t-1$ differences between adjacent time points from each sampling unit.

Tests of No Differences Among Groups

Depending on the results of the test of H_{01}, two tests of the hypothesis H_{02} of no differences among groups are possible.

First, if the parallelism hypothesis is reasonable, the test for differences among groups can be carried out using the sum (or average) of the repeated observations from each subject. In this case,

$$\begin{aligned} \boldsymbol{A}_{(s-1)\times s} &= (\boldsymbol{I}_{s-1}, -\boldsymbol{1}_{s-1}), \\ \boldsymbol{C}_{t\times 1} &= \boldsymbol{1}_t, \\ \boldsymbol{D}_{(s-1)\times 1} &= \boldsymbol{0}_{s-1}. \end{aligned}$$

Note that $\boldsymbol{A}$ is the same as for the test of parallelism (H_{01}). Because the s groups are independent, this test of H_{02} is equivalent to that from a one-way ANOVA on the totals (or means) across time from each subject.

A multivariate test for differences among groups can also be carried out without assuming parallelism. In this case, the null hypothesis is

$$H_{02}: \begin{pmatrix} \mu_{11} \\ \mu_{12} \\ \vdots \\ \mu_{1t} \end{pmatrix} = \begin{pmatrix} \mu_{21} \\ \mu_{22} \\ \vdots \\ \mu_{2t} \end{pmatrix} = \cdots = \begin{pmatrix} \mu_{s1} \\ \mu_{s2} \\ \vdots \\ \mu_{st} \end{pmatrix}.$$

In terms of the general hypothesis H_0: $\boldsymbol{ABC} = \boldsymbol{D}$,

$$\begin{aligned} \boldsymbol{A}_{(s-1)\times s} &= (\boldsymbol{I}_{s-1}, -\boldsymbol{1}_{s-1}), \\ \boldsymbol{C}_{t\times t} &= \boldsymbol{I}_t, \\ \boldsymbol{D}_{(s-1)\times t} &= \begin{pmatrix} 0 & \cdots & 0 \\ \vdots & \ddots & \vdots \\ 0 & \cdots & 0 \end{pmatrix}. \end{aligned}$$

If comparisons among groups for a subset of the t time points are of interest, the columns of $\boldsymbol{C}$ corresponding to the excluded time points can be omitted.

Tests of No Differences Among Time Points

Depending on the results of the test of H_{01}, two tests of H_{03} are possible. If the parallelism hypothesis is reasonable, the test for differences among time points can be carried out using the sum (or average) across groups of the observations at each time point. In this case, the null hypothesis is H_{03}: $\boldsymbol{ABC} = \boldsymbol{D}$, where

$$\begin{aligned} \boldsymbol{A}_{1\times s} &= (1, \ldots, 1) \text{ or } (1/s, \ldots, 1/s), \\ \boldsymbol{C}_{t\times(t-1)} &= \begin{pmatrix} \boldsymbol{I}_{t-1} \\ -\boldsymbol{1}'_{t-1} \end{pmatrix}, \\ \boldsymbol{D}_{1\times(t-1)} &= \boldsymbol{0}'_{t-1}. \end{aligned}$$

This is equivalent to a one-sample T^2 test, as described in Section 3.3.1.

This procedure weights each of the s groups equally and is usually appropriate. However, if unequal group sizes result from the nature of the experimental conditions, it may be desirable to use a weighted average rather than a simple average. In this case, $\boldsymbol{A} = (n_1, \ldots, n_s)$ or $\boldsymbol{A} = (n_1/n, \ldots, n_s/n)$ can be used; note that $\boldsymbol{C}$ and $\boldsymbol{D}$ are unchanged.

The hypothesis H_{03} can also be tested without assuming parallelism:

$$H_{03}: \begin{pmatrix} \mu_{11} \\ \mu_{21} \\ \vdots \\ \mu_{s1} \end{pmatrix} = \begin{pmatrix} \mu_{12} \\ \mu_{22} \\ \vdots \\ \mu_{s2} \end{pmatrix} = \cdots = \begin{pmatrix} \mu_{1t} \\ \mu_{2t} \\ \vdots \\ \mu_{st} \end{pmatrix}.$$

In this case,

$$\begin{aligned} \boldsymbol{A}_{s\times s} &= \boldsymbol{I}_s, \\ \boldsymbol{C}_{t\times(t-1)} &= \begin{pmatrix} \boldsymbol{I}_{t-1} \\ -\boldsymbol{1}'_{t-1} \end{pmatrix}, \\ \boldsymbol{D}_{s\times(t-1)} &= \begin{pmatrix} 0 & \cdots & 0 \\ \vdots & \ddots & \vdots \\ 0 & \cdots & 0 \end{pmatrix}. \end{aligned}$$

If comparisons among time points in a particular group (or subset of groups) are of interest, the rows of $\boldsymbol{A}$ corresponding to the excluded groups can be omitted.

4.3.2 Example

Potthoff and Roy (1964) describe a study conducted at the University of North Carolina Dental School in two groups of children (16 boys and 11 girls). In Section 3.4.2, Hotelling's T^2 statistic was used to compare boys and girls at ages 8, 10, 12, and 14 years with respect to the distance (mm) from the center of the pituitary gland to the pterygomaxillary fissure. Table 3.3 lists the individual measurements as well as the sample means and standard deviations in both groups. The profile analysis methods summarized in Section 4.3.1 can also be used to analyze these data.

Let $\boldsymbol{y}_{b,1},\ldots,\boldsymbol{y}_{b,16}$ and $\boldsymbol{y}_{g,1},\ldots,\boldsymbol{y}_{g,11}$ denote the 4×1 vectors of measurements from the 16 boys and 11 girls in the study. Similarly, let $\boldsymbol{e}_{b,1},\ldots,\boldsymbol{e}_{b,16}$ and $\boldsymbol{e}_{g,1},\ldots,\boldsymbol{e}_{g,11}$ denote the corresponding vectors of residuals. Also, let $\boldsymbol{\mu}_b = (\mu_{b,8},\mu_{b,10},\mu_{b,12},\mu_{b,14})'$ and $\boldsymbol{\mu}_g = (\mu_{g,8},\mu_{g,10},\mu_{g,12},\mu_{g,14})'$ denote the mean profiles for boys and girls, respectively. The profile analysis model is

$$\begin{pmatrix} \boldsymbol{y}'_{b,1} \\ \vdots \\ \boldsymbol{y}'_{b,16} \\ \boldsymbol{y}'_{g,1} \\ \vdots \\ \boldsymbol{y}'_{g,11} \end{pmatrix} = \begin{pmatrix} 1 & 0 \\ \vdots & \vdots \\ 1 & 0 \\ 0 & 1 \\ \vdots & \vdots \\ 0 & 1 \end{pmatrix} \begin{pmatrix} \mu_{b,8} & \mu_{b,10} & \mu_{b,12} & \mu_{b,14} \\ \mu_{g,8} & \mu_{g,10} & \mu_{g,12} & \mu_{g,14} \end{pmatrix} + \begin{pmatrix} \boldsymbol{e}'_{b,1} \\ \vdots \\ \boldsymbol{e}'_{b,16} \\ \boldsymbol{e}'_{g,1} \\ \vdots \\ \boldsymbol{e}'_{g,11} \end{pmatrix},$$

or $\boldsymbol{Y} = \boldsymbol{X}\boldsymbol{B} + \boldsymbol{E}$, where $\boldsymbol{Y}$ and $\boldsymbol{E}$ are 27×4 matrices, $\boldsymbol{X}$ is 27×2, and $\boldsymbol{B}$ is 2×4.

The hypothesis of parallelism is $H_{01}\colon \boldsymbol{ABC} = \boldsymbol{0}'_3$, where $\boldsymbol{A} = (1,-1)$ and

$$\boldsymbol{C} = \begin{pmatrix} 1 & 0 & 0 \\ -1 & 1 & 0 \\ 0 & -1 & 1 \\ 0 & 0 & -1 \end{pmatrix}.$$

Because there are only two groups, the test statistics Λ, V, U, and Θ described in Section 4.2.3 are all equivalent to Hotelling's T^2. As shown in Section 3.4.2, the corresponding F statistic is 2.70. With reference to the $F_{3,23}$ distribution, the p-value of the test of H_{01} is 0.07. Although not statistically significant at the 5% level of significance, there is some evidence that the profiles are not parallel.

For purposes of illustration, the test for differences between boys and girls assuming parallelism is carried out as follows. The null hypothesis is H_{02}: $\boldsymbol{ABC} = 0$, where $\boldsymbol{A} = (1, -1)$ and $\boldsymbol{C} = (1, 1, 1, 1)'$. This is equivalent to a two-sample t test on the totals (or means) from each subject. The F statistic is 9.29 with 1 and 25 df. Because $p = 0.005$, there is evidence that boys and girls differ.

If we do not assume that the profiles over time for boys and girls are parallel, the test for differences between boys and girls is the test of

$$H_{02}\colon \boldsymbol{ABC} = \boldsymbol{0}_4',$$

where $\boldsymbol{A} = (1, -1)$ and $\boldsymbol{C} = \boldsymbol{I}_4$. The test statistic is equivalent to the two-sample Hotelling's T^2 statistic [Equation (3.2)]. As was shown in Section 3.4.2, the F statistic is 3.63. With reference to the $F_{4,22}$ distribution, $p = 0.02$. At the 5% level of significance, one would conclude that the profiles for boys and girls are not the same.

The hypothesis H_{03} of no differences among time points for both boys and girls can also be tested both assuming parallelism and not assuming parallelism. Under the assumption that the profiles for boys and girls are parallel, and weighting each group equally, the test is of H_{03}: $\boldsymbol{ABC} = \boldsymbol{0}_3'$, where $\boldsymbol{A} = (1, 1)$ and

$$\boldsymbol{C} = \begin{pmatrix} 1 & 0 & 0 \\ 0 & 1 & 0 \\ 0 & 0 & 1 \\ -1 & -1 & -1 \end{pmatrix}. \tag{4.2}$$

Because this is equivalent to a one-sample T^2 test, the four test statistics from Section 4.2.3 are equivalent, and the resulting F statistic is 31.69 with 3 and 23 df. Thus, the means at the four time points are highly significantly different ($p < 0.001$).

If we test this same hypothesis without assuming parallelism, the test is of H_{03}: $\boldsymbol{ABC} = \boldsymbol{D}$, where $\boldsymbol{A} = \boldsymbol{I}_2$, $\boldsymbol{C}$ is given by Equation (4.2), and $\boldsymbol{D}$ is a 2×3 matrix with all elements equal to zero. In testing this hypothesis, the statistics Λ, V, U, and Θ from Section 4.2.3 are not equivalent. The value of Wilk's Λ is 0.16. The corresponding F statistic is 11.46 with 6 and 46 df ($p < 0.001$).

It will often be of interest to test whether there are differences among time points within a single group rather than in both groups overall. In boys, this hypothesis is tested using $\boldsymbol{A} = (1, 0)$ and $\boldsymbol{C}$ given by Equation (4.2). All four test statistics yield $F = 31.89$ with 3 and 23 df; thus, there is highly significant evidence of differences among time points for boys ($p < 0.001$). The corresponding $\boldsymbol{A}$ matrix for testing this hypothesis in girls is $\boldsymbol{A} = (0, 1)$. The F statistic is 7.09 with 3 and 23 df, with $p = 0.0015$.

4.4 Growth Curve Analysis

4.4.1 Introduction

Although the profile analysis model is often a convenient framework in which to analyze repeated measurements, it does not make use of the fact that a subject's repeated measurements are ordered. In fact, profile analysis is applicable in very general settings in which there is a multivariate outcome variable for each experimental unit. Because repeated measurements obtained over time are naturally ordered, it may be of interest to characterize trends over time using low-order polynomials. The means at the repeated time points can then be summarized by a few coefficients rather than by the entire vector. When the number of repeated measurements t is large, reduction to a low-order polynomial is very useful. In this case, focus shifts from hypothesis testing to estimation of a substantive model for the responses.

This approach to the analysis of repeated measurements is called growth curve analysis. This extension of the standard MANOVA model was initially proposed by Potthoff and Roy (1964). An alternative formulation was developed by Rao (1965, 1966, 1967) and Khatri (1966). Grizzle and Allen (1969) unify and illustrate the methodology, and Kleinbaum (1973) extends the growth curve analysis approach to accommodate missing data. Timm (1980) gives a review of growth curve methodology, and the books by Kshirsagar and Smith (1995) and Pan and Fang (2001) provide a comprehensive treatment of this topic.

Growth curve analysis is a relatively unused approach due to unfamiliarity with the methodology and lack of readily available software. In addition, Chapter 6 will introduce more flexible alternatives to the traditional growth curve model that are now available. However, with a little work, it is possible to fit growth curve models using standard MANOVA programs.

4.4.2 The Growth Curve Model

As in Section 4.3.1, suppose that repeated measurements at t time points have been obtained from s groups of subjects. Let n_h denote the number of subjects in group h, for $h = 1, \ldots, s$, and let $n = \sum_{h=1}^{s} n_h$ denote the total sample size. Let y_{hij} denote the response at time j from the ith subject in group h for $h = 1, \ldots, s$, $i = 1, \ldots, n_h$, and $j = 1, \ldots, t$. For purposes of illustrating the growth curve model, we will assume that the t time points are the equally spaced values $1, \ldots, t$. It is only necessary, however, to have a common set of time points for each subject.

In growth curve analysis, we assume that the time trend in each group can be described by a $(q-1)$st-degree polynomial, with $q \leq t$. The growth curve model is

$$y_{hij} = \beta_{h0} + \beta_{h1}\, j + \beta_{h2}\, j^2 + \cdots + \beta_{h,q-1}\, j^{q-1} + e_{hij}, \tag{4.3}$$

where e_{hij} is the residual at time j for the ith subject in group h. This model has sq parameters. Although the functional form of the time trend is the same in each of the s groups, the parameters are specific to each group.

Let $\boldsymbol{y}_{hi} = (y_{hi1}, \ldots, y_{hit})'$ denote the vector of observations from subject i in group h, and let $\boldsymbol{e}_{hi} = (e_{hi1}, \ldots, e_{hit})'$ denote the corresponding vector of residuals. Similarly, let $\boldsymbol{Y}$ and $\boldsymbol{E}$ denote the corresponding $n \times t$ matrices of observations and residuals, as described in Section 4.3.1.

The growth curve model is

$$\boldsymbol{Y} = \boldsymbol{XBT} + \boldsymbol{E},$$

where $\boldsymbol{X}$ is an $n \times s$ across-individual design matrix, $\boldsymbol{B}$ is an $s \times q$ parameter matrix, and $\boldsymbol{T}$ is a $q \times t$ within-individual design matrix. We assume that $\operatorname{rank}(T) = q$, where $q \leq t$. Each row $\boldsymbol{y}'_{hi} = (y_{hi1}, \ldots, y_{hit})$ of the data matrix $\boldsymbol{Y}$ is assumed to have an independent multivariate normal distribution with covariance matrix $\boldsymbol{\Sigma}$. Thus, $\mathrm{E}(\boldsymbol{Y}) = \boldsymbol{XBT}$ and

$$\operatorname{Var}\begin{pmatrix} \boldsymbol{y}_{11} \\ \vdots \\ \boldsymbol{y}_{sn_s} \end{pmatrix} = \boldsymbol{I}_n \otimes \boldsymbol{\Sigma}.$$

In terms of Equation (4.3), the matrix of parameters is

$$\boldsymbol{B} = \begin{pmatrix} \beta_{10} & \cdots & \beta_{1,q-1} \\ \beta_{20} & \cdots & \beta_{2,q-1} \\ \vdots & & \vdots \\ \beta_{s0} & \cdots & \beta_{s,q-1} \end{pmatrix},$$

and the design matrices $\boldsymbol{X}$ and $\boldsymbol{T}$ are given by

$$\boldsymbol{X} = \begin{pmatrix} 1 & 0 & \cdots & 0 \\ \vdots & \vdots & \cdots & \vdots \\ 1 & 0 & \cdots & 0 \\ \hline 0 & 1 & \cdots & 0 \\ \vdots & \vdots & \cdots & \vdots \\ 0 & 1 & \cdots & 0 \\ \hline & & \vdots & \\ \hline 0 & 0 & \cdots & 1 \\ \vdots & \vdots & \cdots & \vdots \\ 0 & 0 & \cdots & 1 \end{pmatrix}, \quad \boldsymbol{T} = \begin{pmatrix} 1 & 1 & \cdots & 1 \\ 1 & 2 & \cdots & t \\ 1 & 4 & \cdots & t^2 \\ \vdots & \vdots & \vdots & \vdots \\ 1 & 2^{q-1} & \cdots & t^{q-1} \end{pmatrix}$$

The basic idea of the Potthoff–Roy(1964) approach to growth curve analysis is to transform the growth curve model to the usual MANOVA model used in profile analysis. To accomplish this, let $\boldsymbol{G}$ be a $t \times t$ symmetric, positive-definite matrix satisfying the following conditions:

1. $\boldsymbol{G}$ must be either nonstochastic or independent of $\boldsymbol{Y}$.

2. $\boldsymbol{TG}^{-1}\boldsymbol{T}'$ has rank q.

If both sides of the model $\boldsymbol{Y} = \boldsymbol{XBT} + \boldsymbol{E}$ are postmultiplied by the $t \times q$ matrix $\boldsymbol{G}^{-1}\boldsymbol{T}'(\boldsymbol{TG}^{-1}\boldsymbol{T}')^{-1}$, then

$$\begin{aligned} \boldsymbol{YG}^{-1}\boldsymbol{T}'(\boldsymbol{TG}^{-1}\boldsymbol{T}')^{-1} &= \boldsymbol{XBTG}^{-1}\boldsymbol{T}'(\boldsymbol{TG}^{-1}\boldsymbol{T}')^{-1} \\ &\quad + \boldsymbol{EG}^{-1}\boldsymbol{T}'(\boldsymbol{TG}^{-1}\boldsymbol{T}')^{-1} \end{aligned}$$

or $\boldsymbol{Z} = \boldsymbol{XB} + \boldsymbol{E}^*$, where

$$\boldsymbol{Z} = \boldsymbol{YG}^{-1}\boldsymbol{T}'(\boldsymbol{TG}^{-1}\boldsymbol{T}')^{-1}$$

is an $n \times q$ matrix of transformed dependent variables.

The transformed data matrix $\boldsymbol{Z}$ has mean $\boldsymbol{XB}$. The rows of $\boldsymbol{Z}$ have independent q-variate normal distributions with covariance matrix

$$\boldsymbol{\Sigma}^* = (\boldsymbol{TG}^{-1}\boldsymbol{T}')^{-1}\boldsymbol{TG}^{-1}\boldsymbol{\Sigma}\boldsymbol{G}^{-1}\boldsymbol{T}'(\boldsymbol{TG}^{-1}\boldsymbol{T}')^{-1}.$$

The growth curve model has thus been reduced to the profile analysis model. Standard multivariate linear model theory, as described in Section 4.2, can now be used to estimate $\boldsymbol{B}$ and test hypotheses of the form $\boldsymbol{ABC} = \boldsymbol{D}$. In particular, the unbiased estimator of $\boldsymbol{B}$ is

$$\widehat{\boldsymbol{B}} = (\boldsymbol{X}'\boldsymbol{X})^{-1}\boldsymbol{X}'\boldsymbol{YG}^{-1}\boldsymbol{T}'(\boldsymbol{TG}^{-1}\boldsymbol{T}')^{-1}.$$

Potthoff and Roy (1964) discuss the choice of the matrix $\boldsymbol{G}$. They prove that the minimum variance unbiased estimator of $\boldsymbol{B}$ is

$$\widehat{\boldsymbol{B}} = (\boldsymbol{X}'\boldsymbol{X})^{-1}\boldsymbol{X}'\boldsymbol{Y}\boldsymbol{\Sigma}^{-1}\boldsymbol{T}'(\boldsymbol{T}\boldsymbol{\Sigma}^{-1}\boldsymbol{T}')^{-1}.$$

Therefore, although $\widehat{\boldsymbol{B}}$ is unbiased for any $\boldsymbol{G}$, the optimal choice is $\boldsymbol{G} = \boldsymbol{\Sigma}$. Unfortunately, $\boldsymbol{\Sigma}$ is usually unknown in practice. Potthoff and Roy (1964) suggest using an estimate of $\boldsymbol{\Sigma}$ obtained from an independent experiment. They do not, however, develop the theory for allowing $\boldsymbol{G} = \boldsymbol{S}$, where $\boldsymbol{S}$ is the sample covariance matrix calculated from the data used to estimate $\boldsymbol{B}$.

The computations required prior to using standard MANOVA programs to carry out the analysis become much simpler when $q = t$ (i.e., when the time trend across the t points is described by a $(t-1)$st degree polynomial). Of course, this choice is less interesting because it does not make use of low-order polynomials to describe the data. In this case,

$$\boldsymbol{Z} = \boldsymbol{Y}\boldsymbol{G}^{-1}\boldsymbol{T}'(\boldsymbol{T}\boldsymbol{G}^{-1}\boldsymbol{T}')^{-1} = \boldsymbol{Y}\boldsymbol{G}^{-1}\boldsymbol{T}'(\boldsymbol{T}')^{-1}\boldsymbol{G}\boldsymbol{T}^{-1} = \boldsymbol{Y}\boldsymbol{T}^{-1},$$

so there is no need to choose $\boldsymbol{G}$.

The computations become even simpler if $\boldsymbol{T}$ is chosen to be an orthogonal matrix. In this case, $\boldsymbol{T}^{-1} = \boldsymbol{T}'$. The transformation then becomes $\boldsymbol{Z} = \boldsymbol{Y}\boldsymbol{T}'$, and matrix inversion is not required. Bock (1963) developed this procedure using orthogonal polynomials and Roy–Bargmann (Roy and Bargmann, 1958) step-down F tests.

The choice $q = t$ simplifies the computations but does not provide any reduction to a lower-order polynomial. When $q < t$, the simplest choice of $\boldsymbol{G}$ is the $t \times t$ identity matrix. In this case,

$$\boldsymbol{Z} = \boldsymbol{Y}\boldsymbol{G}^{-1}\boldsymbol{T}'(\boldsymbol{T}\boldsymbol{G}^{-1}\boldsymbol{T}')^{-1} = \boldsymbol{Y}\boldsymbol{T}'(\boldsymbol{T}\boldsymbol{T}')^{-1}.$$

If the time trends are parameterized using orthogonal polynomial coefficients, the transformation further simplifies to $\boldsymbol{Z} = \boldsymbol{Y}\boldsymbol{T}'$. Although this simplifies the calculations and eliminates the need for matrix inversion, it may not be the best choice in terms of power. Information is lost in reducing $\boldsymbol{Y}$ to $\boldsymbol{Z}$ unless $\boldsymbol{G} = \boldsymbol{\Sigma}$ or unless $\boldsymbol{\Sigma} = \sigma^2\boldsymbol{I}_t$.

Rao (1965, 1966, 1967) and Khatri (1966) develop an alternative approach to the growth curve model. To avoid the arbitrary choice of $\boldsymbol{G}$, Khatri (1966) derives the maximum likelihood estimator of $\boldsymbol{B}$. Rao considers the conditional model

$$\mathrm{E}(\boldsymbol{Y}|\boldsymbol{W}) = \boldsymbol{X}\boldsymbol{B} + \boldsymbol{W}\boldsymbol{\Gamma}$$

and derives a covariate-adjusted estimator of $\boldsymbol{B}$. If $q < t$, identical results are obtained from:

1. Khatri's maximum likelihood approach;
2. Rao's covariate-adjusted approach using $t - q$ covariates;

3. Potthoff and Roy's approach using $\boldsymbol{G} = \boldsymbol{S}$.

In addition, when $q < t$, the Potthoff–Roy approach using $\boldsymbol{G} = \boldsymbol{I}$ is equivalent to not using covariates in Rao's conditional model.

Stanek and Koch (1985) show the equivalence of parameter estimates from growth curve models and seemingly unrelated regression (SUR) models (Zellner, 1962). Patel (1986) proposed a multivariate model for repeated measurements designs with time-varying covariates, and Verbyla (1988) showed that Patel's model can be written as an SUR model. Verbyla and Venables (1988) and Park and Woolson (1992) extend the SUR approach to situations where parallel profiles are required and where the data are incomplete, respectively.

4.4.3 Examples

One Sample

Although growth curve analysis is most useful in comparing multiple groups of experimental units, the methodology will first be illustrated using an example involving a single group of subjects.

Table 3.1 and Figure 3.2 display the data from a dental study in which the height of the ramus bone (mm) was measured in 20 boys at ages 8, 8.5, 9, and 9.5 years (Elston and Grizzle, 1962). In Section 3.3.2, the unstructured multivariate approach was used to assess whether the mean ramus bone heights differ across the four ages and whether the relationship between ramus bone height and age is linear. The growth curve model can also be used to analyze these data.

Let $\boldsymbol{y}_i = (y_{i1}, y_{i2}, y_{i3}, y_{i4})'$ denote the vector of ramus bone heights at ages 8, 8.5, 9, and 9.5 years of age for subject i, for $i = 1, \ldots, 20$, and let $\boldsymbol{Y}$ denote the 20×4 data matrix with rows $\boldsymbol{y}_1', \ldots, \boldsymbol{y}_{20}'$. Because there is a single group of subjects, the design matrix $\boldsymbol{X}$ is the 20×1 vector $(1, \ldots, 1)'$.

A simple initial approach is to choose $q = t = 4$ and to use

$$\boldsymbol{T} = \begin{pmatrix} 1/2 & 1/2 & 1/2 & 1/2 \\ -3/\sqrt{20} & -1/\sqrt{20} & 1/\sqrt{20} & 3/\sqrt{20} \\ 1/2 & -1/2 & -1/2 & 1/2 \\ -1/\sqrt{20} & 3/\sqrt{20} & -3/\sqrt{20} & 1/\sqrt{20} \end{pmatrix}. \tag{4.4}$$

This is the 4×4 matrix of standardized orthogonal polynomial coefficients. The numerators of rows 2, 3, and 4 of T are the orthogonal polynomial coefficients for four equally spaced time points (Table 3.2). The entries in each row are standardized by dividing by the sum of the squares of the values. With this choice of $\boldsymbol{T}$,

$$\boldsymbol{Z} = \boldsymbol{Y}\boldsymbol{G}^{-1}\boldsymbol{T}'(\boldsymbol{T}\boldsymbol{G}^{-1}\boldsymbol{T}')^{-1} = \boldsymbol{Y}\boldsymbol{T}^{-1} = \boldsymbol{Y}\boldsymbol{T}'.$$

TABLE 4.1. Results of hypothesis tests from cubic growth curve model for ramus bone heights

Hypothesis	F Statistic	df	p-value
$\beta_0 = 0$	8113.21	1,19	< 0.001
$\beta_1 = 0$	51.83	1,19	< 0.001
$\beta_2 = 0$	0.04	1,19	0.848
$\beta_3 = 0$	0.00	1,19	0.982
$\beta_2 = \beta_3 = 0$	0.02	2,18	0.982

Thus, it is not necessary to choose $\boldsymbol{G}$, and matrix inversion is not required. We will use this model to test whether the nonlinear components of the time effect are statistically significant.

The transformed model is $\boldsymbol{Z} = \boldsymbol{XB} + \boldsymbol{E}^*$, where $\boldsymbol{B} = (\beta_0, \beta_1, \beta_2, \beta_3)$. The elements of $\boldsymbol{B}$ are the constant, linear, quadratic, and cubic effects of age. Table 4.1 displays the F statistics, df, and p-values for tests of various hypotheses of interest. Note that, in this application, the multivariate general linear model test statistics Λ, V, U, and Θ are equivalent. Whereas the constant and linear age effects are highly significant, the quadratic and cubic effects of age are nonsignificant, both individually and jointly.

We will now model the effects of age on ramus height using a linear growth curve model ($q = 2$). Although the computations are easier using standardized orthogonal polynomial coefficients, interpretation of the results is simpler using the matrix

$$\boldsymbol{T} = \begin{pmatrix} 1 & 1 & 1 & 1 \\ 8.0 & 8.5 & 9.0 & 9.5 \end{pmatrix}.$$

We will first use $\boldsymbol{G} = \boldsymbol{I}_4$. In this case,

$$\boldsymbol{Z} = \boldsymbol{Y}\boldsymbol{G}^{-1}\boldsymbol{T}'(\boldsymbol{T}\boldsymbol{G}^{-1}\boldsymbol{T}')^{-1} = \boldsymbol{Y}\boldsymbol{T}'(\boldsymbol{T}\boldsymbol{T}')^{-1}.$$

The transformation is computed as follows:

$$\boldsymbol{T}\boldsymbol{T}' = \begin{pmatrix} 1 & 1 & 1 & 1 \\ 8.0 & 8.5 & 9.0 & 9.5 \end{pmatrix} \begin{pmatrix} 1 & 8.0 \\ 1 & 8.5 \\ 1 & 9.0 \\ 1 & 9.5 \end{pmatrix} = \begin{pmatrix} 4 & 35 \\ 35 & 307.5 \end{pmatrix},$$

$$(\boldsymbol{T}\boldsymbol{T}')^{-1} = \begin{pmatrix} 61.5 & -7 \\ -7 & 0.8 \end{pmatrix},$$

$$\boldsymbol{T}'(\boldsymbol{T}\boldsymbol{T}')^{-1} = \begin{pmatrix} 5.5 & -0.6 \\ 2.0 & -0.2 \\ -1.5 & 0.2 \\ -5.0 & 0.6 \end{pmatrix}.$$

The transformation $\boldsymbol{Z} = \boldsymbol{Y}\boldsymbol{T}'(\boldsymbol{T}\boldsymbol{T}')^{-1}$ thus produces a 20×2 matrix of transformed dependent variables.

TABLE 4.2. Results of linear growth curve model for ramus bone heights using $G = I_4$

Parameter	Estimate	Standard Error	F Statistic	df	p-value
β_0	33.498	2.320	208.41	1,19	< 0.001
β_1	1.896	0.263	51.83	1,19	< 0.001

Table 4.2 displays the results of fitting the model $\boldsymbol{Z} = \boldsymbol{XB} + \boldsymbol{E}^*$, where $\boldsymbol{B} = (\beta_0, \beta_1)$. The resulting linear model is

$$\text{ramus height} = 33.498 + 1.896 \text{ age}.$$

The linear growth curve model could also have been fit using $\boldsymbol{G} = \boldsymbol{S}$, where $\boldsymbol{S}$ is the sample covariance matrix. In this example,

$$\boldsymbol{G} = \boldsymbol{S} = \begin{pmatrix} 6.32997 & 6.18908 & 5.77700 & 5.35579 \\ 6.18908 & 6.44934 & 6.15342 & 5.78526 \\ 5.77700 & 6.15342 & 6.91800 & 6.77421 \\ 5.35579 & 5.78526 & 6.77421 & 7.18316 \end{pmatrix}.$$

The transformation $\boldsymbol{Z} = \boldsymbol{YG}^{-1}\boldsymbol{T}'(\boldsymbol{TG}^{-1}\boldsymbol{T}')^{-1}$ is computed as follows:

$$\boldsymbol{G}^{-1} = \begin{pmatrix} 2.6933 & -2.8416 & 0.0498 & 0.2334 \\ -2.8416 & 4.1461 & -1.5651 & 0.2555 \\ 0.0498 & -1.5651 & 3.8824 & -2.4379 \\ 0.2334 & 0.2555 & -2.4379 & 2.0585 \end{pmatrix},$$

$$\boldsymbol{G}^{-1}\boldsymbol{T}' = \begin{pmatrix} 0.13501 & 0.05932 \\ -0.00513 & 0.85011 \\ -0.07088 & -1.12416 \\ 0.10952 & 1.65380 \end{pmatrix},$$

$$\boldsymbol{TG}^{-1}\boldsymbol{T}' = \begin{pmatrix} 0.16853 & 1.43907 \\ 1.43907 & 13.29412 \end{pmatrix},$$

$$(\boldsymbol{TG}^{-1}\boldsymbol{T}')^{-1} = \begin{pmatrix} 78.42127 & -8.48897 \\ -8.48897 & 0.99414 \end{pmatrix},$$

$$\boldsymbol{G}^{-1}\boldsymbol{T}'(\boldsymbol{TG}^{-1}\boldsymbol{T}')^{-1} = \begin{pmatrix} 10.08419 & -1.08714 \\ -7.61849 & 0.88864 \\ 3.98441 & -0.51587 \\ -5.45011 & 0.71437 \end{pmatrix}.$$

The transformation $\boldsymbol{Z} = \boldsymbol{YG}^{-1}\boldsymbol{T}'(\boldsymbol{TG}^{-1}\boldsymbol{T}')^{-1}$ again produces a 20×2 matrix of transformed dependent variables.

Table 4.3 displays the results of fitting the model $\boldsymbol{Z} = \boldsymbol{XB} + \boldsymbol{E}^*$, where $\boldsymbol{B} = (\beta_0, \beta_1)$. The resulting linear model is

$$\text{ramus height} = 33.390 + 1.906 \text{ age}.$$

TABLE 4.3. Results of linear growth curve model for ramus bone heights using $\boldsymbol{G} = \boldsymbol{S}$

Parameter	Estimate	Standard Error	F Statistic	df	p-value
β_0	33.390	1.980	284.33	1,19	< 0.001
β_1	1.906	0.223	73.12	1,19	< 0.001

Although the parameter estimates are similar to those from the model using $\boldsymbol{G} = \boldsymbol{I}_4$, the standard errors of the estimates are smaller when $\boldsymbol{G} = \boldsymbol{S}$ is used.

Multiple Samples

Potthoff and Roy (1964) describe a study conducted at the University of North Carolina Dental School in two groups of children (16 boys and 11 girls). In Section 3.4.2, Hotelling's T^2 statistic was used to compare boys and girls at ages 8, 10, 12, and 14 years with respect to the distance (mm) from the center of the pituitary gland to the pterygomaxillary fissure. Section 4.3.2 illustrated the analysis of these data using profile analysis methods. Table 3.3 lists the individual measurements as well as the sample means and standard deviations in both groups.

The change in the pituitary–pterygomaxillary distance during growth is important in orthodontal therapy. Thus, growth curve methods are of interest in order to:

1. describe the distance in boys and girls as simple functions of age;

2. compare the functions for boys and girls.

As in the previous example, a useful initial approach is to fit a growth curve model with $q = t = 4$ using standardized orthogonal polynomial coefficients. Because the four measurement times are again equally spaced, the matrix $\boldsymbol{T}$ is given by Equation (4.4). This choice eliminates the need for matrix inversion and/or computation of the pooled covariance matrix $\boldsymbol{S}$ because

$$\boldsymbol{Z} = \boldsymbol{Y}\boldsymbol{G}^{-1}\boldsymbol{T}'(\boldsymbol{T}\boldsymbol{G}^{-1}\boldsymbol{T}')^{-1} = \boldsymbol{Y}\boldsymbol{T}^{-1} = \boldsymbol{Y}\boldsymbol{T}',$$

where $\boldsymbol{Y}$ is the 27×4 data matrix used in the profile analysis model of Section 4.3.2. Using the results of this model, we can then test the significance of the constant, linear, quadratic, and cubic terms to determine the appropriate degree of polynomial to consider in subsequent models.

The transformed model is $\boldsymbol{Z} = \boldsymbol{X}\boldsymbol{B} + \boldsymbol{E}^*$, where

$$\boldsymbol{X} = \begin{pmatrix} 1&1&1&1&1&1&1&1&1&1&1&1&1&1&1&1&0&0&0&0&0&0&0&0&0&0&0 \\ 0&0&0&0&0&0&0&0&0&0&0&0&0&0&0&0&1&1&1&1&1&1&1&1&1&1&1 \end{pmatrix}'$$

TABLE 4.4. Results of hypothesis tests from cubic growth curve model for the dental measurements data

Hypothesis	F Statistic	df	p-value
$\beta_{10} = \beta_{20} = 0$	2066.22	2,25	< 0.001
$\beta_{11} = \beta_{21} = 0$	52.28	2,25	< 0.001
$\beta_{12} = \beta_{22} = 0$	1.27	2,25	0.298
$\beta_{13} = \beta_{23} = 0$	0.21	2,25	0.810
$\beta_{12} = \beta_{13} = \beta_{22} = \beta_{23} = 0$	0.68	4,48	0.611

is 27×2 and $\boldsymbol{B}$ is the 2×4 matrix

$$\boldsymbol{B} = \begin{pmatrix} \beta_{10} & \beta_{11} & \beta_{12} & \beta_{13} \\ \beta_{20} & \beta_{21} & \beta_{22} & \beta_{23} \end{pmatrix}.$$

The elements in the first row of $\boldsymbol{B}$ are the constant, linear, quadratic, and cubic effects of age in boys, and the second row of $\boldsymbol{B}$ contains the corresponding effects for girls.

Table 4.4 displays the F statistics, df, and p-values for tests of various hypotheses of interest. For the tests listed in the first four rows of Table 4.4, the multivariate general linear model test statistics Λ, V, U, and Θ are equivalent. The F statistic reported for the fourth hypothesis (joint quadratic and cubic effects of age) is that from Wilks' Λ. Whereas the joint constant effects and joint linear age effects in boys and girls are highly significant, the nonlinear effects of age are nonsignificant.

Given these results, fitting a linear growth curve model is appropriate. One approach to obtaining the maximum likelihood estimators of the model parameters is using Rao's covariate-adjusted model. Let $\boldsymbol{Z}_1$ be the 27×2 matrix consisting of the first two columns of $\boldsymbol{Z}$ (the constant and linear components), and let $\boldsymbol{Z}_2$ be the 27×2 matrix consisting of the third and fourth columns of $\boldsymbol{Z}$ (the quadratic and cubic components). The Rao covariate-adjusted model is

$$\boldsymbol{Z}_1 = \boldsymbol{X}\boldsymbol{B}_1 + \boldsymbol{Z}_2\boldsymbol{B}_2,$$

where

$$\boldsymbol{B}_1 = \begin{pmatrix} \beta_{10} & \beta_{11} \\ \beta_{20} & \beta_{21} \end{pmatrix}, \quad \boldsymbol{B}_2 = \begin{pmatrix} \beta_{12} & \beta_{13} \\ \beta_{22} & \beta_{23} \end{pmatrix}.$$

This model used the quadratic and cubic effects as covariates.

The maximum likelihood estimates of the parameters of the linear growth curve model can also be obtained from the Potthoff–Roy approach using $\boldsymbol{G} = \boldsymbol{S}$, where

$$\boldsymbol{S} = \begin{pmatrix} 5.41545 & 2.71682 & 3.91023 & 2.71023 \\ 2.71682 & 4.18477 & 2.92716 & 3.31716 \\ 3.91023 & 2.92716 & 6.45574 & 4.13074 \\ 2.71023 & 3.31716 & 4.13074 & 4.98574 \end{pmatrix}.$$

is the pooled sample covariance matrix. In this case, the model is

$$\boldsymbol{Z} = \boldsymbol{X}\boldsymbol{B}_1,$$

where the transformation $\boldsymbol{Z} = \boldsymbol{Y}\boldsymbol{G}^{-1}\boldsymbol{T}'(\boldsymbol{T}\boldsymbol{G}^{-1}\boldsymbol{T}')^{-1}$ is computed as follows:

$$\boldsymbol{T} = \begin{pmatrix} 1/2 & 1/2 & 1/2 & 1/2 \\ -3/\sqrt{20} & -1/\sqrt{20} & 1/\sqrt{20} & 3/\sqrt{20} \end{pmatrix},$$

$$\boldsymbol{G}^{-1} = \boldsymbol{S}^{-1} = \begin{pmatrix} 0.37168 & -0.15407 & -0.19490 & 0.06194 \\ -0.15407 & 0.57220 & 0.05082 & -0.33905 \\ -0.19490 & 0.05082 & 0.43363 & -0.28713 \\ 0.06194 & -0.33905 & -0.28713 & 0.63038 \end{pmatrix},$$

$$\boldsymbol{G}^{-1}\boldsymbol{T}' = \begin{pmatrix} 0.04232 & -0.21691 \\ 0.06495 & -0.24067 \\ 0.00121 & 0.02373 \\ 0.03307 & 0.39293 \end{pmatrix},$$

$$\boldsymbol{T}\boldsymbol{G}^{-1}\boldsymbol{T}' = \begin{pmatrix} 0.07077 & -0.02046 \\ -0.02046 & 0.46821 \end{pmatrix},$$

$$(\boldsymbol{T}\boldsymbol{G}^{-1}\boldsymbol{T}')^{-1} = \begin{pmatrix} 14.31048 & 0.62545 \\ 0.62545 & 2.16312 \end{pmatrix},$$

$$\boldsymbol{G}^{-1}\boldsymbol{T}'(\boldsymbol{T}\boldsymbol{G}^{-1}\boldsymbol{T}')^{-1} = \begin{pmatrix} 0.47002 & -0.44273 \\ 0.77889 & -0.47998 \\ 0.03214 & 0.05208 \\ 0.71894 & 0.87063 \end{pmatrix}.$$

Both models give the same estimates of the constant and linear age effects in boys and girls.

It is easier to interpret the results of the linear growth curve model if the transformation matrix $\boldsymbol{T}$ is on the natural time scale, that is, using

$$\boldsymbol{T} = \begin{pmatrix} 1 & 1 & 1 & 1 \\ 8 & 10 & 12 & 14 \end{pmatrix}.$$

In this case, the vector of transformed dependent variables

$$\boldsymbol{Z} = \boldsymbol{Y}\boldsymbol{G}^{-1}\boldsymbol{T}'(\boldsymbol{T}\boldsymbol{G}^{-1}\boldsymbol{T}')^{-1}$$

is computed as follows:

$$\boldsymbol{G}^{-1}\boldsymbol{T}' = \begin{pmatrix} 0.08465 & -0.03890 \\ 0.12989 & 0.35251 \\ 0.00242 & 0.13271 \\ 0.06613 & 2.48467 \end{pmatrix},$$

$$\boldsymbol{T}\boldsymbol{G}^{-1}\boldsymbol{T}' = \begin{pmatrix} 0.28309 & 2.93099 \\ 2.93099 & 39.59178 \end{pmatrix},$$

TABLE 4.5. Parameter estimates from linear growth curve model using $G = S$

	Boys		Girls	
	Estimate	Standard Error	Estimate	Standard Error
Constant	15.842	0.972	17.425	1.173
Linear age	0.827	0.082	0.476	0.099

$$(TG^{-1}T')^{-1} = \begin{pmatrix} 15.12612 & -1.11979 \\ -1.11979 & 0.10816 \end{pmatrix},$$

$$G^{-1}T'(TG^{-1}T')^{-1} = \begin{pmatrix} 1.32398 & -0.09000 \\ 1.57005 & -0.10733 \\ -0.11203 & 0.01165 \\ -1.78200 & 0.19468 \end{pmatrix}.$$

Table 4.5 displays the parameter estimates from this model. The slopes for boys and girls are significantly different ($p = 0.01$). The intercepts for boys and girls are not significantly different ($p = 0.3$). All hypothesis tests involving slopes, as well as the joint tests of intercepts and slopes, are identical to those from the orthogonal polynomial parameterization.

Finally, the computations for the Potthoff–Roy approach are much simpler with the choice $G = I_4$. In this case, the matrix of transformed dependent variables is given by

$$Z = YG^{-1}T'(TG^{-1}T')^{-1} = YT'(TT')^{-1}.$$

This transformation is computed as follows:

$$TT' = \begin{pmatrix} 1 & 1 & 1 & 1 \\ 8 & 10 & 12 & 14 \end{pmatrix} \begin{pmatrix} 1 & 8 \\ 1 & 10 \\ 1 & 12 \\ 1 & 14 \end{pmatrix} = \begin{pmatrix} 4 & 44 \\ 44 & 504 \end{pmatrix},$$

$$(TT')^{-1} = \begin{pmatrix} 6.30 & -0.55 \\ -0.55 & 0.05 \end{pmatrix},$$

$$T'(TT')^{-1} = \begin{pmatrix} 1.9 & -0.15 \\ 0.8 & -0.05 \\ -0.3 & 0.05 \\ -1.4 & 0.15 \end{pmatrix}.$$

Table 4.6 displays the parameter estimates from this model. The parameter estimates differ slightly between the two models (Tables 4.5 and 4.6). In addition, the standard errors of the parameter estimates using $G = S$ (Table 4.5) are somewhat smaller.

TABLE 4.6. Parameter estimates from linear growth curve model using $\boldsymbol{G} = \boldsymbol{I}$

	Boys		Girls	
	Estimate	Standard Error	Estimate	Standard Error
Constant	16.341	1.019	17.373	1.228
Linear age	0.784	0.086	0.480	0.104

4.5 Problems

4.1 Consider the profile analysis model of Section 4.3.1 for the specific case where $s = 3$ and $t = 4$. Thus, the parameter matrix is

$$\boldsymbol{B} = \begin{pmatrix} \mu_{11} & \mu_{12} & \mu_{13} & \mu_{14} \\ \mu_{21} & \mu_{22} & \mu_{23} & \mu_{24} \\ \mu_{31} & \mu_{32} & \mu_{33} & \mu_{34} \end{pmatrix}.$$

(a) Specify the matrices $\boldsymbol{A}$ and $\boldsymbol{C}$ for testing the hypothesis of parallelism. Compute $\boldsymbol{ABC}$, and verify that this transformation correctly specifies the hypothesis of interest.

(b) Repeat (a) for the hypothesis of no differences among groups (assuming parallelism).

(c) Repeat (a) for the hypothesis of no differences among groups (not assuming parallelism).

(d) Repeat (a) for the hypothesis of no differences among time points (assuming parallelism).

(e) Repeat (a) for the hypothesis of no differences among time points (not assuming parallelism).

4.2 Table 4.7 displays scaled test scores for a cohort of 64 students of the Laboratory School of the University of Chicago (Bock, 1975). These students (36 boys, 28 girls) were tested on the vocabulary section of the Cooperative Reading Tests at grades 8, 9, 10, and 11. Because girls commonly complete their physical growth earlier than boys, these data provide an opportunity to determine whether the same is true of the development of verbal abilities as measured by these vocabulary scores.

(a) Analyze these data using profile analysis methods. In particular, provide answers to the following questions: (1) Are the response profiles parallel for boys and girls? (2) Are there differences between boys and girls? If so, at which grade levels? (3) Are there differences among grade levels?

(b) Analyze these data using growth curve techniques. Compare your results with those from part (a).

TABLE 4.7. Scaled vocabulary test scores from 36 boys and 28 girls

	Boys					Girls			
	Grade					Grade			
ID	8	9	10	11	ID	8	9	10	11
1	1.75	2.60	3.76	3.68	37	1.24	4.90	2.42	2.54
2	0.90	2.47	2.44	3.43	38	5.94	6.56	9.36	7.72
3	0.80	0.93	0.40	2.27	39	0.87	3.36	2.58	1.73
4	2.42	4.15	4.56	4.21	40	−0.09	2.29	3.08	3.35
5	−1.31	−1.31	−0.66	−2.22	41	3.24	4.78	3.52	4.84
6	−1.56	1.67	0.18	2.33	42	1.03	2.10	3.88	2.81
7	1.09	1.50	0.52	2.33	43	3.58	4.67	3.83	5.19
8	−1.92	1.03	0.50	3.04	44	1.41	1.75	3.70	3.77
9	−1.61	0.29	0.73	3.24	45	−0.65	−0.11	2.40	3.53
10	2.47	3.64	2.87	5.38	46	1.52	3.04	2.74	2.63
11	−0.95	0.41	0.21	1.82	47	0.57	2.71	1.90	2.41
12	1.66	2.74	2.40	2.17	48	2.18	2.96	4.78	3.34
13	2.07	4.92	4.46	4.71	49	1.10	2.65	1.72	2.96
14	3.30	6.10	7.19	7.46	50	0.15	2.69	2.69	3.50
15	2.75	2.53	4.28	5.93	51	−1.27	1.26	0.71	2.68
16	2.25	3.38	5.79	4.40	52	2.81	5.19	6.33	5.93
17	2.08	1.74	4.12	3.62	53	2.62	3.54	4.86	5.80
18	0.14	0.01	1.48	2.78	54	0.11	2.25	1.56	3.92
19	0.13	3.19	0.60	3.14	55	0.61	1.14	1.35	0.53
20	2.19	2.65	3.27	2.73	56	−2.19	−0.42	1.54	1.16
21	−0.64	−1.31	−0.37	4.09	57	1.55	2.42	1.11	2.18
22	2.02	3.45	5.32	6.01	58	−0.04	0.50	2.60	2.61
23	2.05	1.80	3.91	2.49	59	3.10	2.00	3.92	3.91
24	1.48	0.47	3.63	3.88	60	−0.29	2.62	1.60	1.86
25	1.97	2.54	3.26	5.62	61	2.28	3.39	4.91	3.89
26	1.35	4.63	3.54	5.24	62	2.57	5.78	5.12	4.98
27	−0.56	−0.36	1.14	1.34	63	−2.19	0.71	1.56	2.31
28	0.26	0.08	1.17	2.15	64	−0.04	2.44	1.79	2.64
29	1.22	1.41	4.66	2.62					
30	−1.43	0.80	−0.03	1.04					
31	−1.17	1.66	2.11	1.42					
32	1.68	1.71	4.07	3.30					
33	−0.47	0.93	1.30	0.76					
34	2.18	6.42	4.64	4.82					
35	4.21	7.08	6.00	5.65					
36	8.26	9.55	10.24	10.58					

4.3 Box (1950) describes an experiment in which 30 rats were randomly assigned to three treatment groups. Group 1 was a control group, group 2 had thyroxin added to their drinking water, and group 3 had thiouracil added to their drinking water. Whereas there were ten rats in each of groups 1 and 3, group 2 consisted of only seven rats (due to an unspecified accident at the beginning of the experiment). The resulting body weights of each of the 27 rats at the beginning of the experiment and at weekly intervals for four weeks were previously considered in Problem 2.4 and are displayed in Table 2.12.

(a) Analyze these data using profile analysis methods. In particular, provide answers to the following questions: (1) Are the response profiles parallel? (2) Are there differences among the three treatment groups? If so, at which time points? (3) Are there differences among time points? If so, for which groups?

(b) Analyze these data using growth curve techniques. Compare your results with those from part (a).

4.4 Koch (1970) discussed an investigation of the effects of a certain compound (ethionine) on absorption of iron in the liver. In this study, 34 male albino rats, each weighing approximately 200 grams, were randomly divided into 17 pairs. One animal in each pair was selected at random to receive an experimental diet containing ethionine, whereas the other was a pair-fed control (that is, the control animal received the same amount of food as was eaten by the corresponding treated animal).

After seven days, the 34 rats were sacrificed, and the liver of each animal was extracted and divided into three parts. The 17 pairs were then randomized to one of two groups. In the eight pairs randomized to group 1, the liver thirds from each animal were randomly assigned to be treated with radioactive iron in a solution of low pH (2.0–3.0), medium pH (4.5–5.5), or high pH (7.0–7.7) at a temperature of 37°C. The same procedure was followed in the nine pairs randomized to group 2, with the exception that the liver portions were treated at 25°C.

The response variable of interest is the amount of iron absorbed by the variously treated liver thirds, which can be assumed to be continuous and normally distributed. Table 4.8 displays the data from this experiment.

(a) Suppose that the data will be analyzed using the multivariate general linear model. Let $\boldsymbol{Y}$ denote the 17×6 data matrix, and consider the model $\mathrm{E}(\boldsymbol{Y}) = \boldsymbol{XB} + \boldsymbol{E}$, where

$$\boldsymbol{X}' = \begin{pmatrix} 1 & 1 & 1 & 1 & 1 & 1 & 1 & 1 & 0 & 0 & 0 & 0 & 0 & 0 & 0 & 0 & 0 \\ 0 & 0 & 0 & 0 & 0 & 0 & 0 & 0 & 1 & 1 & 1 & 1 & 1 & 1 & 1 & 1 & 1 \end{pmatrix}$$

and

$$\boldsymbol{B} = \begin{pmatrix} \mu_{11} & \mu_{12} & \mu_{13} & \mu_{14} & \mu_{15} & \mu_{16} \\ \mu_{21} & \mu_{22} & \mu_{23} & \mu_{24} & \mu_{25} & \mu_{26} \end{pmatrix}.$$

TABLE 4.8. Iron absorption in liver thirds of 17 pairs of albino rats

		Ethionine			Control		
Group	Pair	Low pH (2.0–3.0)	Med. pH (4.5–5.5)	High pH (7.0–7.7)	Low pH (2.0–3.0)	Med. pH (4.5–5.5)	High pH (7.0–7.7)
1	1	2.23	2.59	4.50	1.34	1.40	3.87
(37°)	2	1.14	1.54	3.92	0.84	1.51	2.81
	3	2.63	3.68	10.33	0.68	2.49	8.42
	4	1.00	1.96	8.23	0.69	1.74	3.82
	5	1.35	2.94	2.07	2.08	1.59	2.42
	6	2.01	1.61	4.90	1.16	1.36	2.85
	7	1.64	1.23	6.84	0.96	3.00	4.15
	8	1.13	6.96	6.42	0.74	4.81	5.64
2	9	3.00	6.77	2.95	1.56	4.71	2.64
(25°)	10	4.78	4.97	3.42	2.30	1.60	2.48
	11	0.71	1.46	6.85	1.01	0.67	3.66
	12	1.01	0.96	0.94	1.61	0.71	0.68
	13	1.70	5.59	3.72	1.06	5.21	3.20
	14	1.31	9.56	6.00	1.35	5.12	3.77
	15	2.13	1.08	3.13	1.40	0.95	3.94
	16	2.42	1.58	2.74	1.18	1.56	2.62
	17	1.32	8.09	3.91	1.55	1.68	2.40

Specify matrices $\boldsymbol{A}$ and $\boldsymbol{C}$ for testing the following null hypotheses of the form H_0: $\boldsymbol{ABC} = \boldsymbol{0}$:

1. There is no pH effect for either compound in either group.
2. In group 2, the effect of pH is the same for ethionine as for control.
3. The change in response from low pH to medium pH is the same as the change in response from medium pH to high pH for control animals in group 1.
4. The mean responses in groups 1 and 2 are equal.
5. There is no difference between the mean responses for ethionine and control.
6. The effect of pH is the same in group 1 as in group 2.

(b) Carry out the tests of part (a) and summarize the results.

4.5 Consider the experiment described in Problem 4.4. Could standard growth curve techniques be used to analyze these data? If so, describe briefly the approach you would follow. If not, state why growth curve methodology is inappropriate.

4.6 In an investigation of the effects of various dosages of radiation therapy on psychomotor skills (Danford et al., 1960), 45 cancer patients were trained to operate a psychomotor testing device. Six patients were not given radiation and served as controls, whereas the remainder were treated with dosages of 25–50 R, 75–100 R, or 125–250 R. The resulting psychomotor test scores on the three days following radiation treatment were previously considered in Problem 2.6 and are displayed in Table 2.14.

(a) Analyze these data using profile analysis methods. In particular, provide answers to the following questions: (1) Are the response profiles parallel? (2) Are there differences among the four treatment groups? If so, at which time points? (3) Are there differences among time points? If so, for which groups?

(b) Analyze these data using growth curve techniques. Compare your results with those from part (a).

4.7 Sixty female rats were randomly assigned to one of four dosages of a drug (control, low dose, medium dose, or high dose). The body weights of each animal (grams) at week 0 (just prior to initiation of treatment) and at weekly intervals for 9 weeks were previously considered in Problem 2.8 and are partially displayed in Tables 2.16.

(a) Analyze these data using profile analysis techniques. Regardless of the results of the test of parallelism, report the results for both analyses (assuming parallelism, not assuming parallelism).

(b) Analyze these data using growth curve analysis techniques. Test the fit of the degree of polynomial chosen. Use both the Potthoff–Roy method and the maximum likelihood (covariate-adjusted) method.

(c) Which approach—part (a) or part (b)—gives the most powerful test for differences among dosage groups? Comment, in general, concerning situations in which one method would be preferred over the other.

4.8 Forty male subjects were randomly assigned to one of two treatment groups. The values of the BPRS factor measured before treatment (week 0) and at weekly intervals for eight weeks are displayed in Table 2.10 and were previously considered in Problems 2.2 and 3.12.

(a) Use the method of divided differences to test whether the relationship between BPRS and time is linear. Carry out this test in each of the two groups and also test the joint significance of the nonlinear effects in both groups.

(b) Repeat part (a) using orthogonal polynomial coefficients. Determine the appropriate polynomial order that provides an adequate fit in each of the two groups (and in both groups jointly).

(c) Fit a quadratic growth curve model using standardized orthogonal polynomial coefficients. Use the Potthoff–Roy approach with $\boldsymbol{G} = \boldsymbol{S}$. Test whether the two intercept terms are jointly equal to zero, the two linear terms are jointly equal to zero, the two quadratic terms are jointly equal to zero, and whether the curves for the two groups are equal. Also test the equality of the two intercepts, the two linear terms, and the two quadratic terms, as well as the hypothesis of parallelism.

(d) Repeat part (c) for a model on the natural time scale. Report the estimates of the two curves and summarize the results.

(e) Compare the results with those from Problems 2.2 and 3.12.

4.9 Table 4.9 displays measurements of coronary sinus potassium (MIL equivalents per liter) from four groups of dogs (Grizzle and Allen, 1969). Group 1 was a control group of nine untreated dogs with coronary occlusion. The ten animals in group 2 were given extrinsic cardiac denervation three weeks prior to coronary occlusion, whereas the eight animals in group 3 were similarly treated immediately prior to coronary occlusion. Group 4 consisted of nine dogs treated with bilateral thoracic sympathectomy and stellectomy three weeks prior to coronary occlusion.

(a) Determine the appropriate degree of polynomial that can be adequately fitted to these data.

(b) Based on the results of part (a), fit a growth curve model and test for differences among the four groups.

4.10 Reiczigel (1999) describes an experiment of Sterczer et al. (1996) using two-dimensional ultrasonography to study the effect of cholagogues on changes in gallbladder volume (GBV) in three groups of healthy dogs. Groups 1 and 2 were administered cholechystokynin and clanobutin, respectively. Group 3 was a control group. GBV values were determined immediately before the administration of the test substance and at 10-minute intervals for 120 minutes thereafter. Table 4.10 displays the data.

(a) Use the method of divided differences to test the joint significance of the nonlinear components of the relationship between GBV and time in the three groups.

(b) Repeat part (a) using orthogonal polynomial coefficients. Determine the appropriate polynomial order that provides an adequate fit.

(c) Analyze these data using growth curve model methodology and summarize the results.

TABLE 4.9. Coronary sinus potassium measurements from 36 dogs

		Minutes after Occlusion						
Group	Dog	1	3	5	7	9	11	13
1	1	4.0	4.0	4.1	3.6	3.6	3.8	3.1
	2	4.2	4.3	3.7	3.7	4.8	5.0	5.2
	3	4.3	4.2	4.3	4.3	4.5	5.8	5.4
	4	4.2	4.4	4.6	4.9	5.3	5.6	4.9
	5	4.6	4.4	5.3	5.6	5.9	5.9	5.3
	6	3.1	3.6	4.9	5.2	5.3	4.2	4.1
	7	3.7	3.9	3.9	4.8	5.2	5.4	4.2
	8	4.3	4.2	4.4	5.2	5.6	5.4	4.7
	9	4.6	4.6	4.4	4.6	5.4	5.9	5.6
2	10	3.4	3.4	3.5	3.1	3.1	3.7	3.3
	11	3.0	3.2	3.0	3.0	3.1	3.2	3.1
	12	3.0	3.1	3.2	3.0	3.3	3.0	3.0
	13	3.1	3.2	3.2	3.2	3.3	3.1	3.1
	14	3.8	3.9	4.0	2.9	3.5	3.5	3.4
	15	3.0	3.6	3.2	3.1	3.0	3.0	3.0
	16	3.3	3.3	3.3	3.4	3.6	3.1	3.1
	17	4.2	4.0	4.2	4.1	4.2	4.0	4.0
	18	4.1	4.2	4.3	4.3	4.2	4.0	4.2
	19	4.5	4.4	4.3	4.5	5.3	4.4	4.4
3	20	3.2	3.3	3.8	3.8	4.4	4.2	3.7
	21	3.3	3.4	3.4	3.7	3.7	3.6	3.7
	22	3.1	3.3	3.2	3.1	3.2	3.1	3.1
	23	3.6	3.4	3.5	4.6	4.9	5.2	4.4
	24	4.5	4.5	5.4	5.7	4.9	4.0	4.0
	25	3.7	4.0	4.4	4.2	4.6	4.8	5.4
	26	3.5	3.9	5.8	5.4	4.9	5.3	5.6
	27	3.9	4.0	4.1	5.0	5.4	4.4	3.9
4	28	3.1	3.5	3.5	3.2	3.0	3.0	3.2
	29	3.3	3.2	3.6	3.7	3.7	4.2	4.4
	30	3.5	3.9	4.7	4.3	3.9	3.4	3.5
	31	3.4	3.4	3.5	3.3	3.4	3.2	3.4
	32	3.7	3.8	4.2	4.3	3.6	3.8	3.7
	33	4.0	4.6	4.8	4.9	5.4	5.6	4.8
	34	4.2	3.9	4.5	4.7	3.9	3.8	3.7
	35	4.1	4.1	3.7	4.0	4.1	4.6	4.7
	36	3.5	3.6	3.6	4.2	4.8	4.9	5.0

TABLE 4.10. Gallbladder volume measurements in three groups of six healthy dogs

	Minutes after Treatment												
ID	0	10	20	30	40	50	60	70	80	90	100	110	120
Group 1: Cholechystokynin													
1	17.70	10.35	10.78	11.44	11.20	12.38	12.68	12.30	14.00	14.64	14.96	14.18	16.78
2	17.22	11.30	11.30	13.28	14.08	13.98	14.74	15.63	17.60	17.34	17.38	17.36	17.64
3	14.24	9.20	9.40	9.62	10.10	10.08	9.60	9.70	11.23	11.20	11.96	12.20	13.98
4	39.58	26.88	26.20	29.80	31.50	32.75	34.45	35.64	36.62	38.65	38.56	39.20	39.36
5	13.33	7.15	7.82	7.94	8.40	8.94	9.28	9.95	10.40	10.95	11.70	12.10	12.35
6	16.16	8.36	9.53	9.80	9.64	9.84	10.70	11.26	12.12	12.60	13.98	14.52	14.78
Group 2: Clanobutin													
1	16.35	13.65	13.10	13.58	14.03	15.45	15.58	15.56	15.62	16.10	16.28	16.74	16.25
2	15.65	13.08	12.35	12.76	13.78	13.76	13.54	14.18	14.40	15.16	15.20	15.18	13.40
3	12.68	9.68	10.70	10.98	11.12	11.78	12.02	11.95	12.16	12.25	12.40	12.55	12.54
4	21.88	15.92	15.18	17.04	18.60	18.98	19.26	20.38	21.32	21.03	21.80	21.08	22.65
5	12.78	9.03	9.28	9.54	9.38	9.88	9.94	10.14	10.34	11.50	11.83	11.78	12.08
6	15.58	11.50	11.88	12.06	12.58	12.98	13.00	13.00	13.04	13.18	13.88	13.43	13.85
Group 3: Control													
1	20.75	19.83	19.98	18.84	19.10	19.50	19.75	19.64	20.00	19.13	20.15	19.45	19.43
2	13.88	13.60	13.73	13.16	13.44	13.62	13.86	13.58	14.28	14.10	13.12	13.53	13.42
3	11.92	11.74	11.84	10.90	11.75	11.45	11.98	12.38	11.70	11.48	11.80	11.20	12.03
4	26.38	26.90	27.73	27.73	27.56	28.43	27.54	26.50	27.94	27.58	27.56	27.64	28.83
5	13.30	13.18	13.52	13.43	13.40	13.25	13.28	13.24	13.44	12.98	12.60	13.48	13.08
6	13.80	13.86	13.06	13.76	13.82	13.80	13.86	13.84	13.76	13.82	13.50	13.72	13.70

4.11 Kenward (1987) describes an experiment to compare two treatments for controlling intestinal parasites in calves. There were 30 calves in each of the two groups, and the weight of each calf was determined at 11 measurement times. These data are partially displayed in Table 2.11 and were previously considered in Problems 2.3 and 3.11.

(a) Use the method of divided differences to test whether the relationship between weight and time is linear. Carry out this test in each of the two groups and also test the joint significance of the nonlinear effects in both groups.

(b) Repeat part (a) using orthogonal polynomial coefficients. Determine the appropriate polynomial order that provides an adequate fit in each of the two groups.

(c) Discuss the appropriateness of growth curve methods for analyzing these data.

4.12 Hand and Taylor (1987, pp. 117–125) describe a study of urinary salsolinol excretion levels in two groups of subjects admitted to an alcoholism treatment unit. Group 1 includes six subjects considered to be moderately dependent on alcohol, and group 2 includes eight subjects considered to be severely dependent on alcohol. This study was previously considered in Problem 3.13, and the raw data are displayed in Table 3.11. As in Problem 3.13, carry out the following analyses on log-transformed urinary salsolinol levels.

(a) Use profile analysis methods to test whether the response profiles for the two groups are parallel. Depending on the results of the test of parallelism, use an appropriate profile analysis test to assess whether there are differences between the two groups and differences among the four days.

(b) Fit a cubic growth curve model using standardized orthogonal polynomial coefficients. Determine the appropriate polynomial order that provides an adequate fit in each of the two groups. Discuss the appropriateness of growth curve methods for analyzing these data.

5 Normal-Theory Methods: Repeated Measures ANOVA

5.1 Introduction

The unstructured multivariate approach described in Chapters 3 and 4 makes no assumptions concerning the covariance structure of the vector of repeated measurements from each experimental unit. Although not making covariance structure assumptions may be advantageous, these approaches can result in low power to detect differences of interest. This is due to the fact that a large number of degrees of freedom must be used to estimate the covariance parameters.

For normally distributed responses, it would be natural to use analysis-of-variance (ANOVA) methods if the repeated measurements were independent. A traditional approach to the analysis of repeated measurements is to:

1. perform a standard ANOVA, as if the observations are independent;

2. determine whether additional assumptions or modifications are required to make the analysis valid.

This method is commonly called "repeated measures ANOVA."

Section 5.2 describes the fundamental model and assumptions for repeated measures ANOVA. Section 5.3 demonstrates this approach for one-sample problems, and Section 5.4 describes the use of repeated measures ANOVA for multisample problems. In some settings, the repeated measures ANOVA approach may be a useful alternative to the unstructured multivariate approach because it does not require estimation of the covariance structure. However, the methods to be described in Chapter 6 offer the advantage of allowing parsimonious modeling of the covariance structure without requiring assumptions as strict as those for repeated measures ANOVA.

With the development of these more flexible approaches, repeated measures ANOVA is no longer as useful as it was in the past. Hence, this chapter provides only a brief overview of this methodology.

5.2 The Fundamental Model

Assume that a continuous, normally distributed response variable is measured at each of t time points for each of n experimental units (subjects). Let y_{ij} denote the response from subject i at time j for $i = 1, \ldots, n$, $j = 1, \ldots, t$. The general basis for repeated measures ANOVA is the model

$$y_{ij} = \mu_{ij} + \pi_{ij} + e_{ij}. \tag{5.1}$$

This model has three components. First, μ_{ij} is the mean at time j for individuals randomly selected from the same population as individual i. The second term in Equation (5.1) is π_{ij}, the consistent departure of y_{ij} from μ_{ij} for the ith subject. Under hypothetical repetitions from the same individual, y_{ij} has mean $\mu_{ij} + \pi_{ij}$. The final component of model (5.1) is e_{ij}, the departure of y_{ij} from $\mu_{ij} + \pi_{ij}$ for individual i at time j.

The μ_{ij} parameters are called *fixed* effects because μ_{ij} has a fixed value irrespective of the particular individual. Because π_{ij} varies randomly over the population of individuals, the π_{ij} parameters are called *random* effects. The e_{ij} parameters are random error terms. Because the fundamental model contains both fixed and random effects, it is often called the mixed model. Crowder and Hand (1990, p. 25) refer to μ_{ij} as "an immutable constant of the universe," π_{ij} as "a lasting characteristic of the individual," and e_{ij} as "a fleeting aberration of the moment."

For given j, the means and variances of the random effects π_{ij} are assumed to be as follows:

$$\begin{aligned} \mathrm{E}(\pi_{ij}) &= 0, \\ \mathrm{Var}(\pi_{ij}) &= \sigma^2_{\pi j}. \end{aligned}$$

Thus, any nonzero mean is absorbed in μ_{ij}, and the variance at time j is constant over individuals. In addition, for given j,

$$\begin{aligned} \mathrm{E}(e_{ij}) &= 0, \\ \mathrm{Var}(e_{ij}) &= \sigma^2_{ej}. \end{aligned}$$

Thus, the error variance at time j is constant over individuals.

With respect to the correlation structure of the random effects π_{ij}, it is assumed that

$$\mathrm{Cov}(\pi_{ij}, \pi_{i'j}) = \mathrm{Cov}(\pi_{ij}, \pi_{i'j'}) = 0$$

for $i \neq i'$ and $j \neq j'$ (i.e., that the random effects for different subjects are uncorrelated). A further assumption is that $\mathrm{Cov}(\pi_{ij}, \pi_{ij'}) = \sigma_{\pi jj'}$, so that the within-subject covariances of random effects are the same across subjects.

The error terms e_{ij} are also assumed to be uncorrelated. Thus,

$$\mathrm{Cov}(e_{ij}, e_{i'j'}) = 0$$

if $i \neq i'$ or $j \neq j'$. In addition, the random effects and the error terms are also uncorrelated, so that

$$\mathrm{Cov}(\pi_{ij}, e_{i'j'}) = 0$$

for all i, j, i', j'. A final distributional assumption is that the random effects π_{ij} and the error terms e_{ij} are normally distributed.

The preceding general assumptions are often further simplified. First, the variances $\sigma^2_{\pi j}$ may be assumed to be constant across time points, so that $\mathrm{Var}(\pi_{ij}) = \sigma^2_{\pi}$. Similarly, $\sigma_{\pi jj'}$ is often assumed to be constant for all j, j'. In addition, the variances σ^2_{ej} of the random errors e_{ij} are often assumed to be constant over time; that is, $\mathrm{Var}(e_{ij}) = \sigma^2_e$.

In terms of the observations y_{ij}, $\mathrm{E}(y_{ij}) = \mu_{ij}$ because $\mathrm{E}(\pi_{ij}) = \mathrm{E}(e_{ij}) = 0$. Furthermore,

$$\begin{aligned}
\mathrm{Cov}(y_{ij}, y_{i'j'}) &= \mathrm{E}[(y_{ij} - \mu_{ij})(y_{i'j'} - \mu_{i'j'})] \\
&= \mathrm{E}[(\pi_{ij} + e_{ij})(\pi_{i'j'} + e_{i'j'})] \\
&= \mathrm{E}[\pi_{ij}\pi_{i'j'} + \pi_{ij}e_{i'j'} + \pi_{i'j'}e_{ij} + e_{ij}e_{i'j'}]. \quad (5.2)
\end{aligned}$$

In simplifying Equation (5.2), first observe that

$$\mathrm{E}(\pi_{ij}\pi_{i'j'}) = \begin{cases} \mathrm{Var}(\pi_{ij}) & \text{if } i = i',\ j = j' \\ \mathrm{Cov}(\pi_{ij}, \pi_{i'j'}) & \text{otherwise} \end{cases}.$$

Because

$$\mathrm{E}(\pi_{ij}\pi_{i'j'}) = \begin{cases} \sigma^2_{\pi j} & \text{if } i = i',\ j = j' \\ \sigma_{\pi jj'} & \text{if } i = i',\ j \neq j' \\ 0 & \text{if } i \neq i' \end{cases},$$

then $\mathrm{E}(\pi_{ij}\pi_{i'j'}) = \delta_{ii'}\sigma_{\pi jj'}$, where

$$\delta_{ii'} = \begin{cases} 1 & \text{if } i = i' \\ 0 & \text{otherwise} \end{cases}$$

and $\sigma_{\pi jj} = \sigma^2_{\pi j}$.

Because $\text{Cov}(\pi_{ij}, e_{i'j'}) = 0$ for all i, j, i', j', the second and third terms of Equation (5.2) are

$$\text{E}(\pi_{ij}e_{i'j'}) = 0, \qquad \text{E}(\pi_{i'j'}e_{ij}) = 0.$$

Finally, the fourth term of Equation (5.2) is

$$\text{E}(e_{ij}e_{i'j'}) = \begin{cases} \text{Var}(e_{ij}) & \text{if } i = i',\ j = j' \\ \text{Cov}(e_{ij}, e_{i'j'}) & \text{otherwise} \end{cases},$$

so that

$$\text{E}(e_{ij}e_{i'j'}) = \begin{cases} \sigma^2_{ej} & \text{if } i = i',\ j = j' \\ 0 & \text{otherwise} \end{cases}.$$

This can be written as $\text{E}(e_{ij}e_{i'j'}) = \delta_{ii'}\delta_{jj'}\sigma^2_{ej}$.

Thus, the model specification for the first two moments of y_{ij} is

$$\begin{aligned} \text{E}(y_{ij}) &= \mu_{ij} \\ \text{Cov}(y_{ij}, y_{i'j'}) &= \delta_{ii'}\sigma_{\pi jj'} + \delta_{ii'}\delta_{jj'}\sigma^2_{ej} \\ &= \delta_{ii'}(\sigma_{\pi jj'} + \delta_{jj'}\sigma^2_{ej}). \end{aligned}$$

Observations y_{ij} and $y_{i'j}$ from different individuals ($i \neq i'$) are uncorrelated. The correlation between measurements on the same individual is called an *intraclass correlation* and is given by

$$\text{Corr}(y_{ij}, y_{ij'}) = \frac{\sigma_{\pi jj'}}{[(\sigma_{\pi jj} + \sigma^2_{ej})(\sigma_{\pi j'j'} + \sigma^2_{ej'})]^{1/2}}.$$

In the special case where $\sigma^2_{ej} = \sigma^2_e$ and $\sigma_{\pi jj'} = \sigma^2_\pi$,

$$\rho = \text{Corr}(y_{ij}, y_{ij'}) = \frac{\sigma^2_\pi}{\sigma^2_\pi + \sigma^2_e}.$$

The intraclass correlation coefficient ρ ranges from 0 to 1 as σ^2_π/σ^2_e ranges from 0 to ∞.

5.3 One Sample

5.3.1 Repeated Measures ANOVA Model

Table 1.3 displays the situation where repeated measurements are obtained from a single sample. The repeated measures ANOVA model for this case is

$$y_{ij} = \mu + \pi_i + \tau_j + e_{ij} \tag{5.3}$$

for $i = 1, \ldots, n$ and $j = 1, \ldots, t$. In Equation (5.3), y_{ij} is the response from subject i at time j, μ is the overall mean, π_i is a random effect for subject i

which is constant over all occasions, τ_j is the fixed effect of time j, and e_{ij} is a random error component specific to subject i at time j. The random effects π_i are independent $N(0, \sigma_\pi^2)$, the random errors e_{ij} are independent $N(0, \sigma_e^2)$, and the random effects π_i and the random error terms e_{ij} are independent. The fixed effects τ_j are assumed to satisfy the sum-to-zero constraints $\sum_{j=1}^{t} \tau_j = 0$.

In terms of the parameters of the general model given by Equation (5.1) in Section 5.2,

- $\mu_{ij} = \mu + \tau_j$ (note that the subscript i is unnecessary);
- $\pi_{ij} = \pi_i$ (constant across time points).

The variances and covariances of the observations are

$$\begin{aligned} \text{Var}(y_{ij}) &= \text{Var}(\mu + \pi_i + \tau_j + e_{ij}) = \sigma_\pi^2 + \sigma_e^2, \\ \text{Cov}(y_{ij}, y_{i'j}) &= 0, \text{ for } i \neq i', \\ \text{Cov}(y_{ij}, y_{ij'}) &= \sigma_\pi^2, \text{ for } j \neq j'. \end{aligned}$$

Thus, the covariance matrix of the vector $\boldsymbol{y}_i = (y_{i1}, \ldots, y_{it})'$ is given by

$$\begin{aligned} \boldsymbol{\Sigma} &= \begin{pmatrix} \sigma_\pi^2 + \sigma_e^2 & & \sigma_\pi^2 \\ & \ddots & \\ \sigma_\pi^2 & & \sigma_\pi^2 + \sigma_e^2 \end{pmatrix} \\ &= (\sigma_\pi^2 + \sigma_e^2) \begin{pmatrix} 1 & & \rho \\ & \ddots & \\ \rho & & 1 \end{pmatrix}, \end{aligned} \tag{5.4}$$

where

$$\rho = \frac{\sigma_\pi^2}{\sigma_\pi^2 + \sigma_e^2} = \text{Corr}(y_{ij}, y_{ij'}).$$

Although all random variables in model (5.3) are independent, the repeated observations from a subject are correlated. The resulting covariance matrix given by Equation (5.4) with equal diagonal elements and equal off-diagonal elements is said to have compound symmetry. This covariance structure implies that the correlation between any pair of repeated observations is the same, regardless of the spacing between observations. This assumption is highly restrictive and often unrealistic, especially when the repeated measurements factor is time.

The ANOVA table for model (5.3) is the same as that of the two-way mixed model with one observation per cell and no subject × time interaction. Table 5.1 displays the sum of squares (SS), df, mean square (MS), and expected MS for each source of variation. The sums of squares in Table 5.1 are computed using the observations y_{ij}, the overall mean

$$\overline{y}_{..} = \frac{\sum_{i=1}^{n} \sum_{j=1}^{t} y_{ij}}{nt},$$

TABLE 5.1. Sums of squares, degrees of freedom, mean squares, and expected mean squares for one-sample repeated measures ANOVA

Source	SS	df	MS	E(MS)
Time	$\mathrm{SS_T}$	$t-1$	$\mathrm{MS_T} = \dfrac{\mathrm{SS_T}}{t-1}$	$\sigma_e^2 + n\sigma_\tau^2$
Subjects	$\mathrm{SS_S}$	$n-1$	$\mathrm{MS_S} = \dfrac{\mathrm{SS_S}}{n-1}$	$\sigma_e^2 + t\sigma_\pi^2$
Residual	$\mathrm{SS_R}$	$(n-1)(t-1)$	$\mathrm{MS_R} = \dfrac{\mathrm{SS_R}}{(n-1)(t-1)}$	σ_e^2

the means for each subject over time

$$\overline{y}_{i.} = \frac{\sum_{j=1}^{t} y_{ij}}{t},$$

and the means at each time point over subjects

$$\overline{y}_{.j} = \frac{\sum_{i=1}^{n} y_{ij}}{n}.$$

The sums of squares are then defined as follows:

$$\mathrm{SS_T} = \sum_{i=1}^{n}\sum_{j=1}^{t}(\overline{y}_{.j} - \overline{y}_{..})^2 = n\sum_{j=1}^{t}(\overline{y}_{.j} - \overline{y}_{..})^2, \tag{5.5}$$

$$\mathrm{SS_S} = \sum_{i=1}^{n}\sum_{j=1}^{t}(\overline{y}_{i.} - \overline{y}_{..})^2 = t\sum_{i=1}^{n}(\overline{y}_{i.} - \overline{y}_{..})^2, \tag{5.6}$$

$$\mathrm{SS_R} = \sum_{i=1}^{n}\sum_{j=1}^{t}(y_{ij} - \overline{y}_{i.} - \overline{y}_{.j} + \overline{y}_{..})^2. \tag{5.7}$$

In addition, the symbol σ_τ^2 in the column of expected mean squares of Table 5.1 represents a function of the fixed effects τ_j.

The sums of squares displayed in Table 5.1 can be computed using a standard ANOVA program for a two-way main-effects model with one observation per cell. The null hypothesis that there are no differences among time periods can be tested using the statistic $F = \mathrm{MS_T}/\mathrm{MS_R}$. Provided that the assumptions of the model hold, this test statistic has the $F_{t-1,(n-1)(t-1)}$ distribution if the null hypothesis is true. Linear contrasts of the time period means can also be tested.

If compound symmetry holds, this F statistic provides a more powerful test than the approach using Hotelling's T^2 statistic described in Section 3.3. However, because the F test is anticonservative in the absence of compound symmetry, rejection decisions cannot be trusted.

TABLE 5.2. Sums of squares, degrees of freedom, and expected mean squares for Scheffé's one-sample repeated measures ANOVA model

Source	SS	df	E(MS)
Time	SS_T	$t-1$	$\sigma_e^2 + \sigma_{T\times S}^2 + n\sigma_\tau^2$
Subjects	SS_S	$n-1$	$\sigma_e^2 + t\sigma_\pi^2$
Time × subjects	SS_{TS}	$(n-1)(t-1)$	$\sigma_e^2 + \sigma_{T\times S}^2$

Scheffé (1959) gives an alternative model for the one-way repeated measurements setting. Although y_{ij}, μ, and τ_j are defined as in Equation (5.3), the random error components e_{ij} now include subject × time interaction as well as measurement error. Scheffé assumes that the π_i and e_{ij} components follow a multivariate normal distribution. One important difference is that $\text{Cov}(e_{ij}, e_{ij'}) \neq 0$ and $\text{Cov}(\pi_i, e_{ij}) \neq 0$ in Scheffé's model. Provided that certain assumptions are satisfied, the analysis is the same for both models. This may explain why many textbooks do not make a distinction between the two models.

Table 5.2 displays the sum of squares, degrees of freedom, and expected mean squares for each source of variation in Scheffé's model. The sums of squares SS_T and SS_S are computed as in Equations (5.5) and (5.6). The treatment × subjects sum of squares SS_{TS} is the same as the residual sum of squares SS_R given by Equation (5.7). The statistic $F = MS_T/MS_{TS}$, where

$$MS_{TS} = \frac{SS_{TS}}{(n-1)(t-1)},$$

tests the null hypothesis that the means at the t time points are equal.

5.3.2 Sphericity Condition

Equation (5.4) displays the covariance matrix of the observations y_{ij} from the one-way repeated measures ANOVA model; this structure is called compound symmetry. Although the compound symmetry condition is sufficient for the F statistic used to test the null hypothesis of no differences among time points to have the $F_{t-1,(n-1)(t-1)}$ distribution, it is not necessary. Compound symmetry is a special case of a more general situation, sphericity, under which the F test is valid.

The sphericity condition can be expressed in a number of alternative ways, including:

1. The variances of all pairwise differences between variables are equal; that is,

$$\text{Var}(y_{ij} - y_{ij'}) \text{ is constant for all } j, j'. \tag{5.8}$$

2. $\epsilon = 1$, where

$$\epsilon = \frac{t^2(\overline{\sigma}_{ii} - \overline{\sigma}_{..})^2}{(t-1)(S - 2t\sum \overline{\sigma}_{i.}^2 + t^2\overline{\sigma}_{..}^2)}, \tag{5.9}$$

and $\overline{\sigma}_{ii}$ is the mean of the entries on the main diagonal of $\mathbf{\Sigma}$, $\overline{\sigma}_{..}$ is the mean of all of the elements of $\mathbf{\Sigma}$, $\overline{\sigma}_{i.}$ is the mean of the entries in row i of $\mathbf{\Sigma}$, and S is the sum of the squares of the elements of $\mathbf{\Sigma}$.

If compound symmetry holds, then both $\text{Var}(y_{ij})$ and $\text{Cov}(y_{ij}, y_{ij'})$ are constant for all i and j. Then, because

$$\text{Var}(y_{ij} - y_{ij'}) = \text{Var}(y_{ij}) + \text{Var}(y_{ij'}) - 2\text{Cov}(y_{ij}, y_{ij'}),$$

it is clear that Equation (5.8) is satisfied. There are, however, other situations under which the equivalent conditions of Equations (5.8) and (5.9) hold. Although sphericity is a more general criterion for validity of the F test of the repeated measures ANOVA model, it is difficult to argue substantively for any patterned form of $\mathbf{\Sigma}$ other than compound symmetry. In particular, if the variances are equal, then the covariances must also be equal in order for the sphericity condition to be satisfied (Huynh and Feldt, 1970). Huynh (1978) states that it would be difficult to conceptualize a situation that would give rise to a covariance matrix satisfying the sphericity condition but not having compound symmetry. As a result, Wallenstein (1982) concludes that, for all practical purposes, the required assumption for repeated measures ANOVA should be that of compound symmetry.

Mauchly (1940) gives a test of the sphericity condition. This test, however, has low power for small sample sizes. In addition, for large sample sizes, the test is likely to show significance even though the effect on the F test may be negligible. Mauchly's test for sphericity has also been shown to be sensitive to departures from normality; in particular, it is conservative for light-tailed distributions and anticonservative for heavy-tailed distributions. It is also very sensitive to outliers. Because of these properties, it is not of great practical use.

If the sphericity assumption seems unreasonable, one alternative is to use the unstructured multivariate approach described in Chapter 3. Another possibility is to modify the repeated measures ANOVA approach.

When sphericity does not hold, the F statistic has an approximate

$$F_{\epsilon(t-1),\epsilon(t-1)(n-1)}$$

distribution, where ϵ, given by Equation (5.9), is a function of the actual covariance matrix $\mathbf{\Sigma}$ (Box, 1954). It can be shown that $1/(t-1) \le \epsilon \le 1$.

Several approaches to hypothesis testing have been suggested for the situation where the sphericity assumption is violated. One is to adjust the degrees of freedom of the F statistic by using the lower bound for ϵ. With

$\epsilon = 1/(t-1)$, the $F_{\epsilon(t-1),\epsilon(t-1)(n-1)}$ distribution becomes $F_{1,n-1}$. This test, however, is very conservative.

Greenhouse and Geisser (1959) recommend adjusting the degrees of freedom of the F statistic using the estimator $\widehat{\epsilon}$ computed from the sample covariance matrix $\boldsymbol{S}$ using Equation (5.9). This is the maximum likelihood estimator of ϵ. Adjusting the degrees of freedom using $\widehat{\epsilon}$ tends to overcorrect the degrees of freedom and produce a conservative test. This approach is known to be seriously biased for $\epsilon > 0.75$ and $n < 2t$.

Huynh and Feldt (1976) proposed the estimator

$$\widetilde{\epsilon} = \min\left(1, \frac{n(t-1)\widehat{\epsilon} - 2}{(t-1)(n-1-(t-1)\widehat{\epsilon})}\right).$$

The estimator $\widetilde{\epsilon}$ is based on unbiased estimators of the numerator and denominator of ϵ and is less biased than $\widehat{\epsilon}$. It can be shown that $\widetilde{\epsilon} \geq \widehat{\epsilon}$. Although $\widehat{\epsilon}$ is better for $\epsilon \leq 0.5$, $\widetilde{\epsilon}$ performs better for $\epsilon \geq 0.75$. In practice, however, ϵ is unknown.

Greenhouse and Geisser (1959) suggested the following approach to the use of repeated measures ANOVA.

1. Conduct the univariate F test under the assumption that the repeated measures ANOVA assumptions are satisfied.

2. If this test is not significant, then fail to reject H_0.

3. If this test is significant, then conduct the conservative test using $\epsilon = 1/(t-1)$, which leads to the $F_{1,n-1}$ distribution.

   (a) If the conservative test is significant, then reject H_0.

   (b) If the conservative test is not significant, then estimate ϵ and conduct an approximate test.

Although Greenhouse and Geisser proposed estimating ϵ by $\widehat{\epsilon}$, the somewhat less conservative estimator $\widetilde{\epsilon}$ could also be used.

5.3.3 *Example*

Table 2.1 displays data from a study in which ventilation volumes (l/min) were measured in eight subjects under six different temperatures of inspired dry air (Deal et al., 1979). These data were analyzed using the summary-statistic approach in Section 2.2 and using the unstructured multivariate approach in Section 3.3.2. Let $\mu_1, \ldots, \mu_6$ denote the mean ventilation volumes at temperatures -10, 25, 37, 50, 65, and 80°C, respectively. Under the assumption that ventilation volumes are normally distributed, repeated measures ANOVA can be used to test $H_0\colon \mu_1 = \cdots = \mu_6$.

With reference to Table 5.1, $SS_T = 413.867$ is the sum of squares for temperature and $SS_R = 935.35$. The test statistic is

$$F = \frac{SS_T/(t-1)}{SS_R/[(n-1)(t-1)]} = \frac{413.867/5}{935.35/35} = \frac{82.773}{26.724} = 3.10.$$

Comparison of this value with the $F_{5,35}$ distribution gives $p = 0.02$. At the 5% level of significance, there is sufficient evidence to reject H_0.

The chi-square approximation to Mauchly's (1940) test of the sphericity assumption is 13.44 with 14 df ($p = 0.49$). Although there is insufficient evidence to reject sphericity, this test has low power because the sample size is small. If we follow step 3 of the Greenhouse–Geisser approach by using $\epsilon = 1/(t-1)$, the relevant F distribution is $F_{1,7}$ and the corresponding p-value is 0.12. In this case, we would fail to reject H_0.

Because the conclusions of the standard repeated measures ANOVA test and the conservative test differ, it may be of interest to estimate ϵ. In this example, $\widehat{\epsilon} = 0.5364$, and the resulting p-value is 0.056. The estimator $\widetilde{\epsilon}$ is 0.9012, with resulting p-value 0.025. With $n = 8$ subjects and $t = 6$ time points, $n < 2t$ and hence $\widehat{\epsilon}$ is likely too conservative. The use of the estimator $\widetilde{\epsilon}$ results in the conclusion that the means at the six temperatures are not equal.

Recall that in Section 2.2 the summary-statistic approach indicated that ventilation volume decreased significantly over time. In Section 3.3.2, however, the test of H_0 using the unstructured multivariate approach was not statistically significant at the 5% level of significance.

5.4 Multiple Samples

5.4.1 Repeated Measures ANOVA Model

Suppose that repeated measurements at t time points are obtained from s groups of subjects. Let n_h denote the number of subjects in group h, and let $n = \sum_{h=1}^{s} n_h$. Let y_{hij} denote the response at time j from the ith subject in group h for $h = 1, \ldots, s$, $i = 1, \ldots, n_h$, and $j = 1, \ldots, t$. Table 1.2 displays the general data layout for this setting.

There are at least three models for this situation, all resulting in the same ANOVA table. The simplest is

$$y_{hij} = \mu + \gamma_h + \tau_j + (\gamma\tau)_{hj} + \pi_{i(h)} + e_{hij}. \tag{5.10}$$

In model (5.10), μ is the overall mean and γ_h is the fixed effect of group h, with $\sum_{h=1}^{s} \gamma_h = 0$. In addition, τ_j is the fixed effect of time j, with $\sum_{j=1}^{t} \tau_j = 0$, and $(\gamma\tau)_{hj}$ is the fixed effect for the interaction of the hth group with the jth time. The constraints on the interaction param-

TABLE 5.3. Sums of squares, degrees of freedom, and expected mean squares for multisample repeated measures ANOVA

Source	SS	df	E(MS)
Group	SS_G	$s-1$	$\sigma_e^2 + t\sigma_\pi^2 + D_G$
Subjects(Group)	$SS_{S(G)}$	$n-s$	$\sigma_e^2 + t\sigma_\pi^2$
Time	SS_T	$t-1$	$\sigma_e^2 + D_T$
Group × Time	SS_{GT}	$(s-1)(t-1)$	$\sigma_e^2 + D_{GT}$
Residual	SS_R	$(n-s)(t-1)$	σ_e^2

eters are

$$\sum_{h=1}^{s}(\gamma\tau)_{hj} = \sum_{j=1}^{t}(\gamma\tau)_{hj} = 0.$$

The parameters $\pi_{i(h)}$ are random effects for the ith subject in the hth group. The $\pi_{i(h)}$ are assumed to be independently normally distributed with mean zero and variance σ_π^2. Finally, the e_{hij} parameters are independent random error terms, with $e_{hij} \sim N(0, \sigma_e^2)$.

In terms of the parameters of the general model given by Equation (5.1) in Section 5.2,

- $\mu_{ij} = \mu + \gamma_h + \tau_j + (\gamma\tau)_{hj}$;
- $\pi_{ij} = \pi_{i(h)}$;
- $e_{ij} = e_{hij}$.

Table 5.3 displays the sum of squares (SS), df, and expected MS for each source of variation. In the column of expected mean squares, the quantities labeled D_G, D_T, and D_{GT} represent differences among groups, differences among time points, and the group × time interaction, respectively.

The sums of squares in Table 5.3 are based on the following decomposition of the deviations $y_{hij} - \overline{y}_{...}$ of each observation about the overall mean:

$$\begin{aligned} y_{hij} - \overline{y}_{...} &= (\overline{y}_{h..} - \overline{y}_{...}) + (\overline{y}_{hi.} - \overline{y}_{h..}) + (\overline{y}_{..j} - \overline{y}_{...}) \\ &\quad + (\overline{y}_{h.j} - \overline{y}_{h..} - \overline{y}_{..j} + \overline{y}_{...}) + (y_{hij} - \overline{y}_{h.j} - \overline{y}_{hi.} + \overline{y}_{h..}), \end{aligned}$$

where

$$\overline{y}_{...} = \frac{\sum_{h=1}^{s}\sum_{i=1}^{n_h}\sum_{j=1}^{t} y_{hij}}{nt}$$

is the overall mean,

$$\overline{y}_{h..} = \frac{\sum_{i=1}^{n_h}\sum_{j=1}^{t} y_{hij}}{n_h t}$$

is the mean for group h,

$$\overline{y}_{..j} = \frac{\sum_{h=1}^{s} \sum_{i=1}^{n_h} y_{hij}}{n}$$

is the mean at time j,

$$\overline{y}_{h.j} = \frac{\sum_{i=1}^{n_h} y_{hij}}{n_h}$$

is the mean for group h at time j, and

$$\overline{y}_{hi.} = \frac{\sum_{j=1}^{t} y_{hij}}{t}$$

is the mean for the ith subject in group h.

The sums of squares are then defined as follows:

$$\begin{aligned}
\mathrm{SS_G} &= \sum_{h=1}^{s} \sum_{i=1}^{n_h} \sum_{j=1}^{t} (\overline{y}_{h..} - \overline{y}_{...})^2 = t \sum_{h=1}^{s} n_h (\overline{y}_{h..} - \overline{y}_{...})^2, \\
\mathrm{SS_{S(G)}} &= \sum_{h=1}^{s} \sum_{i=1}^{n_h} \sum_{j=1}^{t} (\overline{y}_{hi.} - \overline{y}_{h..})^2 = t \sum_{h=1}^{s} \sum_{i=1}^{n_h} (\overline{y}_{hi.} - \overline{y}_{h..})^2, \\
\mathrm{SS_T} &= \sum_{h=1}^{s} \sum_{i=1}^{n_h} \sum_{j=1}^{t} (\overline{y}_{..j} - \overline{y}_{...})^2 = n \sum_{j=1}^{t} (\overline{y}_{..j} - \overline{y}_{...})^2, \\
\mathrm{SS_{GT}} &= \sum_{h=1}^{s} \sum_{i=1}^{n_h} \sum_{j=1}^{t} (\overline{y}_{h.j} - \overline{y}_{h..} - \overline{y}_{..j} + \overline{y}_{...})^2, \\
\mathrm{SS_R} &= \sum_{h=1}^{s} \sum_{i=1}^{n_h} \sum_{j=1}^{t} (y_{hij} - \overline{y}_{h.j} - \overline{y}_{hi.} + \overline{y}_{h..})^2.
\end{aligned}$$

Note that $\mathrm{SS_G}$, $\mathrm{SS_T}$, and $\mathrm{SS_{GT}}$ are equal to the sums of squares from a two-factor ANOVA model (assuming that all nt observations are independent) with effects for group, time, and the group × time interaction. The residual sum of squares $\mathrm{SS_R}$ is due to the subject effect nested within the cross-classification of group × time.

The F statistic for testing for differences among groups is given by

$$F = \frac{\mathrm{MS_G}}{\mathrm{MS_{S(G)}}} = \frac{\mathrm{SS_G}/(s-1)}{\mathrm{SS_{S(G)}}/(n-s)}$$

with $s-1$ and $n-s$ df. This test requires the assumption that the within-group covariance matrices are equal. In general, this assumption is required for all tests of between-subjects effects.

The F statistic for testing differences among time points is given by

$$F = \frac{\mathrm{MS_T}}{\mathrm{MS_R}} = \frac{\mathrm{SS_T}/(t-1)}{\mathrm{SS_R}/[(n-s)(t-1)]}$$

TABLE 5.4. Logarithms of times (seconds) to dissolve for four groups of tablets

		Fraction Remaining					
Group	Tablet	0.90	0.70	0.50	0.30	0.25	0.10
1	1	2.56	2.77	2.94	3.14	3.18	3.33
	2	2.64	2.89	3.09	3.26	3.33	3.47
	3	2.94	3.18	3.33	3.50	3.50	3.66
	4	2.56	2.83	3.04	3.22	3.26	3.37
	5	2.64	2.77	2.94	3.14	3.22	3.30
	6	2.56	2.77	2.94	3.14	3.18	3.26
2	1	2.56	2.83	3.07	3.26	3.33	3.51
	2	2.44	2.74	3.02	3.20	3.28	3.44
	3	2.34	2.67	2.91	3.16	3.22	3.39
	4	2.41	2.71	2.94	3.16	3.21	3.36
3	1	2.46	2.83	3.09	3.32	3.37	3.54
	2	2.60	2.93	3.21	3.40	3.46	3.62
	3	2.48	2.84	3.12	3.35	3.41	3.58
	4	2.49	2.82	3.05	3.29	3.37	3.52
4	1	2.40	2.67	2.94	3.20	3.26	3.47
	2	2.64	2.94	3.18	3.40	3.45	3.66
	3	2.40	2.64	2.86	3.09	3.16	3.38

with $t-1$ and $(n-s)(t-1)$ df. Similarly, the F statistic for testing the significance of the group × time interaction is given by

$$F = \frac{\text{MS}_{\text{GT}}}{\text{MS}_{\text{R}}} = \frac{\text{SS}_{\text{GT}}/[(s-1)(t-1)]}{\text{SS}_{\text{R}}/[(n-s)(t-1)]}$$

with $(s-1)(t-1)$ and $(n-s)(t-1)$ df. Both of these tests require the assumption that the within-group covariance matrices are equal and that the sphericity condition is satisfied. In general, these assumptions are required for all tests of within-subjects effects.

An alternative repeated measures ANOVA model for this setting includes an additional random effect for the subject × time interaction. This effect is usually assumed to be uncorrelated with the random subject effect. Although the expected mean squares for this model are different from those displayed in Table 5.3, the sums of squares and test statistics are identical.

5.4.2 *Example*

Crowder (1996) presents data from an experiment comparing dissolution times of pills. Table 5.4 displays the logarithms of the times, in seconds, for each pill to reach fractions remaining of 0.9, 0.7, 0.5, 0.3, 0.25, and 0.10. The four groups correspond to different storage conditions. Under the assumption that the logarithms of the times are normally distributed, repeated

TABLE 5.5. ANOVA table for drug dissolution data

Source	SS	df	MS	F	p-value
Group	0.2038	3	0.0679	0.87	0.4798
Subjects(Group)	1.0108	13	0.0778		
Fraction	10.0388	5	2.0078	3187.45	< 0.001
Group × Fraction	0.2045	15	0.0136	21.64	< 0.001
Residual	0.0409	65	0.0006		

measures ANOVA can be used to test for effects due to group, fraction remaining, and the interaction between group and fraction remaining.

Table 5.5 displays the ANOVA table for this example. Under the assumptions that the within-group covariance matrices are equal and that the sphericity condition is satisfied, there is a highly significant interaction effect between group and fraction remaining. Thus, the shapes of the profiles are not the same across the four groups.

The test of sphericity, however, is rejected. The chi-square approximation to Mauchly's (1940) criterion is 37.21 with 14 df ($p < 0.001$). The Greenhouse–Geisser estimate of ϵ is $\widehat{\epsilon} = 0.454$, and the Huynh–Feldt estimator is $\widetilde{\epsilon} = 0.683$. In this example, the adjusted tests of the fraction and group × fraction effects based on both $\widehat{\epsilon}$ and $\widetilde{\epsilon}$ yield $p < 0.001$.

The dissolution times (and their logarithms) for the type of data displayed in Table 5.4 are strictly increasing. Thus, the test of the effect of the repeated measures factor (fraction remaining) is not of great interest because it is likely to be highly significant. An alternative approach to the analysis of such dissolution data is to use repeated measures ANOVA on the first differences of the log-transformed times (Mauger et al., 1986).

5.5 Problems

5.1 Consider the $t \times t$ compound symmetric covariance matrix $\mathbf{\Sigma}$ with main diagonal elements σ^2 and off-diagonal elements $\rho\sigma^2$. Show that

$$\epsilon = \frac{t^2(\overline{\sigma}_{ii} - \overline{\sigma}_{..})^2}{(t-1)(S - 2t\sum \overline{\sigma}_{i.}^2 + t^2\overline{\sigma}_{..}^2)}$$

is equal to 1, where $\overline{\sigma}_{ii}$ is the mean of the entries on the main diagonal of $\mathbf{\Sigma}$, $\overline{\sigma}_{..}$ is the mean of all elements of $\mathbf{\Sigma}$, $\overline{\sigma}_{i.}$ is the mean of the entries in row i of $\mathbf{\Sigma}$, and S is the sum of the squares of the elements of $\mathbf{\Sigma}$.

5.2 Determine whether these covariance matrices satisfy the sphericity condition:

$$\text{(a) } \mathbf{\Sigma} = \begin{pmatrix} 5 & 2.5 & 5 \\ & 10 & 7.5 \\ & & 15 \end{pmatrix}. \qquad \text{(b) } \mathbf{\Sigma} = \begin{pmatrix} 5 & 2.5 & 7.5 \\ & 15 & 12.5 \\ & & 25 \end{pmatrix}.$$

TABLE 5.6. Weights of 13 male mice from birth to weaning

	Day						
Mouse	3	6	9	12	15	18	21
1	.190	.388	.621	.823	1.078	1.132	1.191
2	.218	.393	.568	.729	.839	.852	1.004
3	.211	.394	.549	.700	.783	.870	.925
4	.209	.419	.645	.850	1.001	1.026	1.069
5	.193	.362	.520	.530	.641	.640	.751
6	.201	.361	.502	.530	.657	.762	.888
7	.202	.370	.498	.650	.795	.858	.910
8	.190	.350	.510	.666	.819	.879	.929
9	.219	.399	.578	.699	.709	.822	.953
10	.225	.400	.545	.690	.796	.825	.836
11	.224	.381	.577	.756	.869	.929	.999
12	.187	.329	.441	.525	.589	.621	.796
13	.278	.471	.606	.770	.888	1.001	1.105

5.3 Table 5.6 displays the weights of 13 male mice measured at intervals of three days over the 21 days from birth to weaning (Rao, 1987).

(a) Use both the unstructured multivariate approach and repeated measures ANOVA to test the null hypothesis that the means at all seven of the measurement times are equal. Which of the two analyses do you prefer? Why?

(b) Based on your preferred method of analysis from part (a), test the null hypothesis that the relationship between weight and measurement day is linear.

5.4 Problem 3.6 describes a study in which response times of the eyes to a stimulus were measured (Crowder and Hand, 1990, p. 30). The variable of interest was the time lag (milliseconds) between the stimulus (a light flash) and the electrical response at the back of the cortex. In seven student volunteers, recordings were made for left and right eyes through lenses of powers 6/6, 6/18, 6/36, and 6/60. Table 3.6 displays the data. Use repeated measures ANOVA to assess the effects of eye, lens strength, and eye $\times$ lens strength interaction.

5.5 Problem 3.8 describes a study of 12 hospitalized patients who underwent a dietary treatment regimen during which plasma ascorbic acid levels were recorded on each of seven occasions during a 16-week period. There were two measurements prior to treatment (weeks 1 and 2), three during treatment (weeks 6, 10, and 14), and two after (weeks 15 and 16) the treatment regimen. Table 3.8 displays the data.

(a) Test the null hypothesis that the means at weeks 1, 2, 6, 10, 14, 15, and 16 are equal by the unstructured multivariate approach and repeated measures ANOVA. Which of the two analyses do you prefer? Why?

(b) Use repeated measures ANOVA to test the significance of the effects due to phase (before treatment, during treatment, after treatment).

5.6 Cole and Grizzle (1966) describe an experiment in which 16 mongrel dogs were divided into four groups. Groups 1 and 2 received morphine sulphate intravenously, and groups 3 and 4 received intravenous trimethaphan. In addition, the dogs in groups 2 and 4 were treated so that their supplies of available histamine were depleted at the time of treatment, whereas groups 1 and 3 had intact histamine supplies. Table 5.7 displays blood histamine levels (μg/ml) at minutes 1, 3, and 5 of treatment. (Note that Cole and Grizzle replaced a missing value at 5 minutes for the second dog in group 2 with the value 0.11.) Before completing the following analyses, transform the responses by taking the base 10 logarithm to maintain consistency with the results reported by Cole and Grizzle (1966).

(a) Ignore the factorial structure of the experiment and use repeated measures ANOVA to assess the effects of group, time, and the group $\times$ time interaction.

(b) Use repeated measures ANOVA to assess the effects of treatment, histamine supply, time, and the two-way and three-way interactions of these effects.

5.7 Table 5.8 lists repeated measurements of total cholesterol amounts measured every four weeks for 24 weeks in 12 subjects treated with a drug and 11 subjects treated with a placebo (Hirotsu, 1991). Use repeated measures ANOVA to assess the effects of group, week, and the group $\times$ week interaction.

5.8 Table 3.3 lists the data from a study conducted at the University of North Carolina Dental School in which the distance (mm) from the center of the pituitary gland to the pterygomaxillary fissure was measured at ages 8, 10, 12, and 14 in 16 boys and 11 girls (Potthoff and Roy, 1964). Use repeated measures ANOVA to test the significance of the effects of sex, year, and the sex $\times$ year interaction. Comment on the validity of this methodology for these data as well as on its usefulness relative to the analysis approaches illustrated in Sections 3.4.2, 4.3.2, and 4.4.3.

5.9 Box (1950) describes an experiment in which 30 rats were randomly assigned to three treatment groups. Group 1 was a control group, group 2 had thyroxin added to their drinking water, and group 3 had thiouracil added to their drinking water. Whereas there were ten rats in each of

TABLE 5.7. Blood histamine levels in four groups of dogs

		Histamine		Minute		
Group	Treatment	Supply	Dog	1	3	5
1	Morphine	Intact	1	0.20	0.10	0.08
			2	0.06	0.02	0.02
			3	1.40	0.48	0.24
			4	0.57	0.35	0.24
2	Morphine	Depleted	1	0.09	0.13	0.14
			2	0.11	0.10	0.11
			3	0.07	0.07	0.07
			4	0.07	0.06	0.07
3	Trimethaphan	Intact	1	0.62	0.31	0.22
			2	1.05	0.73	0.60
			3	0.83	1.07	0.80
			4	3.13	2.06	1.23
4	Trimethaphan	Depleted	1	0.09	0.09	0.08
			2	0.09	0.09	0.10
			3	0.10	0.12	0.12
			4	0.05	0.05	0.05

groups 1 and 3, group 2 consisted of only seven rats (due to an unspecified accident at the beginning of the experiment). The resulting body weights of each of the 27 rats at the beginning of the experiment and at weekly intervals for four weeks were previously considered in Problems 2.4 and 4.3 and are displayed in Table 2.12. Use repeated measures ANOVA to test the significance of the effects of treatment group, week, and treatment × week interaction. Comment on the validity of this methodology for these data as well as on its usefulness relative to the approaches of Problems 2.4 and 4.3.

5.10 Groves et al. (1998) discuss a randomized, double-blind clinical trial comparing the antispastic efficacy of two drugs. In this study, 26 patients with cerebral lesions were randomly assigned to treatment with tizanidine (T) or diazepam (D). One of the outcome variables in the study was total muscle strength. This is computed as the sum of 32 upper- and lower-limb measurements, each of which is a rating on a six-point ordinal scale from 0 (normal strength) to 5 (no voluntary movement). The total muscle-strength score ranges from 0 to 160, with lower scores indicating increased strength. Table 5.9 displays total muscle-strength measurements at baseline (week 0) and at weeks 2, 4, and 6 of treatment. Use repeated measures ANOVA to test the significance of the effects of treatment, time, and the treatment × time interaction.

TABLE 5.8. Total cholesterol measurements from 23 subjects

		Week					
Group	Subject	4	8	12	16	20	24
Drug	1	317	280	275	270	274	266
	2	186	189	190	135	197	205
	3	377	395	368	334	338	334
	4	229	258	282	272	264	265
	5	276	310	306	309	300	264
	6	272	250	250	255	228	250
	7	219	210	236	239	242	221
	8	260	245	264	268	317	314
	9	284	256	241	242	243	241
	10	365	304	294	287	311	302
	11	298	321	341	342	357	335
	12	274	245	262	263	235	246
Placebo	1	232	205	244	197	218	233
	2	367	354	358	333	338	355
	3	253	256	247	228	237	235
	4	230	218	245	215	230	207
	5	190	188	212	201	169	179
	6	290	263	291	312	299	279
	7	337	337	383	318	361	341
	8	283	279	277	264	269	271
	9	325	257	288	326	293	275
	10	266	258	253	284	245	263
	11	338	343	307	274	262	309

TABLE 5.9. Total muscle-strength scores from 26 subjects

Subject	Treatment	Week 0	2	4	6
1	T	58	54	52	52
2	D	56	52	52	52
3	D	54	54	54	54
4	D	61	61	61	61
5	T	15	15	15	15
6	T	63	63	63	63
7	D	19	19	16	16
8	T	28	28	28	28
9	T	62	56	54	54
10	T	58	58	58	58
11	D	62	50	50	50
12	D	54	52	52	52
13	T	108	108	100	100
14	D	52	52	52	52
15	D	38	36	36	36
16	T	26	26	26	26
17	T	26	26	26	26
18	D	48	48	48	48
19	D	24	20	20	20
20	T	40	40	40	40
21	D	58	58	58	58
22	T	24	24	24	24
23	T	64	64	64	64
24	T	12	12	12	12
25	T	46	46	46	46
26	D	54	54	54	54

TABLE 5.10. Body weights (g) of 15 guinea pigs

		Week					
Group	ID	1	3	4	5	6	7
Control	1	455	460	510	504	436	466
	2	467	565	610	596	542	587
	3	445	530	580	597	582	619
	4	485	542	594	583	611	612
	5	480	500	550	528	562	576
Low dose	6	514	560	565	524	552	597
	7	440	480	536	484	567	569
	8	495	570	569	585	576	677
	9	520	590	610	637	671	702
	10	503	555	591	605	649	675
High dose	11	496	560	622	622	632	670
	12	498	540	589	557	568	609
	13	478	510	568	555	576	605
	14	545	565	580	601	633	649
	15	472	498	540	524	532	583

5.11 In an investigation of the effects of various dosages of radiation therapy on psychomotor skills (Danford et al., 1960), 45 cancer patients were trained to operate a psychomotor testing device. Six patients were not given radiation and served as controls, and the remainder were treated with dosages of 25–50 R, 75–100 R, or 125–250 R. The resulting psychomotor test scores on the three days following radiation treatment were previously considered in Problems 2.6 and 4.6 and are displayed in Table 2.14. Use repeated measures ANOVA to test the significance of the effects of radiation dosage, day, and the radiation dosage $\times$ day interaction. Comment on the validity of this methodology for these data.

5.12 Crowder and Hand (1990) describe a seven-week study of the effect of a vitamin E diet supplement on the growth of 15 guinea pigs. In addition to a control group, low and high doses of vitamin E were studied (with five animals assigned to each of the three groups). All animals were given a growth-inhibiting substance during week 1, and treatment was initiated at the beginning of week 5. Table 5.10 displays the body weights, in grams, of each animal at the end of weeks 1, 3, 4, 5, 6, and 7. Use repeated measures ANOVA to assess whether the growth profiles of the three groups differ.

5.13 Table 4.7 displays scaled test scores for a cohort of 64 students of the Laboratory School of the University of Chicago (Bock, 1975). These data were previously considered in Problem 4.2. Use repeated measures ANOVA to assess whether there are differences between boys and girls and among grade levels, and whether the effects of grade level are the same for boys and girls.

5.14 Hand and Taylor (1987, pp. 117–125) describe a study of urinary salsolinol excretion levels in two groups of subjects admitted to an alcoholism treatment unit. Group 1 includes six subjects considered to be moderately dependent on alcohol, and group 2 includes eight subjects considered to be severely dependent on alcohol. This study was previously considered in Problems 3.13 and 4.12; Table 3.11 displays the raw data. Analyze the log-transformed urinary salsolinol levels using repeated measures ANOVA. Test the significance of the effects of group, day, and the group $\times$ day interaction.

6 Normal-Theory Methods: Linear Mixed Models

6.1 Introduction

Chapters 3, 4, and 5 have considered the situation in which a normally distributed outcome variable is measured repeatedly from each subject or experimental unit. The analysis of such data must account for the dependence among a subject's multiple measurements. "Classical" methodology is based either on multivariate normal models with general covariance structure (Chapters 3 and 4) or on univariate repeated measures ANOVA (Chapter 5). In practice, however, repeated measurements studies are characterized by:

- variation among experimental units with respect to the number and timing of observations;
- missing data;
- time-dependent covariates.

Such features make the classical multivariate procedures difficult (or impossible) to apply.

This chapter considers an alternative approach based on the linear mixed model. The theoretical base of linear mixed models is well-established, and the methodology has applications in many areas not involving repeated measurements. McLean et al. (1991) provide a general introduction to linear mixed models, and Ware (1985) gives an overview of their application to the analysis of repeated measurements.

The linear mixed models approach to repeated measurements views the analysis as a univariate regression analysis of responses with correlated errors. One major advantage of this methodology is that it accommodates the complexities of typical longitudinal data sets. The mixed model approach permits specification of models determined by subject matter considerations rather than by limitations of the statistical methodology. It also allows explicit modeling and analysis of variation between subjects and within subjects.

The use of linear mixed model methodology for the analysis of repeated measurements is becoming increasingly common due to the development of widely available software. In particular, the MIXED procedure of SAS (SAS Institute, 1999) is often used. Hedeker and Gibbons (1996b) also provide software for fitting the linear mixed model to repeated measurements.

Section 6.2 describes the linear mixed model, and Section 6.3 discusses its application to repeated measurements. Section 6.4 presents three examples of the use of the linear mixed model in analyzing repeated measurements data. Finally, Section 6.5 gives some comments and cautions concerning the use of this methodology.

6.2 The Linear Mixed Model

6.2.1 *The Usual Linear Model*

Let $\boldsymbol{y} = (y_1, \ldots, y_n)'$ be an $n \times 1$ vector of independent observations. The usual linear model is

$$\boldsymbol{y} = \boldsymbol{X\beta} + \boldsymbol{\epsilon},$$

where $\boldsymbol{\beta}$ is a $p \times 1$ vector of unknown parameters, $\boldsymbol{X}$ is an $n \times p$ model matrix, and $\boldsymbol{\epsilon} = (\epsilon_1, \ldots, \epsilon_n)'$ is an $n \times 1$ vector of independent errors. The components of $\boldsymbol{\epsilon}$ are independent with mean 0 and constant variance σ^2.

The focus is to model the mean of $\boldsymbol{y}$ in terms of the unknown parameters $\boldsymbol{\beta}$, which are estimated using ordinary least squares. One generalization of the usual linear model is to allow ϵ_i to have mean zero and variance σ_i^2; a further generalization is to assume that $\boldsymbol{\epsilon}$ has mean vector $\mathbf{0}_n$ and arbitrary covariance matrix $\boldsymbol{\Sigma}$. These generalizations are sometimes referred to as weighted least squares and generalized least squares, respectively.

6.2.2 *The Mixed Model*

The linear mixed model is

$$\boldsymbol{y} = \boldsymbol{X\beta} + \boldsymbol{Z\gamma} + \boldsymbol{\epsilon}. \tag{6.1}$$

As in Section 6.2.1, $\boldsymbol{y}$ is an $n \times 1$ vector of observations, $\boldsymbol{X}$ is an $n \times p$ model matrix, $\boldsymbol{\beta}$ is a $p \times 1$ vector of unknown parameters, and $\boldsymbol{\epsilon}$ is an $n \times 1$ vector of errors. In addition, $\boldsymbol{Z}$ is a given $n \times q$ matrix, and $\boldsymbol{\gamma}$ is an unobservable random vector of dimensions $q \times 1$.

The random components of model (6.1) are the vectors $\boldsymbol{\gamma}$ and $\boldsymbol{\epsilon}$. The following assumptions are made concerning these random vectors:

- $\mathrm{E}(\boldsymbol{\gamma}) = \boldsymbol{0}_q$;
- $\mathrm{Var}(\boldsymbol{\gamma}) = \boldsymbol{B}$;
- $\mathrm{E}(\boldsymbol{\epsilon}) = \boldsymbol{0}_n$;
- $\mathrm{Var}(\boldsymbol{\epsilon}) = \boldsymbol{W}$.

In addition, the vectors $\boldsymbol{\gamma}$ and $\boldsymbol{\epsilon}$ are assumed to be uncorrelated. Note that in this model the elements of $\boldsymbol{\epsilon}$ are not necessarily assumed to be independent but are allowed to have arbitrary covariance matrix. In the linear mixed model, both the mean of $\boldsymbol{y}$,

$$\mathrm{E}(\boldsymbol{y}) = \boldsymbol{X\beta},$$

and the variance of $\boldsymbol{y}$,

$$\mathrm{Var}(\boldsymbol{y}) = \boldsymbol{ZBZ}' + \boldsymbol{W},$$

can be modeled.

The elements of $\boldsymbol{B}$ and $\boldsymbol{W}$ are assumed to be known functions of an unknown parameter vector $\boldsymbol{\theta} = (\theta_1, \ldots, \theta_m)'$. The parameter space for the model is taken to be $\{(\boldsymbol{\beta}, \boldsymbol{\theta}): \boldsymbol{\theta} \in \boldsymbol{\Omega}\}$, where $\boldsymbol{\Omega}$ is the set of $\boldsymbol{\theta}$ values for which $\mathrm{Var}(\boldsymbol{y})$ is positive-definite. When $\boldsymbol{W} = \sigma^2\boldsymbol{I}$ and $\boldsymbol{Z} = 0$, the mixed model reduces to the standard linear model.

6.2.3 Parameter Estimation

Estimation of the random effects (variance components) of model (6.1) has been a longstanding problem. Common practice for balanced analysis of variance (ANOVA) was to equate mean squares to their expectations. Henderson (1953) developed widely used analogous techniques for unbalanced data. In the past, maximum likelihood (ML) estimation of the fixed effects and variance components was not commonly used due to computational difficulties. This required the numerical solution of a constrained nonlinear optimization problem. Harville (1977) reviewed previous work, unified the methodology, and described iterative ML algorithms for obtaining parameter estimates.

In addition to computational difficulties, ML estimates of variance components are biased downward. Patterson and Thompson (1971) proposed the alternative restricted maximum likelihood (REML) approach; this is also sometimes called residual maximum likelihood. The REML estimation approach applies ML estimation techniques to the likelihood function associated with a set of "error contrasts" rather than to that associated with the original observations. This accounts for the loss of degrees of freedom resulting from estimation of the fixed effects and gives less biased estimates of the variance components. The bias issue is especially important when the number of parameters is not small relative to the total number of observations. The REML approach yields the standard ANOVA-based estimates in balanced random and mixed ANOVA models (unlike ML estimation).

As an example, consider the estimation of σ^2 in the usual linear model $\boldsymbol{y} = \boldsymbol{X\beta} + \boldsymbol{\epsilon}$, where $\boldsymbol{y}$ is the $n \times 1$ data vector, $\boldsymbol{X}$ is an $n \times p$ model matrix of rank p, and $\boldsymbol{\epsilon} \sim N_n(\boldsymbol{0}_n, \sigma^2 \boldsymbol{I}_n)$. The MLE of σ^2 is

$$\widetilde{\sigma}^2 = \frac{(\boldsymbol{y} - \boldsymbol{X}\widehat{\boldsymbol{\beta}})'(\boldsymbol{y} - \boldsymbol{X}\widehat{\boldsymbol{\beta}})}{n},$$

where $\widehat{\boldsymbol{\beta}} = (\boldsymbol{X}'\boldsymbol{X})^{-1}\boldsymbol{X}'\boldsymbol{y}$. The REML estimate of σ^2 is the minimum variance unbiased estimator

$$\widehat{\sigma}^2 = \frac{(\boldsymbol{y} - \boldsymbol{X}\widehat{\boldsymbol{\beta}})'(\boldsymbol{y} - \boldsymbol{X}\widehat{\boldsymbol{\beta}})}{n-p}.$$

The bias of the MLE is

$$\mathrm{E}(\widetilde{\sigma}^2 - \sigma^2) = -\sigma^2\left(\frac{p}{n}\right),$$

which is negative and worsens as p increases.

6.2.4 Background on REML Estimation

As mentioned in Section 6.2.3, REML estimation applies maximum likelihood estimation techniques to the likelihood function associated with a set of "error contrasts" rather than to that associated with the original observations. An error contrast is a linear combination $\boldsymbol{a}'\boldsymbol{y}$ of the elements of $\boldsymbol{y}$ such that $\mathrm{E}(\boldsymbol{a}'\boldsymbol{y}) = 0$ for any $\boldsymbol{\beta}$ (i.e., if $\boldsymbol{a}'\boldsymbol{X} = \boldsymbol{0}_p'$).

As an example, let $\boldsymbol{S} = \boldsymbol{I}_n - \boldsymbol{P}_{\boldsymbol{X}}$, where $\boldsymbol{P}_{\boldsymbol{X}} = \boldsymbol{X}(\boldsymbol{X}'\boldsymbol{X})^{-1}\boldsymbol{X}'$ is the orthogonal projection matrix onto the column space of $\boldsymbol{X}$. The expected value of $\boldsymbol{Sy}$ is

$$\mathrm{E}(\boldsymbol{Sy}) = (\boldsymbol{I}_n - \boldsymbol{P}_{\boldsymbol{X}})\boldsymbol{X\beta} = \boldsymbol{X\beta} - \boldsymbol{X\beta} = \boldsymbol{0}_n.$$

Each element of $\boldsymbol{Sy}$ is an error contrast. It is a well-known result from linear models theory that although $\boldsymbol{S}$ is $n \times n$ its rank is $n - p$. Thus, there are some redundancies among the elements of $\boldsymbol{Sy}$.

A natural question is:

- How many essentially different error contrasts can be included in a single set?

One can show that any set of error contrasts contains at most $n-p$ linearly independent error contrasts, where the error contrasts $\boldsymbol{a}_1'\boldsymbol{y},\ldots,\boldsymbol{a}_k'\boldsymbol{y}$ are linearly independent if $\boldsymbol{a}_1,\ldots,\boldsymbol{a}_k$ are linearly independent vectors.

Let $\boldsymbol{A}$ be an $n \times (n-p)$ matrix such that $\boldsymbol{A}'\boldsymbol{A} = \boldsymbol{I}_{n-p}$ and $\boldsymbol{A}\boldsymbol{A}' = \boldsymbol{I}_n - \boldsymbol{P}_{\boldsymbol{X}}$. One can show that $\boldsymbol{w} = \boldsymbol{A}'\boldsymbol{y}$ is a vector of $n-p$ linearly independent error contrasts. (It is not, however, the only such vector.)

The REML approach applies maximum likelihood estimation techniques to $\boldsymbol{w} = \boldsymbol{A}'\boldsymbol{y}$ rather than to $\boldsymbol{y}$. Under the assumed model,

$$\boldsymbol{y} \sim N_n(\boldsymbol{X\beta}, \boldsymbol{V}),$$

where $\boldsymbol{V} = \boldsymbol{ZBZ}' + \boldsymbol{W}$. Then,

$$\boldsymbol{w} \sim N_{n-p}(\boldsymbol{0}_{n-p}, \boldsymbol{A}'\boldsymbol{V}\boldsymbol{A}).$$

It is natural to ask whether the estimator $\widehat{\boldsymbol{\theta}}$ obtained by maximizing

$$f_{\boldsymbol{W}}(\boldsymbol{w};\boldsymbol{\theta}),$$

the likelihood function associated with the vector $\boldsymbol{w}$ of error contrasts, is the same as that obtained by maximizing the likelihood function associated with any other vector of $n-p$ linearly independent error contrasts. One can show that if $\boldsymbol{u} = \boldsymbol{C}'\boldsymbol{y}$ is any vector of $n-p$ linearly independent error contrasts, the likelihood function associated with $\boldsymbol{u}$ is a scalar multiple of $f_{\boldsymbol{W}}(\boldsymbol{w};\boldsymbol{\theta})$ that does not depend on $\boldsymbol{\theta}$.

Apart from an additive constant that does not depend on $\boldsymbol{\theta}$, the log-likelihood function $L_R(\boldsymbol{\theta};\boldsymbol{y})$ associated with any vector of $n-p$ linearly independent error contrasts is

$$L_R(\boldsymbol{\theta};\boldsymbol{y}) = -\frac{1}{2}\Big[\log|\boldsymbol{V}| + \log|\boldsymbol{X}'\boldsymbol{V}^{-1}\boldsymbol{X}| + (\boldsymbol{y}-\boldsymbol{X}\widehat{\boldsymbol{\beta}})'\boldsymbol{V}^{-1}(\boldsymbol{y}-\boldsymbol{X}\widehat{\boldsymbol{\beta}})\Big],$$

where $\widehat{\boldsymbol{\beta}} = (\boldsymbol{X}'\boldsymbol{V}^{-1}\boldsymbol{X})^{-1}\boldsymbol{X}'\boldsymbol{V}^{-1}\boldsymbol{y}$. In comparison, the log-likelihood function for $\boldsymbol{y}$ is

$$L_M(\boldsymbol{\theta};\boldsymbol{y}) = -\frac{1}{2}\log|\boldsymbol{V}| - \frac{1}{2}(\boldsymbol{y}-\boldsymbol{X}\widehat{\boldsymbol{\beta}})'\boldsymbol{V}^{-1}(\boldsymbol{y}-\boldsymbol{X}\widehat{\boldsymbol{\beta}}).$$

The only difference is that $L_R(\boldsymbol{\theta};\boldsymbol{y})$ has the additional term

$$-\frac{1}{2}\log|\boldsymbol{X}'\boldsymbol{V}^{-1}\boldsymbol{X}|.$$

The estimator $\widehat{\boldsymbol{\theta}}$ is an REML estimator of $\boldsymbol{\theta}$ if $L_R(\boldsymbol{\theta};\boldsymbol{y})$ attains its maximum value at $\boldsymbol{\theta} = \widehat{\boldsymbol{\theta}}$.

Special cases of the REML approach were considered by earlier authors. Anderson and Bancroft (1952) and Russell and Bradley (1958) developed REML estimation approaches for some specific balanced ANOVA models.

Thompson (1962) extended these results to all balanced ANOVA models. In the usual linear model (Section 6.2.1), the REML equations have a unique solution that coincides with the minimum variance unbiased estimator

$$\widehat{\sigma}^2_{\text{REML}} = \frac{(\boldsymbol{y} - \boldsymbol{X}\widehat{\boldsymbol{\beta}})'(\boldsymbol{y} - \boldsymbol{X}\widehat{\boldsymbol{\beta}})}{n-p}.$$

In balanced mixed and random ANOVA models, the REML equations have an explicit unique solution coinciding with the ANOVA estimate. In general, however, the problem of obtaining an REML estimate of $\boldsymbol{\theta}$ requires iterative methods of maximizing the nonlinear function $L_R(\boldsymbol{\theta}; \boldsymbol{y})$ subject to the constraint $\boldsymbol{\theta} \in \boldsymbol{\Omega}$. Algorithms such as Newton–Raphson and the method of scoring can be used.

6.3 Application to Repeated Measurements

Let $\boldsymbol{y}_i = (y_{i1}, \ldots, y_{it_i})'$ be the $t_i \times 1$ vector of responses from subject i for $i = 1, \ldots, n$. The general linear mixed model for longitudinal data is

$$\boldsymbol{y}_i = \boldsymbol{X}_i\boldsymbol{\beta} + \boldsymbol{Z}_i\boldsymbol{\gamma}_i + \boldsymbol{\epsilon}_i, \qquad i = 1, \ldots, n, \tag{6.2}$$

where $\boldsymbol{X}_i$ is a $t_i \times b$ model (design) matrix for subject i, $\boldsymbol{\beta}$ is a $b \times 1$ vector of regression coefficients, $\boldsymbol{\gamma}_i$ is a $g \times 1$ vector of random effects for subject i, $\boldsymbol{Z}_i$ is a $t_i \times g$ design matrix for the random effects, and $\boldsymbol{\epsilon}_i$ is a $t_i \times 1$ vector of within-subject errors.

The $\boldsymbol{\gamma}_i$ vectors are assumed to be independent $N_g(\boldsymbol{0}_g, \boldsymbol{B})$, and the $\boldsymbol{\epsilon}_i$ vectors are assumed to be independent $N_{t_i}(\boldsymbol{0}_{t_i}, \boldsymbol{W}_i)$. In addition, the $\boldsymbol{\gamma}_i$ and $\boldsymbol{\epsilon}_i$ vectors are assumed to be independent.

Thus, the vectors $\boldsymbol{y}_1, \ldots, \boldsymbol{y}_n$ are independent $N_{t_i}(\boldsymbol{X}_i\boldsymbol{\beta}, \boldsymbol{V}_i)$, where

$$\boldsymbol{V}_i = \boldsymbol{Z}_i\boldsymbol{B}\boldsymbol{Z}_i' + \boldsymbol{W}_i.$$

The matrices $\boldsymbol{X}_i$, $\boldsymbol{Z}_i$, and $\boldsymbol{W}_i$ are subject-specific.

This model is very general because subjects can have varying numbers of observations and because the observation times can differ among subjects. The within-subject covariance matrix $\boldsymbol{W}_i$ is assumed to depend on i only through its dimension t_i; that is, any unknown parameters in $\boldsymbol{W}_i$ do not depend on i. A wide variety of covariance structures for $\boldsymbol{\gamma}_i$ and $\boldsymbol{\epsilon}_i$ can be considered. In particular, the MIXED procedure of SAS (SAS Institute, 1999) implements more than 20 distinct covariance structures, and additional possibilities are described by Byrne and Arnold (1983), Jennrich and Schluchter (1986), Muñoz et al. (1992), Zimmerman and Núñez Antón (1997), Pourahmadi (1999), and Núñez Antón and Zimmerman (2000).

The general linear mixed model for repeated measures has been studied by several authors. Although essentially similar, the various approaches differ in terms of motivation and notation, assumptions concerning the random effects, and methods of obtaining ML and REML parameter estimates. Some of the main references are Laird and Ware (1982), Jennrich and Schluchter (1986), Laird et al. (1987), Diggle (1988), Lindstrom and Bates (1988), Jones and Boadi-Boateng (1991), and Jones (1993).

Laird and Ware (1982) consider the linear mixed model as a two-stage random-effects model. In the first stage, they assume that the model for the ith subject is

$$\boldsymbol{y}_i = \boldsymbol{X}_i\boldsymbol{\beta} + \boldsymbol{Z}_i\boldsymbol{\gamma}_i + \boldsymbol{\epsilon}_i.$$

The vectors $\boldsymbol{\epsilon}_1, \ldots, \boldsymbol{\epsilon}_n$ are assumed to be independent $N(\boldsymbol{0}_{t_i}, \boldsymbol{W}_i)$. The vector of regression coefficients $\boldsymbol{\beta}$ and the subject-specific vectors $\boldsymbol{\gamma}_i$ are considered to be fixed.

In the second stage, $\boldsymbol{\gamma}_1, \ldots, \boldsymbol{\gamma}_n$ are assumed to be independent $N(\boldsymbol{0}_g, \boldsymbol{B})$ and $\boldsymbol{\gamma}_i$ and $\boldsymbol{\epsilon}_i$ are assumed independent. Thus, $\boldsymbol{y}_1, \ldots, \boldsymbol{y}_n$ are independent $N(\boldsymbol{X}_i\boldsymbol{\beta}, \boldsymbol{Z}_i\boldsymbol{B}\boldsymbol{Z}_i' + \boldsymbol{W}_i)$. Laird and Ware (1982) call this the conditional independence model if $\boldsymbol{W}_i = \sigma^2\boldsymbol{I}_{t_i}$. In this case, the t_i responses $y_{i1}, \ldots, y_{it_i}$ are independent, conditional on $\boldsymbol{\gamma}_i$.

Laird and Ware (1982) discuss Bayesian and non-Bayesian formulations of the model. The EM algorithm is used to obtain ML and REML parameter estimates. In this formulation, unobservable random parameters are estimated, not missing data.

Jennrich and Schluchter (1986) approach the model from a different perspective. They consider the problem of how to analyze unbalanced or incomplete repeated measures. They use a general linear model for expected responses and arbitrary structural models for the within-subject variances and covariances. The Jennrich and Schluchter (1986) model is $\boldsymbol{y}_i = \boldsymbol{X}_i\boldsymbol{\beta} + \boldsymbol{\epsilon}_i$, where $\boldsymbol{\epsilon}_1, \ldots, \boldsymbol{\epsilon}_n$ are independent $N_{t_i}(\boldsymbol{0}_{t_i}, \boldsymbol{\Sigma}_i)$. The covariance matrix $\boldsymbol{\Sigma}_i$ is assumed to be a function of a vector $\boldsymbol{\theta}$ of q unknown covariance parameters.

The motivation for the Jennrich and Schluchter (1986) formulation of the model is that estimation of the vector of regression parameters $\boldsymbol{\beta}$ is of primary interest. Efficiency, however, may be improved by modeling $\boldsymbol{\Sigma}_i$ parsimoniously. This is especially important when sample sizes are small and the data are unbalanced. The ability to model $\boldsymbol{\Sigma}_i$ allows examination of alternative covariance structures.

Jennrich and Schluchter (1986) consider specifically an important special case that they call the incomplete data model. This is useful when a fixed number t of measurements are to be obtained from each subject but not all responses are observed. In this case, each $\boldsymbol{\Sigma}_i$ is a submatrix of a $t \times t$ matrix $\boldsymbol{\Sigma} = \boldsymbol{\Sigma}(\boldsymbol{\theta})$. Table 6.1 displays several important structural models for $\boldsymbol{\Sigma}$ in the incomplete data model. Note that in the Jennrich and Schluchter formulation, the use of the covariance model

$$\boldsymbol{\Sigma}_i = \boldsymbol{Z}_i\boldsymbol{B}\boldsymbol{Z}_i' + \boldsymbol{W}_i$$

TABLE 6.1. Covariance structures in the incomplete data model

Structure	q	Description
Independent observations	1	$\boldsymbol{\Sigma} = \sigma^2 \boldsymbol{I}_t$
Compound symmetry	2	$\boldsymbol{\Sigma} = \sigma^2 \boldsymbol{I}_t + \sigma_b^2 \boldsymbol{1}_t \boldsymbol{1}_t'$
Random effects (g effects)	$1 + g(g+1)/2$	$\boldsymbol{\Sigma} = \boldsymbol{ZBZ}' + \sigma^2 \boldsymbol{I}_t$
First-order autoregressive	2	$\sigma_{ij} = \sigma^2 \rho^{\lvert i-j \rvert}$
Toeplitz (banded)	t	$\sigma_{ij} = \theta_k,\ k = \lvert i-j \rvert + 1$
Unstructured	$t(t+1)/2$	$\sigma_{ij} = \sigma_{ji}$

yields the linear mixed model as a special case.

Jennrich and Schluchter describe Newton–Raphson and Fisher scoring algorithms for obtaining ML estimates. The Newton–Raphson method uses the score vector and Hessian matrix to iteratively compute new estimates of $\boldsymbol{\beta}$ and $\boldsymbol{\theta}$ from current values. The Fisher scoring algorithm replaces the Hessian matrix by its expectation; this is often more robust than Newton–Raphson to poor starting values. They also develop a generalized EM (GEM) algorithm for computing REML estimates. In this algorithm, the likelihood is increased (rather than maximized) at each M step. The GEM algorithm is restricted to the incomplete data model but has the advantage of being able to fit covariance matrices with large numbers of parameters.

Jennrich and Schluchter (1986) describe how to compute standard error estimates from the inverse of the Fisher information matrix (when Fisher scoring is used) and from the empirical information matrix (when Newton–Raphson is used). They conclude that standard error estimates from the empirical information matrix are preferable when the data are incomplete. Although their GEM algorithm does not produce standard errors for the elements of $\boldsymbol{\theta}$, these can be obtained by taking a single Newton–Raphson or Fisher scoring step after convergence.

Jennrich and Schluchter (1986) also compare computational algorithms. The Newton–Raphson algorithm has a quadratic convergence rate and generally converges in a small number of iterations (but with a higher cost per iteration). The GEM algorithm has the lowest cost per iteration but may require a large number of iterations. The Fisher scoring algorithm is intermediate in terms of cost per iteration and number of iterations; the cost per iteration is often not much less than Newton–Raphson, but it can require a much higher number of iterations. They conclude that when q, the number of covariance parameters, is small, the Newton–Raphson algorithm is preferred because this method is not restricted to the incomplete data model and because convergence is generally fast. With large q, however, as when fitting an unstructured covariance matrix to more than ten time points, only the GEM algorithm is feasible.

Laird et al. (1987) study the use of the EM algorithm for ML and REML estimation in model (6.2). They consider both the incomplete data model of Jennrich and Schluchter (1986) and the random-effects model of Laird and Ware (1982). In the incomplete data model, the EM algorithm requires an iterative M step within each iteration (or the use of Jennrich and Schluchter's GEM algorithm). The covariates for both observed and missing observations must be specified. The choice affects the rate, but not the point, of convergence. In the random-effects model, the observed data are the measurements actually collected, and the total data set consists of the observed data plus unobservable random parameters and error terms. Thus, there are no missing data in the traditional statistical sense.

Laird et al. (1987) conclude that the random-effects model is more general and includes the incomplete data model as a special case. This avoids specification of covariates for missing observations and eliminates the need for GEM or iterations within each M step (in a broad class of models). Dempster et al. (1981) and Laird et al. (1987) provide computing formulas for ML and REML estimation using the EM algorithm; Laird et al. (1987) also discuss the choice of starting values for the EM iterations and give two methods of speeding convergence of the EM algorithm.

Diggle (1988) considers the model

$$\boldsymbol{y}_i = \boldsymbol{X}_i\boldsymbol{\beta} + \boldsymbol{\epsilon}_i,$$

where $\boldsymbol{\epsilon}_i \sim N(\boldsymbol{0}_{t_i}, \boldsymbol{\Sigma}_i)$ and

$$\boldsymbol{\Sigma}_i = \tau^2\boldsymbol{I} + \nu^2\boldsymbol{J} + \sigma^2\boldsymbol{R}(\boldsymbol{t}_i).$$

In this model, $\boldsymbol{J}$ is a square matrix with elements of 1, $\boldsymbol{t}_i = (t_{i1}, \ldots, t_{in_i})'$ is the vector of measurement times for subject i, and $\boldsymbol{R}(\boldsymbol{t})$ is a symmetric matrix with (k,l)th element equal to $\exp(-\alpha|t_k - t_l|^c)$, where $c = 1$ or 2. The case $c = 1$ corresponds to the continuous-time analog of a first-order autoregressive process, whereas $c = 2$ provides a smoother process (Bartlett, 1966, Chapter 5). Thus, the within-subject covariance structure has four parameters: τ^2, ν^2, σ^2, and α. The parameters are estimated using ML and REML, and the empirical semivariogram of residuals is used to suggest an appropriate correlation structure.

Lindstrom and Bates (1988) consider the special case of model (6.2) when $\boldsymbol{W}_i = \sigma^2\boldsymbol{I}_{t_i}$. They develop efficient implementations of Newton–Raphson and EM algorithms for ML estimation and make improvements to Jennrich and Schluchter's (1986) ML algorithm to speed convergence and ensure a positive-definite covariance matrix for the random effects at each iteration. Lindstrom and Bates (1988) also compare the Newton–Raphson and EM algorithms in fitting models to two data sets: one with 11 subjects and an average of 28 observations/subject, and the other with 74 subjects and an average of 11 observations/subject. They conclude that the Newton–Raphson algorithm is generally preferable based on the number of iterations and the average time per iteration.

Jones and Boadi-Boateng (1991) and Jones (1993) consider model (6.2) when each subject is observed at different and unequally spaced time points.

The repeated measurements from each subject are assumed to be either uncorrelated or to have a continuous-time first-order autoregressive structure. Jones proposes an alternative method of estimation in which a state space representation of the model is used, the likelihood is calculated using the Kalman filter, and ML estimates are obtained using a nonlinear optimization program. An advantage of this approach is that the likelihood can be calculated recursively without using large $(t_i \times t_i)$ matrices.

Weiss and Lazaro (1992) discuss graphical methods that are useful in conjunction with linear mixed models. They study the use of parallel plots (Draper, 1987; Laird and Lange, 1987; Wegman, 1990) for examining the raw data and residuals from models fit to repeated measurements. These plots are useful in determining how well a particular model fits the data and in identifying outlying observations.

6.4 Examples

6.4.1 Two Groups, Four Time Points, No Missing Data

Potthoff and Roy (1964) describe a study conducted at the University of North Carolina Dental School in two groups of children (16 boys and 11 girls). In Section 3.4.2, Hotelling's T^2 statistic was used to compare boys and girls at ages 8, 10, 12, and 14 years with respect to the distance (mm) from the center of the pituitary gland to the pterygomaxillary fissure. Sections 4.3.2 and 4.4.3 illustrated the analysis of these data using profile analysis and growth curve methods, respectively. Table 3.3 lists the individual measurements as well as the sample means and standard deviations in both groups.

Jennrich and Schluchter (1986) fit several types of linear models to these data. Although REML estimation might be preferred, the results that follow are based on the use of ML estimation to match their results.

Jennrich and Schluchter's first model is

$$y_{hij} = \beta_{hj} + \epsilon_{hij},$$

where y_{hij} is the distance at time j for subject i in group h for $h = 1$ for males, $h = 2$ for females, and $j = 8, 10, 12, 14$. The vectors of residuals

$$\epsilon_{hi} = (\epsilon_{hi8}, \ldots, \epsilon_{hi,14})'$$

are assumed to be independent with common unstructured covariance matrix $\boldsymbol{W}$. In this model, the parameter estimates $\widehat{\beta}_{hj}$ are the sample means in group h at time j. The estimated covariance matrix is

$$\widehat{\boldsymbol{W}} = \begin{pmatrix} 5.0143 & 2.5156 & 3.6206 & 2.5095 \\ 2.5156 & 3.8748 & 2.7103 & 3.0714 \\ 3.6206 & 2.7103 & 5.9775 & 3.8248 \\ 2.5095 & 3.0714 & 3.8248 & 4.6164 \end{pmatrix}. \tag{6.3}$$

Using the MIXED procedure of SAS (SAS Institute, 1999), the likelihood ratio (LR) statistic (-2 log likelihood) is $-2\text{LL} = 416.51$.

Model 2 assumes a linear relationship between distance and age, with separate lines for boys and girls:

$$y_{hij} = \alpha_h + \beta_h j + \epsilon_{hij} \tag{6.4}$$

for $h = 1, 2$ and $j = 8, 10, 12, 14$. As in Model 1, the residual vectors ϵ_{hi} are assumed to be independent with common unstructured covariance matrix $\boldsymbol{W}$. This model is equivalent to the Potthoff–Roy growth curve model with $\boldsymbol{G} = \boldsymbol{S}$, as described in Section 4.4.2.

Because the -2LL statistic from Model 1 is equivalent to that from a model parameterized with separate linear, quadratic, and cubic age effects for each sex, the LR test can be used to compare the fit of Model 2 with that of Model 1. For Model 2, $-2\text{LL} = 419.48$; thus, the LR statistic comparing these models is

$$419.48 - 416.51 = 2.97.$$

Because Model 1 has 18 parameters (eight fixed effects and ten variance parameters) and Model 2 has 14 parameters (four fixed effects and ten variance parameters), the LR statistic has an asymptotic chi-square distribution with $18 - 14 = 4$ degrees of freedom (df). Because $p = 0.56$, the assumption of a linear relationship for each sex seems reasonable.

Model 3 again assumes a linear relationship between distance and age but with a common slope for boys and girls. Thus, the model is

$$y_{hij} = \alpha_h + \beta j + \epsilon_{hij}$$

for $h = 1, 2$ and $j = 8, 10, 12, 14$. As in Models 1 and 2, the residual vectors ϵ_{hi} are assumed to be independent with common unstructured covariance matrix $\boldsymbol{W}$. The LR statistic comparing Models 2 and 3 is

$$426.15 - 419.48 = 6.68$$

with $14-13 = 1$ df and $p = 0.01$. Because the slopes for boys and girls differ significantly, all subsequent models will use the same model for the means as Model 2 [Equation (6.4)]; the goal will be to examine the adequacy of restricted covariance structures.

One possible reduced covariance structure is a banded covariance matrix. In this example, $t = 4$, and the covariance matrix $\boldsymbol{W}$ for Model 4 has four parameters:

$$\boldsymbol{W} = \begin{pmatrix} \theta_1 & \theta_2 & \theta_3 & \theta_4 \\ \theta_2 & \theta_1 & \theta_2 & \theta_3 \\ \theta_3 & \theta_2 & \theta_1 & \theta_2 \\ \theta_4 & \theta_3 & \theta_2 & \theta_1 \end{pmatrix}.$$

The estimated covariance matrix from Model 4 is

$$\widehat{W} = \begin{pmatrix} 4.9438 & 3.0506 & 3.4053 & 2.3421 \\ 3.0506 & 4.9438 & 3.0506 & 3.4053 \\ 3.4053 & 3.0506 & 4.9438 & 3.0506 \\ 2.3421 & 3.4053 & 3.0506 & 4.9438 \end{pmatrix}.$$

The LR test comparing Model 4 with Model 2 is

$$424.64 - 419.48 = 5.17$$

with $14 - 8 = 6$ df and $p = 0.52$. Thus, the banded covariance model appears to provide an adequate fit relative to the unstructured covariance matrix.

Model 5 considers the first-order autoregressive (AR–1) covariance structure. In this model, the covariance matrix $\boldsymbol{W}$ has elements $w_{ij} = \sigma^2 \rho^{|i-j|}$ for $i, j = 1, \ldots, 4$. The estimated covariance parameters are $\widehat{\sigma}^2 = 4.8910$ and $\widehat{\rho} = 0.6071$. Thus, the estimated covariance matrix from Model 5 is

$$\widehat{W} = \begin{pmatrix} 4.8910 & 2.9696 & 1.8030 & 1.0947 \\ 2.9696 & 4.8910 & 2.9696 & 1.8030 \\ 1.8030 & 2.9696 & 4.8910 & 2.9696 \\ 1.0947 & 1.8030 & 2.9696 & 4.8910 \end{pmatrix}. \tag{6.5}$$

The LR test comparing Model 5 with Model 2 is

$$440.68 - 419.48 = 21.2$$

with $14 - 6 = 8$ df and $p = 0.007$. Thus, the AR–1 structure does not provide an adequate fit. Comparison of the estimate of $\boldsymbol{W}$ from the AR–1 model [Equation (6.5)] with that from the unstructured covariance model [Equation (6.3)] shows that the covariance estimates between ages 8 and 12, between ages 10 and 14, and between ages 8 and 14 are underestimated by the AR–1 model.

Models 1–5 are all of the form

$$\boldsymbol{y}_i = \boldsymbol{X}_i \boldsymbol{\beta} + \boldsymbol{\epsilon}_i,$$

where the error vectors $\boldsymbol{\epsilon}_i$ are independently distributed with mean vector $\mathrm{E}(\boldsymbol{\epsilon}_i) = \boldsymbol{0}_4$ and arbitrary covariance matrix $\mathrm{Var}(\boldsymbol{\epsilon}_i) = \boldsymbol{W}$. Although $\boldsymbol{W}$ was parameterized using as few as two parameters (Model 5) and as many as ten parameters (Models 1, 2, and 3), no additional random effects were included in these models.

Model 6 is a random coefficients model with a random intercept and slope for each subject and independent random errors. The model is

$$y_{hij} = a_{hi} + b_{hi} j + \epsilon_{hij},$$

where

$$\begin{pmatrix} a_{hi} \\ b_{hi} \end{pmatrix} \sim N_2\left(\begin{pmatrix} \alpha_h \\ \beta_h \end{pmatrix}, \boldsymbol{B} \right)$$

and the random errors ϵ_{hij} are independent $N(0, \sigma^2)$. The covariance matrix $\boldsymbol{B}$ of the random effects is unstructured with variances σ_α^2 and σ_β^2 and covariance $\sigma_{\alpha\beta}$.

The estimated intercept and slope parameters from Model 6 are

$$\begin{aligned} \text{Males}: &\quad \widehat{\alpha}_1 = 16.34, \quad \widehat{\beta}_1 = 0.784; \\ \text{Females}: &\quad \widehat{\alpha}_2 = 17.37, \quad \widehat{\beta}_2 = 0.480. \end{aligned}$$

The estimated matrix of random effects is

$$\widehat{\boldsymbol{B}} = \begin{pmatrix} \widehat{\sigma}_\alpha^2 & \widehat{\sigma}_{\alpha\beta} \\ \widehat{\sigma}_{\alpha\beta} & \widehat{\sigma}_\beta^2 \end{pmatrix} = \begin{pmatrix} 4.55691 & -0.19825 \\ -0.19825 & 0.02376 \end{pmatrix},$$

and the estimate of the residual variance is $\widehat{\sigma}^2 = 1.716$.

Model 7 is the random intercept model with independent random errors. The model is

$$y_{hij} = a_{hi} + \beta_h j + \epsilon_{hij},$$

where the intercepts a_{hi} are independent $N(\alpha_h, \sigma_\alpha^2)$ and the random errors ϵ_{hij} are independent $N(0, \sigma^2)$. The estimated intercept and slope parameters from Model 7 are the same as those from Model 6. The estimated random effects are $\widehat{\sigma}_\alpha^2 = 3.0306$ and $\widehat{\sigma}^2 = 1.8746$.

The LR statistic comparing Models 6 and 7 is

$$428.64 - 427.81 = 0.83$$

with $8 - 6 = 2$ df and $p = 0.66$. Thus, the random intercept model provides an adequate fit. Note that the LR statistic may not have an asymptotic χ^2 distribution in situations where hypothesized parameters are on the boundaries of the parameter space, as is the case when testing whether variance components are equal to zero.

The random intercept model (Model 7) is equivalent to the model

$$y_{hij} = \alpha_h + \beta_h j + \epsilon_{hij},$$

where the vectors of residuals ϵ_{hi} are independent $N_4(\mathbf{0}_4, \boldsymbol{W})$ with

$$\boldsymbol{W} = \begin{pmatrix} \sigma^2 & \rho\sigma^2 & \rho\sigma^2 & \rho\sigma^2 \\ \rho\sigma^2 & \sigma^2 & \rho\sigma^2 & \rho\sigma^2 \\ \rho\sigma^2 & \rho\sigma^2 & \sigma^2 & \rho\sigma^2 \\ \rho\sigma^2 & \rho\sigma^2 & \rho\sigma^2 & \sigma^2 \end{pmatrix}$$

(Model 8). This matrix of variances and covariances has the compound symmetry structure given by Equation (5.4) of Section 5.3.1.

The estimate of $\boldsymbol{W}$ from Model 8 is

$$\widehat{\boldsymbol{W}} = \begin{pmatrix} 4.9052 & 3.0306 & 3.0306 & 3.0306 \\ 3.0306 & 4.9052 & 3.0306 & 3.0306 \\ 3.0306 & 3.0306 & 4.9052 & 3.0306 \\ 3.0306 & 3.0306 & 3.0306 & 4.9052 \end{pmatrix}.$$

The estimated fixed effects and the -2LL statistic are identical to those from the random intercept model (Model 7).

The LR statistic comparing Model 8 (equivalently, Model 7) with Model 2 is

$$428.64 - 419.48 = 9.16$$

with $14 - 6 = 8$ df and $p = 0.33$. Thus, the compound symmetry covariance structure provides an adequate fit for these data.

The only simpler model (Model 9) is

$$y_{hij} = \alpha_h + \beta_h j + \epsilon_{hij},$$

where the ϵ_{hij} random variables are independent $N(0, \sigma^2)$. Model 9 assumes that the repeated measurements from each experimental unit are independent. The LR test comparing Model 9 with Model 2 is

$$478.24 - 419.48 = 58.8$$

with $14 - 5 = 9$ df and $p < 0.001$. Thus, this assumption is not reasonable. Although Models 2, 4, 6, 7, and 8 all fit the data, compound symmetry (Model 8, equivalent to Model 7) requires only six parameters and is most parsimonious.

In attempting to choose the "best" covariance structure, the LR test can be used when two models with the same fixed-effects parameters are fit to the data using ML or REML estimation and one model is a constrained version of the other. Potential problems of using the LR test to compare covariance models include:

1. Parameters may be on the boundary of the parameter space.

2. The models being compared may not be nested.

Two other model selection criteria are Akaike's (1973) information criterion (AIC) and Schwarz's (1978) Bayesian information criterion (BIC). Both the AIC and the BIC penalize the log-likelihood for the number of parameters and/or number of observations.

Most statistical references define the AIC as

$$\text{AIC} = -2\text{LL} + 2p,$$

where p is the number of model parameters. Similarly, the BIC is usually defined as

$$\text{BIC} = -2\text{LL} + p\log(n),$$

TABLE 6.2. Model selection using AIC and BIC

Model	Covariance Structure	AIC	BIC
2	Unstructured	−219.739	−233.149
4	Banded	−216.322	−221.686
5	AR–1	−222.341	−225.023
6	Random intercept and slope	−217.903	−223.267
8	Compound symmetry	−216.320	−219.002
9	Simple	−240.121	−241.462

where n is the number of observations. The model with the smallest AIC (BIC) is deemed best. The BIC has an increased penalty for overfitting compared with the AIC, and the two criteria may not agree as to which model is best. Jones (1993, pp. 46–47) recommends the use of the AIC as follows:

> "I prefer to use AIC with the slight variation that models that are within two units of the lowest AIC are considered to be competitive models for the best. From the competitive models, the one with the fewest parameters is usually selected. This version of AIC has some theoretical justification (Duong, 1984)."

As implemented in the MIXED procedure of SAS (SAS Institute, 1999), the AIC and BIC can be used to compare models with the same fixed effects but different covariance structures. Because Models 2, 4, 5, 6, 8, and 9 all fit a linear relationship between distance and age with separate lines for boys and girls, the alternative covariance structures can be compared. Table 6.2 displays the values of the AIC and BIC for these models. The MIXED procedure uses the definitions

$$
\begin{aligned}
\text{AIC} &= \text{LL} - q, \\
\text{BIC} &= \text{LL} - (q/2)\log(n),
\end{aligned}
$$

where q is the effective number of covariance parameters (those not estimated to be on a boundary constraint). Thus, the model with the largest AIC (BIC) is deemed best. In this example, both criteria identify the compound symmetry covariance structure (equivalent to the random intercept model) as the "best" covariance model.

6.4.2 Three Groups, 24 Time Points, No Missing Data

In a randomized, double-blind, parallel group, placebo-controlled study, patients with postoperative pain were randomly assigned to one of three groups: treatment A (41 patients), treatment B (41 patients), or placebo (40 patients). Subjects enrolled in the study received a single dose of their assigned treatment when they reported moderate to severe postoperative

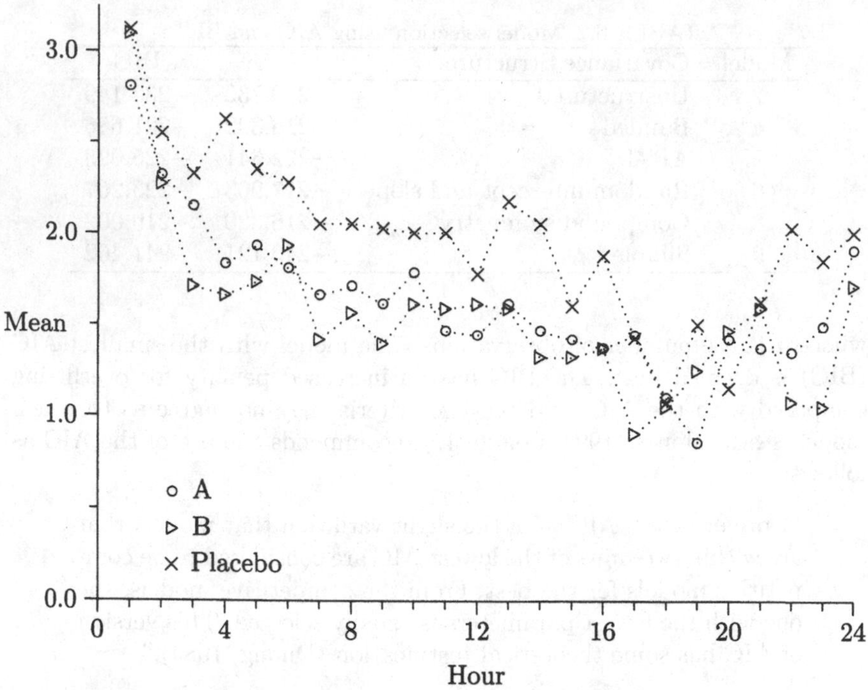

FIGURE 6.1. Mean rescue medication use by treatment group

pain. The primary outcome variable was the quantity of rescue medication used; this was recorded at hourly intervals for 24 hours after dosing. Table 6.3 displays the data from the first ten subjects in each of the three treatment groups.

Because the outcome variable is a count of the number of rescue medications received, the use of normal-theory methods may not be the most appropriate for these data. The analysis plan of the study protocol, however, specified the use of linear model methods to compare the three treatments with respect to the amount of rescue medication taken over the 24-hour interval. Although the protocol stated that the specific comparisons of interest were treatment A versus placebo and treatment B versus placebo, the choice of covariance model was not specified.

Figure 6.1 displays the mean rescue medication use at each hour in each of the three groups. Beginning at hour 2 and continuing through the first 16 hours, the mean rescue medication use is consistently higher in the placebo group than in either of the two treatment groups. In all three groups, the relationship between rescue medication use and time appears to be nonlinear.

The analysis of these data is complicated by the fact that there are 24 repeated measurements per subject. One is therefore limited in the types of covariance structures that can be considered. For example, it will not be

TABLE 6.3. Hourly use of rescue medications for postoperative pain: First ten subjects in each of the three treatment groups

ID	Hour 1	2	3	4	5	6	7	8	9	10	11	12	13	14	15	16	17	18	19	20	21	22	23	24
Group A																								
4	1	0	1	0	0	0	0	0	2	1	0	0	0	0	0	0	0	0	0	0	1	0	1	1
6	1	0	1	1	0	1	0	1	0	1	0	0	1	0	1	0	0	0	0	0	0	0	0	0
12	3	1	1	0	2	0	0	0	1	0	0	0	0	0	0	0	0	1	0	2	0	2	1	0
13	1	0	2	1	1	0	0	1	0	0	0	1	1	0	1	0	1	0	0	0	0	0	1	0
14	2	5	6	3	3	1	2	2	4	6	3	3	2	1	4	1	1	1	0	4	2	4	2	4
19	2	2	3	1	4	2	3	3	4	2	2	3	2	1	2	2	2	1	1	1	2	1	0	1
22	3	2	1	2	1	3	2	4	8	4	3	3	2	6	1	5	4	5	4	2	3	3	5	5
29	1	3	0	3	2	1	1	1	1	1	2	1	2	1	2	2	1	1	0	1	2	3	1	2
30	0	0	0	0	0	0	0	0	3	0	0	0	0	0	0	0	0	0	0	0	2	0	0	0
34	4	4	6	7	4	5	5	5	3	4	3	3	5	2	2	0	0	0	0	0	0	1	1	3
Group B																								
3	0	0	0	0	0	0	0	1	0	1	0	0	0	0	0	0	0	0	0	0	0	0	0	0
5	4	1	1	1	1	1	0	3	1	0	3	2	2	1	0	0	1	0	3	2	2	0	2	2
8	3	2	1	2	2	2	2	0	0	4	2	0	2	0	0	0	0	0	3	1	1	0	1	6
11	1	3	4	3	3	7	2	2	2	2	0	3	3	1	2	1	1	2	2	4	4	4	1	0
15	4	6	3	2	7	3	2	2	5	5	5	6	3	0	3	2	0	2	2	1	3	3	2	3
20	2	2	0	0	0	0	0	1	1	1	0	0	0	2	0	0	1	2	0	0	0	0	0	0
24	1	0	0	0	2	1	1	0	0	1	0	0	0	1	1	0	0	0	1	0	0	0	0	0
25	3	3	0	1	1	1	2	0	1	1	0	1	2	1	1	1	1	0	0	1	2	1	1	5
26	8	0	0	0	0	0	0	0	0	0	0	0	0	0	0	0	0	0	0	0	0	2	1	1
31	0	0	0	0	0	0	0	2	2	2	2	3	1	0	1	2	1	0	1	0	4	1	2	1
Group C																								
1	1	2	2	1	2	3	1	2	2	3	0	2	4	2	1	1	1	1	0	1	1	1	0	3
7	5	4	2	2	1	4	3	4	5	1	5	4	5	5	2	4	2	2	1	0	3	6	1	2
16	4	5	6	5	5	4	4	5	4	3	3	4	2	4	5	3	0	2	3	2	3	3	2	2
17	2	0	0	1	0	0	2	0	0	1	0	0	0	1	1	0	1	0	1	1	0	1	1	1
21	3	2	1	2	1	1	0	1	0	1	1	0	0	1	2	4	1	0	2	0	1	1	0	1
23	1	0	2	4	0	2	1	0	0	1	1	1	0	1	2	1	0	1	4	3	1	3	1	0
27	3	1	0	1	1	1	0	1	1	1	1	2	1	2	0	3	1	0	1	1	3	2	3	3
28	2	3	4	4	1	0	0	2	1	0	0	1	2	0	1	1	1	0	1	1	0	1	1	1
32	2	1	1	2	3	2	0	0	1	0	2	0	0	0	0	0	0	0	0	1	0	1	0	0
33	2	1	1	1	4	1	5	1	2	3	2	1	1	2	1	3	1	0	1	0	2	0	3	0

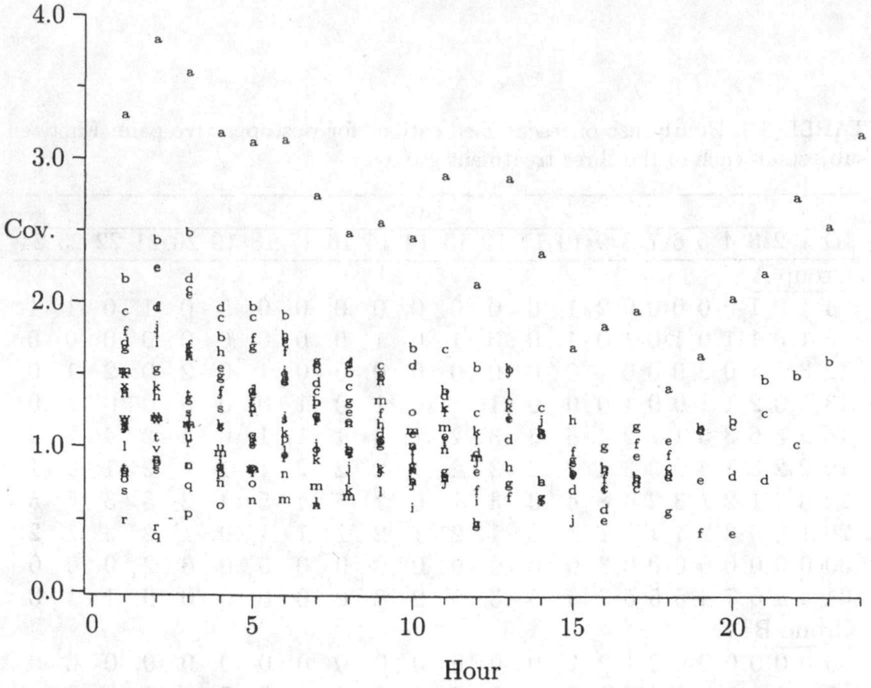

FIGURE 6.2. Variances and covariances of rescue medication use by hour

feasible to compare the adequacy of a reduced covariance model relative to the "full" (unstructured) model because the unstructured covariance model is a 24×24 covariance matrix with 300 parameters.

Figure 6.2 displays the estimated variances and covariances at hours 1–24. These are computed using the data from all 122 subjects combined. At each hour, the variance is plotted with the symbol "a." The one-lag covariance between hour h and hour $h+1$ is denoted by "b," the covariance between hour h and hour $h+2$ by "c," and so on. Thus, whereas 23 symbols are plotted at hour 1, at hour 24 only the variance is plotted. One key observation from Figure 6.2 is that the variances do not appear to be constant over time.

Let $\boldsymbol{y}_i = (y_{i1}, \ldots, y_{i,24})'$ denote the vector of repeated measurements from subject i for $i = 1, \ldots, 122$, and let $\boldsymbol{V}_i = \boldsymbol{Z}_i \boldsymbol{B} \boldsymbol{Z}_i' + \boldsymbol{W}_i$ denote the covariance matrix of $\boldsymbol{y}_i$. One parsimonious covariance model that could be considered in the analysis of these data is the AR–1 model. In this case, the (k, k') element of $\boldsymbol{V}_i$ is

$$v_{kk'} = \sigma^2 \rho^{|k-k'|}.$$

A second potential model adds an additional random error term to the AR–1 structure. In this case,

$$v_{kk'} = \sigma^2 \rho^{|k-k'|} + \sigma_e^2.$$

TABLE 6.4. Results from analyses of rescue medication data

	Covariance Structure		
	AR–1	AR–1 plus Random Error	Random Intercept and Slope
Treatment effect p-value	0.010	0.189	0.198
A − Placebo			
Estimate	−0.329	−0.339	−0.304
S.E.	0.138	0.243	0.229
p-value	0.018	0.163	0.185
B − Placebo			
Estimate	−0.399	−0.419	−0.395
S.E.	0.138	0.243	0.229
p-value	0.004	0.085	0.085
AIC	−4942.2	−4775.0	−4798.9
BIC	−4945.0	−4779.3	−4804.5

A four-parameter covariance model is the random-effects model with a random intercept and slope. In this model,

$$B = \begin{pmatrix} \sigma_\alpha^2 & \sigma_{\alpha\beta} \\ \sigma_{\alpha\beta} & \sigma_\beta^2 \end{pmatrix}, \qquad W_i = \sigma^2 \boldsymbol{I}_{24}.$$

Using each of these three assumed covariance structures, preliminary models showed that the effect of time was nonlinear and that the profiles for the three treatment groups were parallel. Thus, the final model included main effects for treatment group, linear time, and quadratic time. The parameters of this model were estimated using REML for each of the three assumed covariance structures. Table 6.4 displays the p-values of the 2 df test that there is no treatment effect. Table 6.4 also displays the estimated mean differences between treatment A and placebo and between treatment B and placebo, as well as the standard errors and p-values from the tests that the differences are equal to zero.

The test of the treatment effect is significant ($p = 0.01$) using the AR–1 covariance model but not significant with the two other covariance models. Although the estimated mean differences between each of the two treatment groups and the placebo group are of roughly the same magnitude, the standard errors of the estimated differences are much larger in the three-parameter (AR–1 plus random error) and four-parameter (random intercept and slope) covariance models than in the two-parameter model (AR–1).

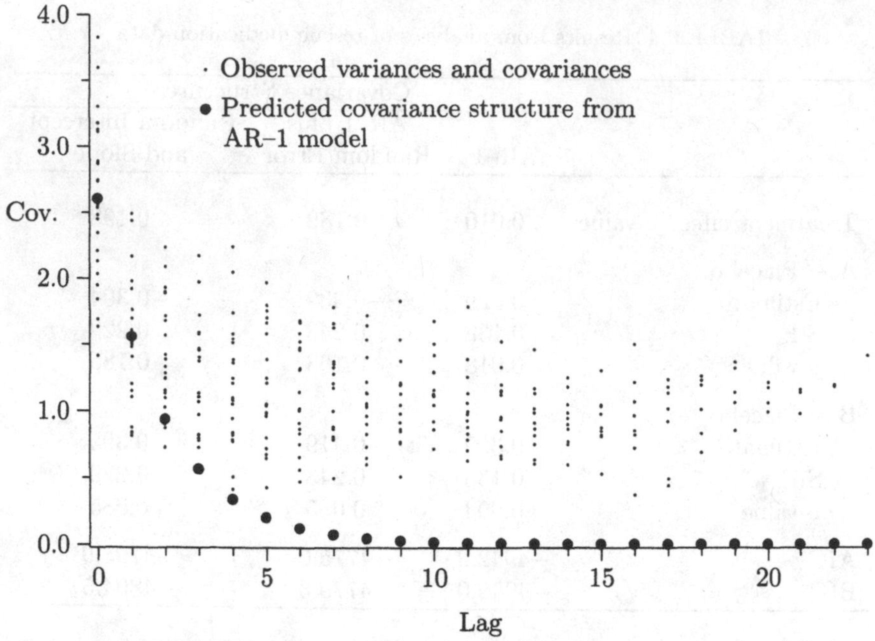

FIGURE 6.3. Variances and covariances of rescue medication use by lag: AR–1 covariance model

The last two rows of Table 6.4 display the AIC and BIC criteria for these three covariance structure models. Both of these criteria would select the "AR–1 plus random error" covariance structure as the "best" model.

Because this example has a common set of time points for all subjects and no missing data, the estimated variances and covariances from each of the three covariance structure models can be displayed graphically. Figure 6.3 displays the observed variances and covariances as well as the predicted covariance structure from the AR–1 covariance model. The observed variances and covariances are the same as those plotted in Figure 6.2. In Figure 6.3, however, the horizontal axis is the lag between observations instead of the hour. Thus, the variances at hours 1–24 are plotted at lag 0, the covariances between measurements one hour apart are plotted at lag 1, and so on. Although the predicted variance (lag 0) and the predicted covariance for lag 1 approximate the average of the corresponding observed quantities reasonably well, the predicted covariances at higher lags are much smaller than the observed covariances.

Figure 6.4 similarly displays the observed variances and covariances as well as the predicted covariance structure from the "AR–1 plus random error" covariance model. The addition of the random error term provides a much-improved approximation to the empirical covariance structure.

Finally, Figure 6.5 displays the observed variances and covariances as well as the predicted covariance structure from the random intercept and

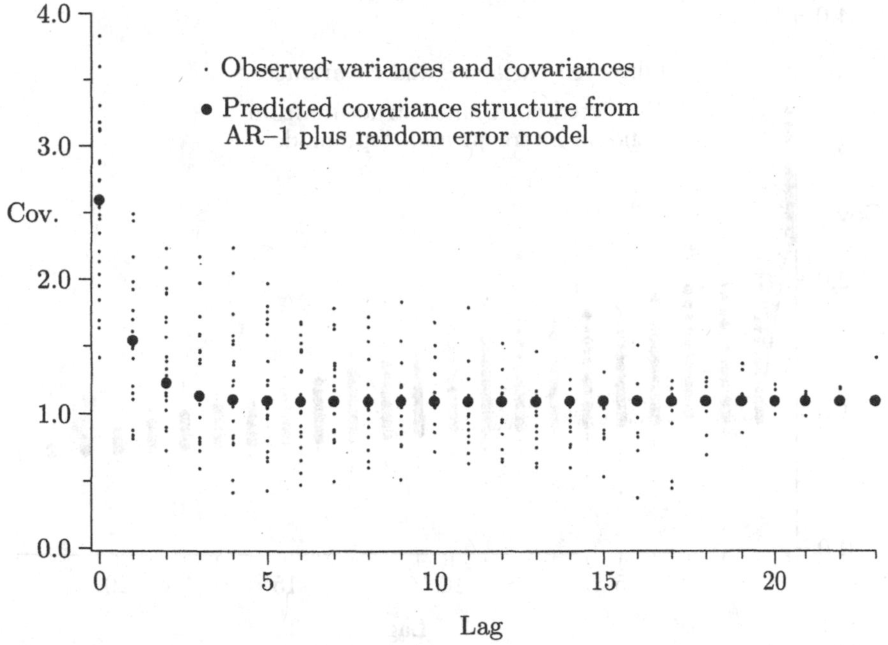

FIGURE 6.4. Variances and covariances of rescue medication use by lag: AR–1 plus random error covariance structure

slope model. In this model, the predicted variances and covariances depend not only on the lag but also on the time point. Figure 6.6 displays this covariance structure using time, rather than lag, on the horizontal axis, as in Figure 6.2. The random intercept and slope model provides considerable flexibility in modeling the covariance structure.

6.4.3 Four Groups, Unequally Spaced Repeated Measurements, Time-Dependent Covariate

Jones and Boadi-Boateng (1991) discuss the analysis of data from 619 subjects with and without a single hereditary kidney disease and with and without hypertension. Table 6.5 displays the sample sizes in the four groups of subjects. The response variable of interest is the reciprocal of serum creatinine (SCR); the values of this variable range from 0.028 to 2.5. The explanatory variables are group and patient age (which ranges from 18 to 84 years). Observations were taken at arbitrary times from each subject, and the number of observations per subject ranges from 1 to 22. Table 6.6 lists the data from the first 50 subjects.

Jones and Boadi-Boateng (1991) fit a model assuming a linear relationship between SCR and age, with separate lines for each of the four groups. Thus, there are eight fixed coefficients (intercept and slope for each of the four groups). In this example, the structural (fixed effects) part of the

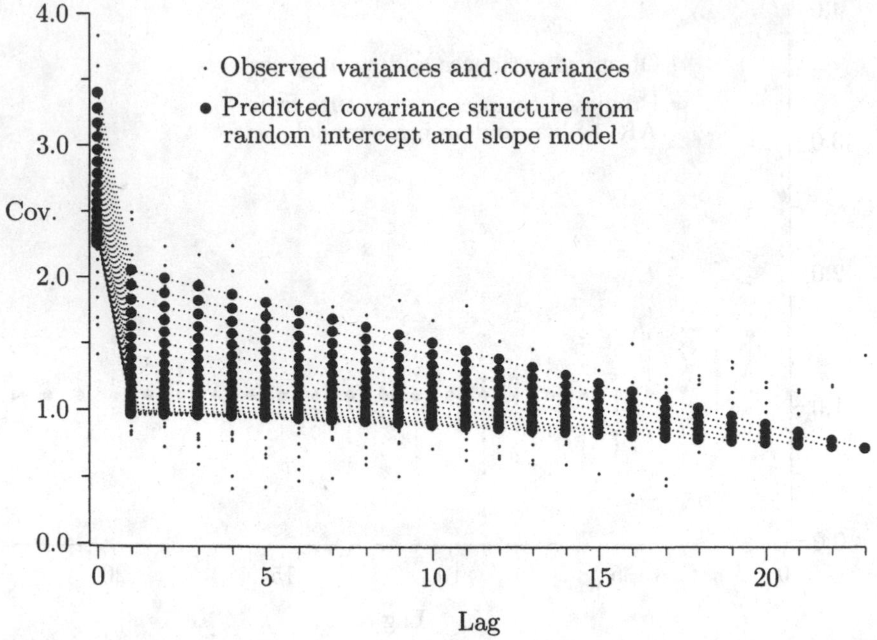

FIGURE 6.5. Variances and covariances of rescue medication use by lag: Random intercept and slope covariance structure

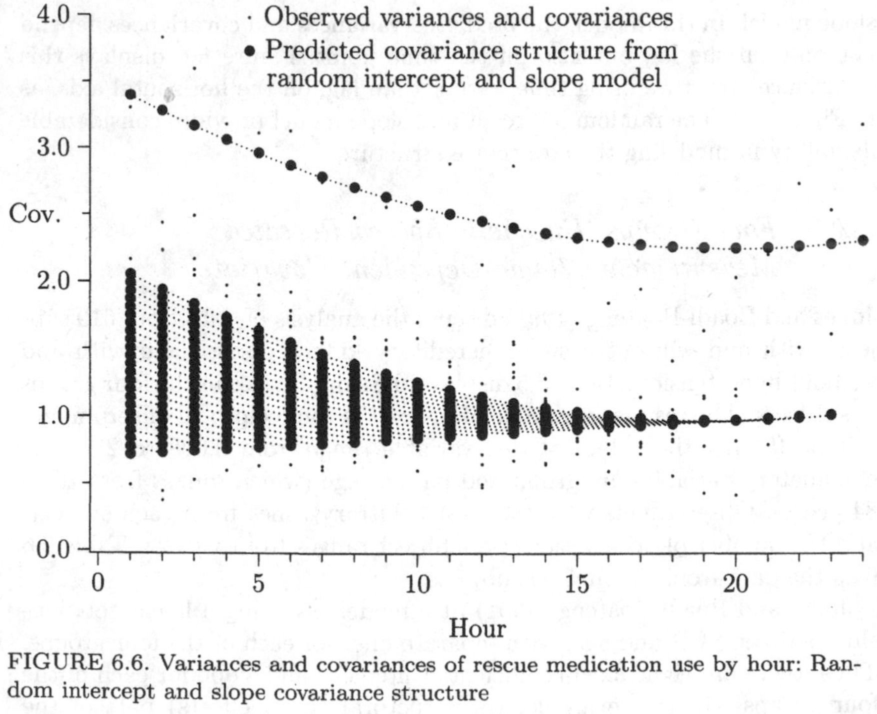

FIGURE 6.6. Variances and covariances of rescue medication use by hour: Random intercept and slope covariance structure

TABLE 6.5. Measurements of serum creatinine reciprocals from 619 subjects: Sample sizes in the four groups

Group	Kidney Disease	Hypertensive	Sample Size
1	Yes	Yes	294
2	Yes	No	103
3	No	Yes	73
4	No	No	149

model will be parameterized with an intercept and slope for group 1 and incremental intercept and slope parameters in each of groups 2–4.

With respect to the covariance structure, Jones and Boadi-Boateng use a model with six parameters. First, they assume a random intercept and slope for each subject so that the matrix $\boldsymbol{Z}_i$ from Equation (6.2) is

$$\boldsymbol{Z}_i = \begin{pmatrix} 1 & t_{i1} \\ \vdots & \vdots \\ 1 & t_{in_i} \end{pmatrix},$$

where subject i has n_i repeated measurements. The covariance matrix of the random effects is

$$\boldsymbol{B} = \begin{pmatrix} \sigma_\alpha^2 & \sigma_{\alpha\beta} \\ \sigma_{\alpha\beta} & \sigma_\beta^2 \end{pmatrix}.$$

The random intercept and slope model is often used in conjunction with the within-subject covariance structure assuming independence of observations (i.e., with $\boldsymbol{W}_i = \sigma^2 \boldsymbol{I}_{n_i}$). In their analysis, Jones and Boadi-Boateng (1991) instead assume that the within-subject covariance structure is a continuous-time AR–1 process with observational error. A continuous-time AR–1 process has correlation function

$$\rho(\tau) = e^{-\phi|\tau|},$$

where τ is the time interval between two observations and ϕ is the positive continuous-time autoregression coefficient. A continuous-time AR–1 process sampled at equally spaced intervals of time produces a discrete-time AR–1 process (Pandit and Wu, 1983).

If observations are sometimes obtained at time points that are quite close together, or if replicate observations are obtained at the same time point from a given subject, the AR–1 structure alone would require the observations to be very similar (or exactly the same if they are replicates). The addition of an observational error parameter σ_0^2 to the AR–1 structure (Jones, 1981) is often more realistic because this allows replicates to be different. Thus, the matrix $\boldsymbol{W}_i$ from Equation (6.2) has diagonal elements $\sigma^2 + \sigma_0^2$ and off-diagonal elements $\sigma^2 e^{-\phi|\tau|}$, where τ is the spacing

TABLE 6.6. Serum creatinine reciprocals from 619 subjects: First 50 subjects

ID	Grp	Age	SCR	ID	Grp	Age	SCR	ID	Grp	Age	SCR
1	1	35.765	0.182	20	1	44.397	1.429	39	2	42.116	1.250
1	1	37.990	0.088	20	1	49.884	1.111	40	1	53.552	1.250
2	2	24.997	1.429	21	2	23.420	1.667	40	1	67.677	0.769
2	2	27.441	1.111	21	2	31.086	1.429	40	1	73.541	0.526
2	2	30.524	1.429	21	2	36.720	1.250	40	1	74.776	0.385
3	1	51.083	0.156	22	4	21.509	2.000	40	1	75.863	0.400
3	1	52.386	0.116	22	4	41.511	1.429	40	1	75.959	0.400
3	1	52.805	0.087	22	4	43.699	1.250	41	4	64.512	1.250
3	1	52.997	0.067	23	3	26.623	1.250	41	4	70.371	1.250
4	4	51.255	0.667	23	3	39.450	0.769	41	4	71.713	1.250
5	4	18.355	1.250	23	3	40.865	0.833	41	4	73.027	1.250
5	4	19.619	1.000	23	3	42.864	0.833	42	1	58.398	0.625
6	4	28.956	1.250	23	3	45.703	0.833	42	1	63.893	0.526
7	4	26.062	2.000	23	3	46.697	0.769	42	1	65.196	0.303
7	4	32.799	1.429	23	3	47.535	0.714	42	1	66.612	0.370
7	4	33.714	1.429	24	4	39.636	0.769	43	1	40.764	1.250
7	4	35.346	1.429	25	4	22.242	1.000	43	1	53.175	0.145
7	4	39.918	1.429	25	4	36.140	0.909	43	1	54.456	0.154
7	4	45.960	1.250	26	3	18.393	1.111	44	1	54.385	0.087
8	4	54.152	0.625	26	3	26.346	0.833	44	1	54.505	0.093
8	4	59.781	1.111	26	3	38.741	0.833	45	1	53.279	1.250
9	4	45.128	1.429	27	4	30.182	0.667	45	1	60.088	0.833
9	4	52.632	1.111	28	3	20.252	1.429	45	1	66.546	0.588
9	4	54.987	1.429	28	3	34.404	1.429	45	1	66.872	0.714
9	4	56.304	1.111	29	4	40.572	0.769	45	1	67.896	0.588
10	4	29.262	1.111	30	3	22.201	1.250	45	1	71.943	0.625
10	4	48.923	1.250	30	3	34.664	0.909	45	1	72.096	0.556
11	3	47.773	1.111	30	3	40.408	0.909	45	1	72.197	0.250
12	2	31.305	1.000	31	3	26.752	0.909	46	3	55.880	1.000
13	2	25.697	0.833	31	3	33.180	0.909	46	3	57.725	1.111
13	2	31.305	1.111	32	3	24.657	0.769	46	3	61.777	1.667
14	4	32.638	1.111	32	3	30.204	1.111	47	1	46.702	1.111
15	4	30.645	1.429	33	1	27.176	0.909	47	1	53.555	1.250
15	4	36.487	0.833	34	4	21.098	1.111	47	1	60.244	1.000
16	4	24.372	1.000	34	4	24.805	2.000	47	1	66.669	0.714
16	4	27.600	1.000	35	4	21.443	1.429	48	3	58.094	1.667
16	4	33.550	1.000	36	2	22.787	1.250	48	3	64.520	1.111
17	2	25.906	1.667	36	2	44.559	0.714	48	3	64.556	1.250
17	2	32.104	2.000	37	1	19.663	0.909	49	3	65.730	1.000
18	4	30.242	1.111	38	2	29.916	0.909	49	3	72.025	1.429
19	4	24.027	1.250	38	2	36.879	0.833	50	4	64.205	1.000
20	1	30.034	1.429	39	2	26.765	1.250	50	4	70.606	1.000

TABLE 6.7. Parameter estimates from the analysis of serum creatinine reciprocals from 619 subjects

Group	Parameter	Estimate	Standard Error	p-value
1	intercept	1.4060	0.0553	< 0.001
	slope	−0.0185	0.0013	< 0.001
2	intercept increment	0.0839	0.1033	0.417
	slope increment	0.0033	0.0029	0.264
3	intercept increment	−0.3594	0.1133	0.002
	slope increment	0.0179	0.0026	< 0.001
4	intercept increment	−0.1782	0.0863	0.039
	slope increment	0.0148	0.0023	< 0.001

between observations. The complete covariance model then has six parameters $(\sigma_\alpha^2, \sigma_{\alpha\beta}, \sigma_\beta^2, \sigma^2, \tau, \sigma_0^2)$.

Although Jones and Boadi-Boateng (1991) obtain ML estimates of the parameters using the Kalman filter to evaluate the likelihood, which is then maximized using a nonlinear optimization program, ML and REML estimates can also be obtained using general-purpose programs such as the MIXED procedure (SAS Institute, 1999). Table 6.7 displays REML estimates of the fixed effects as well as estimated standard errors and p-values from the tests that the specified parameter is equal to zero. In all four groups, the serum creatinine reciprocal is estimated to decrease as age increases. The rate of decrease is greatest in group 1 and is nearly zero in group 3. The rates of decrease in groups 1 and 2 are similar. The intercept is greatest in group 2, followed by groups 1, 4, and 3.

6.5 Comments

6.5.1 *Use of the Random Intercept and Slope Model*

The random intercept and slope model with

$$\boldsymbol{B} = \begin{pmatrix} \sigma_\alpha^2 & \sigma_{\alpha\beta} \\ \sigma_{\alpha\beta} & \sigma_\beta^2 \end{pmatrix}$$

and $\boldsymbol{W}_i = \sigma^2 \boldsymbol{I}$, where $\boldsymbol{I}$ is an identity matrix with dimensions equal to the number of repeated measurements from the ith subject, is often used. This model is both intuitively appealing and also enables one to model the covariance structure using only four parameters. However, the random intercept and slope model has a potential shortcoming in that the covariance matrix of the vector $\boldsymbol{y}_i$ of observations from subject i is nonstationary.

In the case where measurements are obtained from each subject at the equally spaced time points $j = 1, \ldots, t$, general expressions for the variances and covariances of the observations y_{ij} are:

$$\begin{aligned}\text{Var}(y_{ij}) &= \sigma_\alpha^2 + 2j\sigma_{\alpha\beta} + j^2\sigma_\beta^2 + \sigma^2,\\ \text{Cov}(y_{ij}, y_{ij'}) &= \sigma_\alpha^2 + (j+j')\sigma_{\alpha\beta} + jj'\sigma_\beta^2.\end{aligned}$$

Thus, if $\sigma_{\alpha\beta} > -\sigma_\beta^2$, then $\text{Var}(y_{ij})$ will increase monotonically over time. In terms of the correlation coefficient

$$\rho = \frac{\sigma_{\alpha\beta}}{\sigma_\alpha \sigma_\beta},$$

this condition is

$$\rho > -\frac{\sigma_\beta}{\sigma_\alpha}.$$

In many applications, however, the variances of observations are constant, or nearly constant, over time.

The general relationships for arbitrary time point j are as follows:

- if $j > -\sigma_{\alpha\beta}/\sigma_\beta^2$, the variances $\text{Var}(y_{ij})$ increase after time j;
- if $j < -\sigma_{\alpha\beta}/\sigma_\beta^2$, the variances $\text{Var}(y_{ij})$ decrease up to time j.

Only if $\sigma_{\alpha\beta} = -0.5(2j+1)\sigma_\beta^2$ are the jth and $(j+1)$st variances equal; in this case, all subsequent variances increase over time, and all previous variances decrease over time. These consequences of the random intercept and slope model do not appear to be widely known and also appear not to be realistic in many applications.

In Section 6.4.1, Model 6 is the random intercept and slope model. The estimated matrix of random effects is

$$\widehat{\boldsymbol{B}} = \begin{pmatrix} 4.55691 & -0.19825 \\ -0.19825 & 0.02376 \end{pmatrix}.$$

The features observed in this example occur in many applications of this model, namely,

- $\widehat{\sigma}_{\alpha\beta}$ is negative.
- $\widehat{\sigma}_\beta^2$ is close to zero.

If the time points are relabeled 1, 2, 3, 4 instead of 8, 10, 12, 14, the estimated matrix of random effects is

$$\widehat{\boldsymbol{B}} = \begin{pmatrix} 3.03319 & -0.11140 \\ -0.11140 & 0.09504 \end{pmatrix}.$$

Because $-\widehat{\sigma}_{\alpha\beta}/\widehat{\sigma}_{\beta}^2 = 0.11140/0.09504 = 1.17$, the variances increase from time 2 (age 10) onward (and possibly also from time 1). The resulting estimated covariance matrix of the observations $\boldsymbol{y}_{hi} = (y_{hi1}, \ldots, y_{hi4})'$ is

$$\begin{pmatrix} 4.6216 & 2.8891 & 2.8727 & 2.8563 \\ 2.8891 & 4.6839 & 3.0464 & 3.1251 \\ 2.8727 & 3.0464 & 4.9363 & 3.3938 \\ 2.8563 & 3.1251 & 3.3938 & 5.3787 \end{pmatrix}.$$

The estimated variances increase monotonically over time. In comparison, the pooled estimate of the covariance matrix of $\boldsymbol{y}_{hi}$ is

$$\begin{pmatrix} 5.4155 & 2.7168 & 3.9102 & 2.7102 \\ 2.7168 & 4.1848 & 2.9272 & 3.3172 \\ 3.9102 & 2.9272 & 6.4557 & 4.1307 \\ 2.7102 & 3.3172 & 4.1307 & 4.9857 \end{pmatrix}.$$

Unlike the structure imposed by the random intercept and slope model, the empirical variances show no consistent pattern across the four time points.

Although intuitively appealing, the random intercept and slope model is not the best-fitting one for this example. This conclusion is consistent with the results presented in Section 6.4.1. Note, however, that the assumptions of the random intercept and slope model appear to provide an adequate model for the example of Section 6.4.2.

6.5.2 Effects of Choice of Covariance Structure on Estimates and Tests

In the first example (Section 6.4.1), the number of time points was small, the time points were equally spaced, there were no missing data, and all covariates were categorical. In such cases, one can readily carry out likelihood ratio tests to compare the fit of alternative covariance models. When the number of time points is large (as in the example of Section 6.4.2) or when the time points at which the repeated measurements are obtained vary from subject to subject (as in the example of Section 6.4.3), it is not possible to compare the fit of a reduced covariance model to that of the unstructured model. In such situations, the choice of covariance model can have a substantial effect on the results of the analysis.

As an example, the final model for the serum creatinine data of Section 6.4.3 had eight fixed effects and six random effects. The fixed effects were an intercept and slope for group 1 and incremental intercept and slope parameters in each of groups 2–4. The covariance model consisted of a random intercept and slope for each subject (three parameters), plus a three-parameter within-subject covariance structure (continuous-time AR–1 process with observational error).

To illustrate the effect of the choice of covariance model on the analysis results, the same fixed-effects model (separate lines in each of the four groups) was fit using nine alternative covariance structure models:

1. continuous time AR–1 with observational error (three parameters);
2. continuous time AR–1 (two parameters);
3. compound symmetry (two parameters);
4. random intercept and slope plus continuous time AR–1 with observational error (six parameters);
5. random intercept and slope plus continuous time AR–1 (five parameters);
6. random intercept and slope plus independent within-subject errors (four parameters);
7. random intercept plus continuous time AR–1 with observational error (four parameters);
8. random intercept plus continuous time AR–1 (three parameters);
9. random intercept plus independent within-subject errors (two parameters).

Figure 6.7 plots the parameter estimates for the age effect in group 1 and the intercept and age increments in groups 2–4. The parameterization is the same as was described in Section 6.4.3. The plot symbols 1–9 correspond to the nine covariance models just listed.

The estimated slopes (age effects) are not greatly affected by the choice of covariance model. There is, however, considerable variability in the estimates of the intercept increments in groups 2–4. In particular, four of the nine estimated intercept increments in group 2 are positive, whereas the remaining estimates are negative.

Figure 6.8 similarly displays the p-values from the tests that the incremental effects in groups 2–4 are equal to zero. With reference to the conventional $\alpha = 0.05$ level of significance, the intercept increments in groups 2 and 4, as well as the age increment in group 2, are highly statistically significant under some covariance models and very nonsignificant under others.

This example illustrates the importance of carefully selecting a reasonable covariance model. Even in situations where the conclusions are not affected as dramatically as in this example, the choice of an appropriately parsimonious covariance structure can improve the efficiency of inferences concerning the mean structure and provide better estimates of standard errors of estimated parameters (Diggle et al., 1994). In some settings, as

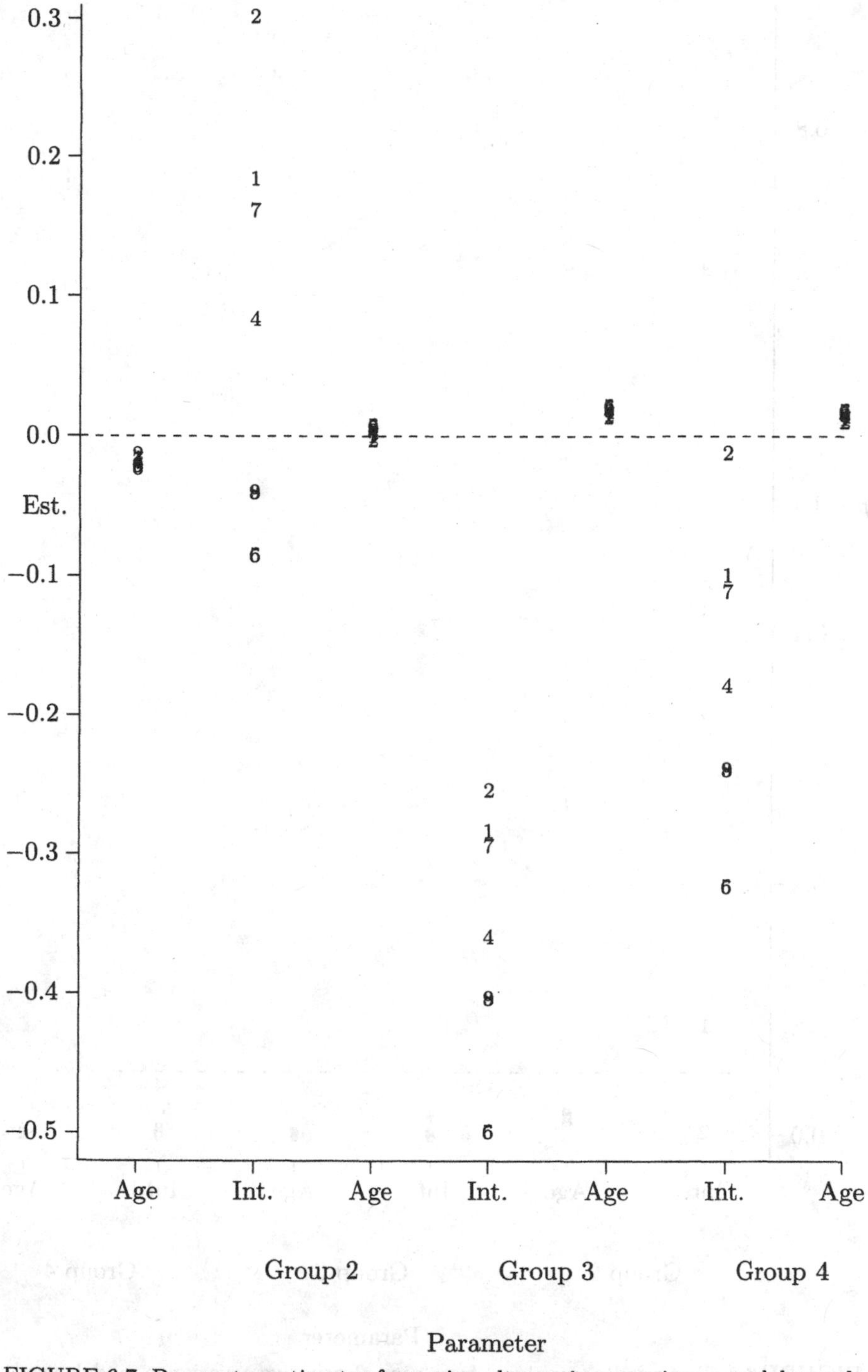

FIGURE 6.7. Parameter estimates from nine alternative covariance models used in the analysis of serum creatinine reciprocals from 619 subjects

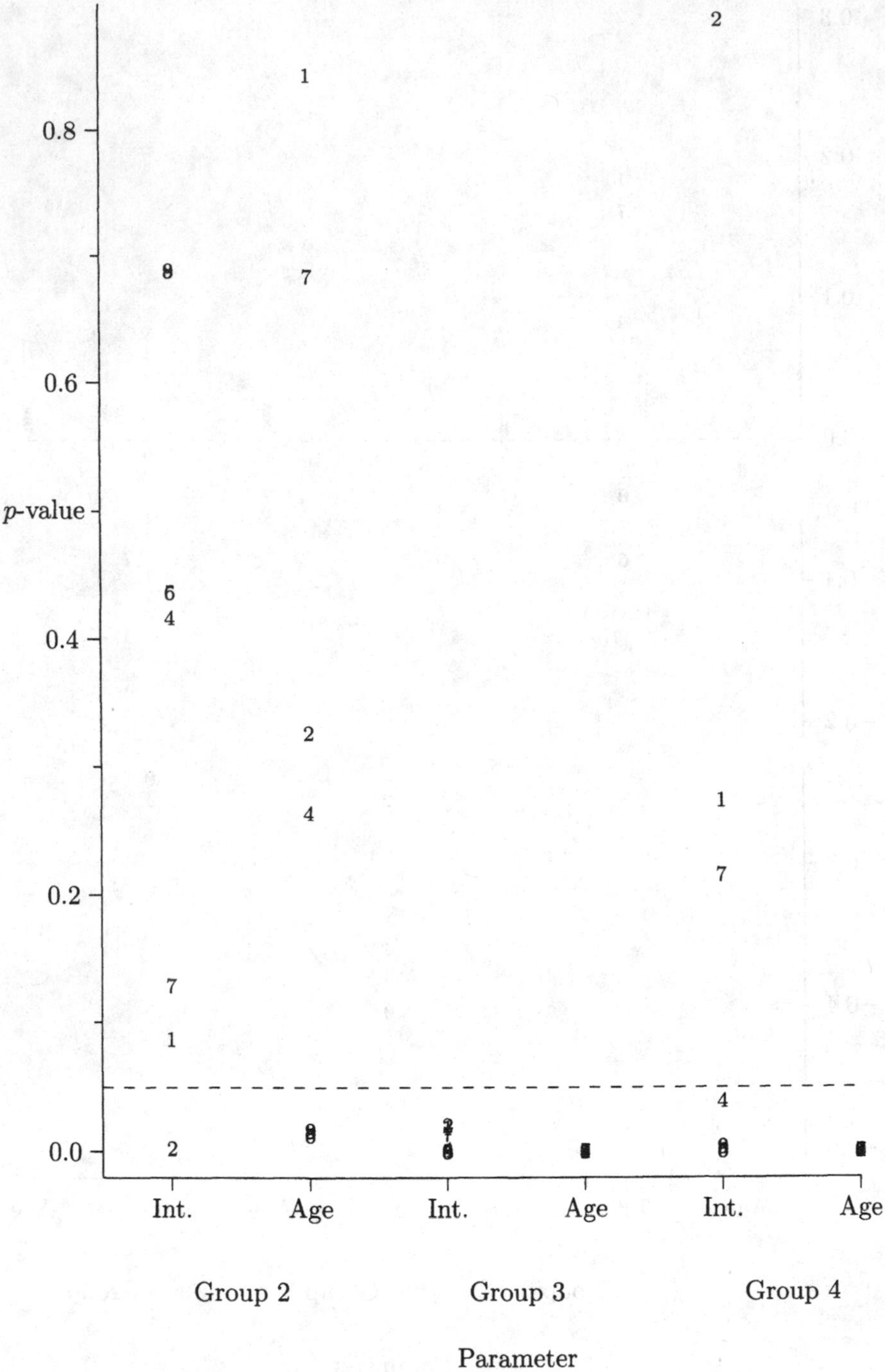

FIGURE 6.8. Test results (p-values) from nine alternative covariance models used in the analysis of serum creatinine reciprocals from 619 subjects

in the examples of Sections 6.4.1 and 6.4.2, likelihood ratio tests and measures such as the AIC and BIC are useful tools for choosing an appropriate covariance model. In this context, Diggle (1988) recommends that a model for the mean structure first be fit and that it is preferable to overfit, rather than underfit, this model. The fit of reduced covariance models can then be investigated relative to an initial, more general covariance structure. Diggle et al. (1994) and Dawson et al. (1997) review other methods, including scatterplot matrices, for assessing the correlation structure of repeated measurements data. Zimmerman (2000) describes and illustrates the use of another graphical diagnostic, the Partial-Regression-on-Intervenors Scatterplot Matrix (PRISM).

6.5.3 Performance of Linear Mixed Model Test Statistics and Estimators

Overall et al. (1999), Ahn et al. (2000), and Park et al. (2001) have investigated the performance of linear mixed model test statistics and estimators in simulation studies. In the Park et al. (2001) study, the properties of three types of test statistics were compared:

1. unstructured multivariate approach using Wilks' Λ;
2. linear mixed model approach using ML estimation;
3. linear mixed model approach using REML estimation.

The case of two groups and four time points was considered. The model for the mean in group h at time j was $\mu_{hj} = \beta_{h0} + \beta_{h1} j$, where

$$\beta_{20} = \beta_{10} + \delta_0, \qquad \beta_{21} = \beta_{11} + \delta_1.$$

The parameter δ_0 is the intercept difference, and δ_1 is the slope difference. Two hypotheses were of interest:

- equality of groups ($H_0\colon \delta_0 = \delta_1 = 0$);
- parallelism ($H_0\colon \delta_1 = 0$).

This scenario is similar to the example of Section 6.4.1.

Data were generated from five correlation models: AR–1 with $\rho = 0.3$ and $\rho = 0.7$, compound symmetry with $\rho = 0.3$ and $\rho = 0.7$, and an unstructured covariance model. The unstructured covariance model was the 4×4 covariance matrix given by Equation (6.3) in Section 6.4.1.

The linear mixed model analyses were carried out using four assumed correlation structures: independence, AR–1, compound symmetry, and unstructured. Sample sizes of 15 and 25 observations/group and several values of (δ_0, δ_1) were considered; 1000 replications were carried out for each combination of factors.

Figure 6.9 displays the empirical sizes of the test of equality of group effects. The horizontal axis lists the total sample size and true correlation structure under which the data were generated. The proportion of 1000 replications for which the null hypothesis was rejected is displayed on the vertical axis. In these simulations, the parameters δ_0 and δ_1 were both equal to zero.

In this simulation study, the unstructured multivariate approach tends to have test sizes closest to the nominal 5% level. The linear mixed model approach tends to yield anticonservative tests. For a given assumed correlation structure, the sizes of the REML tests are smaller (closer to the nominal level) than those of the ML tests. Whereas the unstructured multivariate approach is robust to the true correlation structure, the performance of the linear mixed model tests depends highly on the structures of the true and assumed correlation models. It is somewhat surprising that the unstructured multivariate approach is preferred, even in a four-parameter model with a 4×4 covariance matrix and a total sample size of only 30 subjects.

Figure 6.10 similarly displays the empirical sizes of the test of parallelism. In these simulations, δ_1 was equal to zero. The results for testing parallelism are somewhat different from those for testing group effects. A possible reason is that the test for parallelism is based on the differences among adjacent responses, which might be less sensitive to the correlation structure than the responses themselves. The unstructured multivariate approach tends to have test sizes closest to the nominal 5% level. The linear mixed model approach tends to yield anticonservative tests. For a given assumed correlation structure, the sizes of REML tests are smaller (closer to the nominal level) than those of ML tests. The linear mixed model ML and REML tests assuming independence are conservative.

Finally, Figure 6.11 displays empirical powers of the tests of parallelism for total sample sizes of $n = 30$ (top panel) and $n = 50$ (bottom panel). The horizontal axis lists the values of δ_1 and the true correlation model under which the data were generated. The proportion of 1000 replications for which the null hypothesis was rejected is displayed on the vertical axis. Because the tests based on the linear mixed model are often anticonservative when the null hypothesis is true, it is not surprising that they also tend to sometimes reject more often when the null hypothesis is false. Still, the tests based on the use of the unstructured multivariate model perform well.

6.6 Problems

6.1 Suppose that repeated measurements are obtained at time points $1, \ldots, t$ for each of n subjects. Consider the mixed model

$$\boldsymbol{y}_i = \boldsymbol{X}\boldsymbol{\beta} + \boldsymbol{Z}\boldsymbol{\gamma}_i + \boldsymbol{\epsilon}_i$$

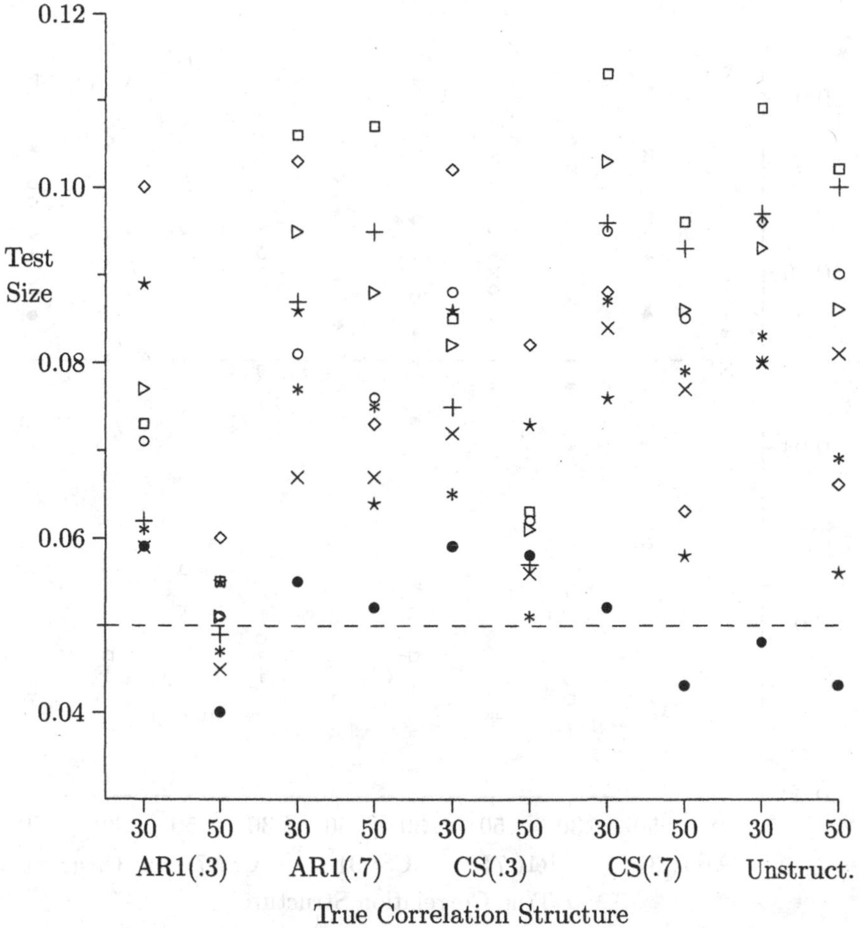

Unstructured multivariate approach: ●
Mixed linear model approach:

Assumed Correlation Structure	ML	REML
Independence	□	+
AR–1	○	×
Compound symmetry	▷	*
Unstructured	◇	★

FIGURE 6.9. Empirical sizes of tests of equality of group effects

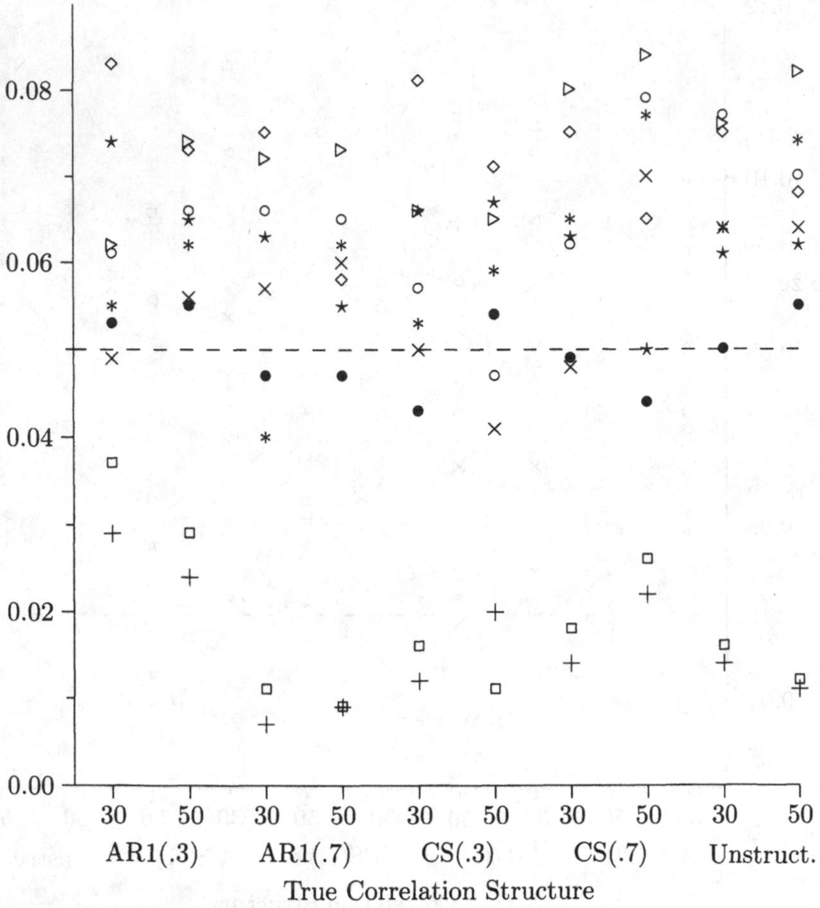

Unstructured multivariate approach: ●
Mixed linear model approach:

Assumed Correlation Structure	ML	REML
Independence	□	+
AR–1	○	×
Compound symmetry	▷	*
Unstructured	◇	★

FIGURE 6.10. Empirical sizes of tests of parallelism

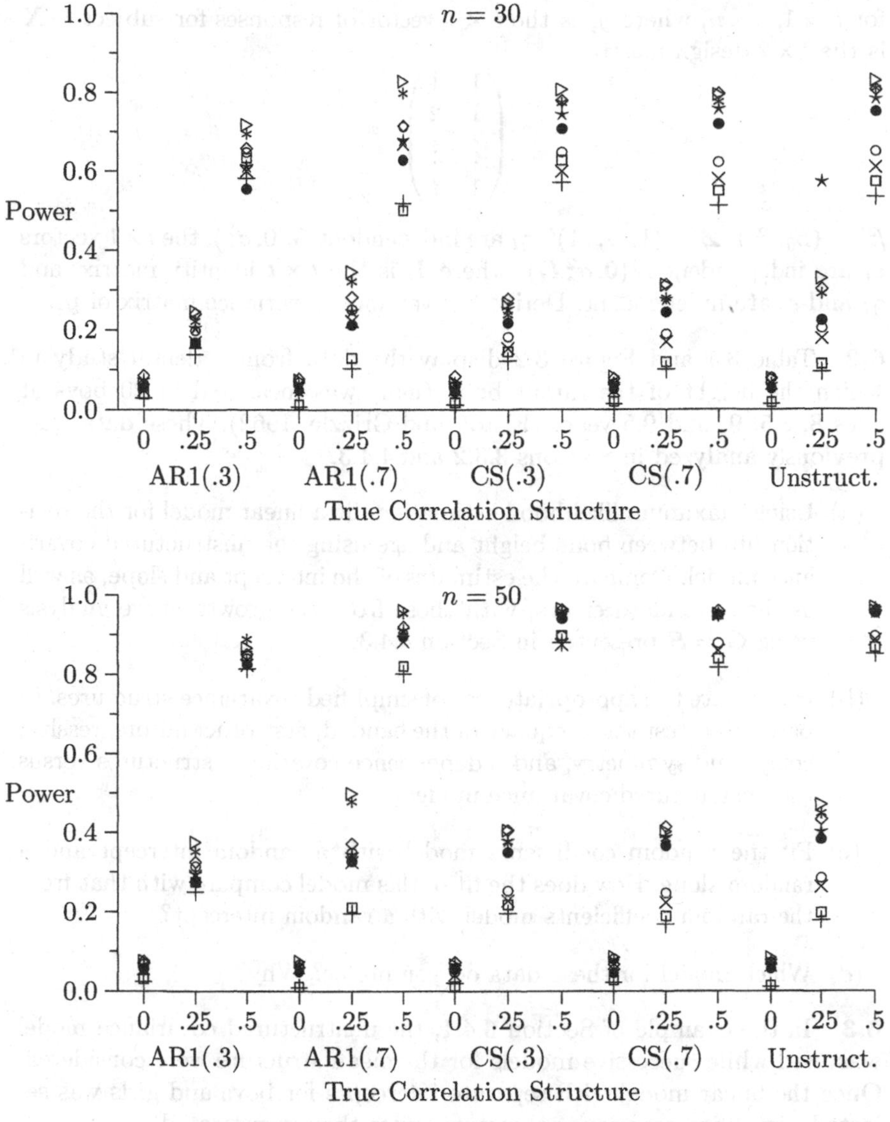

Unstructured multivariate approach: ●
Mixed linear model approach:

Assumed Correlation Structure	ML	REML
Independence	□	+
AR–1	○	×
Compound symmetry	▷	*
Unstructured	◇	★

FIGURE 6.11. Empirical powers of tests of parallelism

for $i = 1, \ldots, n$, where $\boldsymbol{y}_i$ is the $t \times 1$ vector of responses for subject i, $\boldsymbol{X}$ is the $t \times 2$ design matrix

$$\begin{pmatrix} 1 & 1 \\ 1 & 2 \\ \vdots & \vdots \\ 1 & t \end{pmatrix},$$

$\boldsymbol{\beta}' = (\beta_0, \beta_1)$, $\boldsymbol{Z} = (1, \ldots, 1)'$, γ_i are independent $N(0, \sigma^2)$, the $t \times 1$ vectors $\boldsymbol{\epsilon}_i$ are independent $N(\boldsymbol{0}, \sigma_e^2 \boldsymbol{I}_t)$, where $\boldsymbol{I}_t$ is the $t \times t$ identity matrix, and γ_i and $\boldsymbol{\epsilon}_i$ are independent. Derive the variance–covariance matrix of $\boldsymbol{y}_i$.

6.2 Table 3.1 and Figure 3.2 display the data from a dental study in which the height of the ramus bone (mm) was measured in 20 boys at ages 8, 8.5, 9, and 9.5 years (Elston and Grizzle, 1962). These data were previously analyzed in Sections 3.3.2 and 4.4.3.

(a) Using maximum likelihood estimation, fit a linear model for the relationship between bone height and age using the unstructured covariance model. Compare the estimates of the intercept and slope, as well as their standard errors, with those from the growth curve analysis using $\boldsymbol{G} = \boldsymbol{S}$ presented in Section 4.4.3.

(b) Investigate the appropriateness of simplified covariance structures. In particular, test the adequacy of the banded, first-order autoregressive, compound symmetry, and independence covariance structures versus the unstructured covariance model.

(c) Fit the random coefficients model with a random intercept and a random slope. How does the fit of this model compare with that from the random coefficients model with a random intercept?

(d) Which model for these data do you prefer? Why?

6.3 In the example of Section 6.4.1, the unstructured covariance model was used while successive models for the mean structure were considered. Once the linear model with separate intercepts for boys and girls was selected, simplified covariance structures were then investigated.

(a) Using the model with a separate mean at each time point for each sex (Model 1 from Section 6.4.1), investigate the appropriateness of simplified covariance structures. In particular, test the adequacy of the banded, first-order autoregressive, compound symmetry, and independence covariance structures versus the unstructured covariance model.

(b) Repeat part (a) using REML estimation instead of maximum likelihood.

6.4 Patel (1991) discusses the analysis of a randomized, double-blind clinical trial comparing two treatments for rheumatoid arthritis. Table 6.8 displays grip-strength measurements at baseline and at visits 1, 2, and 3 following the initiation of treatment for the 67 subjects included in this trial. Because grip strengths are expected to be higher in males than in females, sex is a stratification factor. Use linear mixed model methods to test whether grip strength is affected by treatment.

6.5 In a randomized, multicenter, double-blind, placebo-controlled trial of botulinum toxin type B (BotB) in patients with cervical dystonia, eligible subjects from nine U.S. sites were randomized to one of three groups: placebo (36 subjects), 5000 units of BotB (36 subjects), or 10,000 units of BotB (37 subjects). The primary outcome variable was the total score on the Toronto Western Spasmodic Torticollis Rating Scale (TWSTRS-Total). The TWSTRS-Total, which measures severity, pain, and disability of cervical dystonia, is a numerical score ranging from 0 to 87; high scores indicate impairment. The TWSTRS-Total was administered at baseline (week 0) and at weeks 2, 4, 8, 12, and 16 following treatment. Table 6.9 displays the age (years), sex, and TWSTRS-Total scores for the first 35 subjects.

(a) Using the unstructured covariance model, fit a fifth-order polynomial model to the data from each of the three groups.

(b) Using the structural model of part (a), investigate whether the covariance structure can be simplified to a more parsimonious covariance model.

(c) Using the covariance model from part (b), fit an appropriate reduced model for the effect of time.

(d) Using the model from part (c), test for parallelism of the profiles for the three groups and, if appropriate, simplify your model.

(e) Based on your final model, test the null hypothesis that the estimated TWSTRS-Total means at week 4 are equal for the three groups. Also compare each of the two BotB groups to the placebo group.

6.6 Table 4.7 displays scaled test scores for a cohort of 64 students of the Laboratory School of the University of Chicago (Bock, 1975). These data were previously considered in Problems 4.2 and 5.13.

(a) Use the unstructured covariance model to fit a cubic polynomial model with separate coefficients for boys and girls.

(b) Using the structural model of part (a), investigate whether the covariance structure can be simplified to a more parsimonious covariance model.

TABLE 6.8. Grip-strength measurements from 67 subjects in a clinical trial comparing two treatments for rheumatoid arthritis

			Visit							Visit			
ID	Sex	Trt.	0	1	2	3	ID	Sex	Trt.	0	1	2	3
1	M	2	120	130	150	120	41	M	2	200	245	290	280
2	F	1	80	80	86	80	42	M	1	300	300	300	300
3	F	2	60	80	60	60	43	M	2	172	170	170	146
4	F	1	64	80	80	70	44	M	1	238	278	170	158
5	F	1	40	60	.	.	45	M	2	158	140	152	150
6	F	2	50	70	70	70	46	F	1	110	82	98	110
7	F	2	80	75	90	90	47	M	2	150	220	168	139
8	F	1	40	50	30	40	48	F	1	180	165	150	160
9	F	1	70	90	110	90	49	F	2	55	60	65	55
10	F	2	80	100	80	90	50	F	1	155	150	170	185
13	F	2	80	60	65	70	51	F	2	130	130	160	125
15	F	1	70	80	95	110	52	F	1	55	105	70	88
17	F	2	58	50	80	80	53	M	2	135	155	215	170
18	F	1	70	80	86	.	54	M	1	200	230	220	240
19	F	1	70	60	70	80	55	F	2	115	95	105	110
20	F	2	60	60	80	60	56	M	2	75	170	220	240
21	F	1	50	80	90	90	57	M	1	130	155	170	125
22	F	2	80	90	120	130	58	M	2	150	200	185	163
23	F	2	60	90	94	100	59	F	1	95	90	90	116
24	F	1	40	60	60	65	61	M	2	155	101	93	120
25	M	2	300	300	300	300	62	F	2	135	120	144	135
26	M	1	175	161	210	230	63	F	1	90	135	95	.
27	M	1	165	215	245	265	64	F	1	145	140	164	.
28	M	2	179	232	285	.	65	F	2	60	85	85	.
29	M	1	175	134	215	139	67	F	2	40	45	76	75
30	F	2	75	131	95	105	70	F	1	34	51	87	.
31	M	2	209	260	200	125	71	F	2	104	107	.	.
34	M	1	178	165	140	175	72	F	2	60	60	55	58
35	M	1	220	220	189	158	73	M	2	190	240	210	173
36	M	2	200	200	200	232	74	M	1	215	230	243	245
37	F	2	150	108	160	160	75	M	2	265	275	255	270
38	M	1	90	146	140	130	76	M	1	207	220	.	.
39	M	2	300	300	300	300	79	M	1	225	220	250	235
40	F	1	140	156	140	150							

TABLE 6.9. TWSTRS-total scores from 109 patients with cervical dystonia: First 35 subjects

					Week					
Site	ID	Treatment	Age	Sex	0	2	4	8	12	16
1	1	5000U	65	F	32	30	24	37	39	36
1	2	10000U	70	F	60	26	27	41	65	67
1	3	5000U	64	F	44	20	23	26	35	35
1	4	Placebo	59	F	53	61	64	62	.	.
1	5	10000U	76	F	53	35	48	49	41	51
1	6	10000U	59	F	49	34	43	48	48	51
1	7	5000U	72	M	42	32	32	43	42	46
1	8	Placebo	40	M	34	33	21	27	32	38
1	9	5000U	52	F	41	32	34	35	37	36
1	10	Placebo	47	M	27	10	31	32	6	14
1	11	10000U	57	F	48	41	32	35	57	51
1	12	Placebo	47	F	34	19	21	24	28	28
2	1	Placebo	70	F	49	47	44	48	44	44
2	2	5000U	49	F	46	35	45	49	53	56
2	3	10000U	59	F	56	44	48	54	49	60
2	4	5000U	64	M	59	48	56	55	57	58
2	5	10000U	45	F	62	60	60	64	67	66
2	6	Placebo	66	F	50	53	52	57	61	54
2	7	10000U	49	F	42	42	43	33	37	43
2	8	Placebo	54	F	53	56	52	54	55	51
2	9	5000U	47	F	67	64	65	64	62	64
2	10	Placebo	31	M	44	40	32	36	42	43
2	11	10000U	53	F	65	58	55	.	56	60
2	12	5000U	61	M	56	54	52	48	52	53
2	13	Placebo	40	M	30	33	25	29	32	32
2	14	5000U	67	M	47	.	54	43	46	50
3	1	10000U	54	F	50	43	51	46	49	53
3	2	Placebo	41	F	34	29	27	21	22	22
3	3	5000U	66	M	39	41	33	39	37	37
3	4	Placebo	68	F	43	31	29	28	33	38
3	5	10000U	41	F	46	26	29	33	45	56
3	6	5000U	77	M	52	44	47	50	50	49
3	7	10000U	41	M	38	19	20	27	29	32
3	8	Placebo	56	M	33	38	40	48	49	44
3	9	5000U	46	F	28	16	11	7	13	21

(c) Using the covariance model from part (b), fit an appropriate reduced model for comparing the profiles over time for boys and girls.

6.7 Forty male subjects were randomly assigned to one of two treatment groups. The values of the BPRS factor measured before treatment (week 0) and at weekly intervals for eight weeks are displayed in Table 2.10 and were previously considered in Problems 2.2, 3.12, and 4.8.

(a) Using maximum likelihood estimation and the unstructured covariance model, fit a quadratic model with separate intercepts, linear terms, and quadratic terms in the two treatment groups. Test equality of intercepts, equality of linear terms, equality of quadratic terms, joint equality of linear and quadratic terms, and joint equality of treatments.

(b) Fit an appropriate reduced model based on the results of part (a). Compare the fit of this model to the model from part (a) using a likelihood ratio test.

(c) Investigate the appropriateness of simplified covariance structures for your model from part (b). In particular, test the adequacy of the banded, first-order autoregressive, compound symmetry, and independence covariance structures versus the unstructured covariance model.

6.8 Parkinson's disease is a neurodegenerative disease associated with aging. The treatment regimen most commonly used to alleviate the signs and symptoms of Parkinson's disease is levodopa. Although levodopa is an effective treatment, its continued use often causes adverse effects on motor function and mental state. Therefore, it is of interest to develop alternative treatments that will enable decreased use of levodopa.

In a clinical trial conducted to determine whether use of an experimental dopamine D_2 agonist can replace the use of levodopa, 25 patients with Stage II through IV Parkinson's disease were randomized to one of five groups: placebo, 8.4 mg, 16.8 mg, 33.5 mg, or 67 mg of the experimental drug. The primary outcome variable was the daily levodopa usage (mg). Table 6.10 displays the data from days 1 to 14 of this study.

(a) The study protocol specified that the five groups would be compared with respect to the predicted mean daily levodopa use at day 14 from a linear mixed model. The model was to incorporate separate mean parameters for each of study days 1, 2, and 3 and a linear regression for study days 4–14. The covariance model was to include a random intercept (at day 4) and slope for each subject. Based on these specifications, test whether the predicted mean daily levodopa use at day 14 is the same for the five groups; also compare each of the four experimental drug dosages to the placebo group.

TABLE 6.10. Levodopa usage of 25 patients with Parkinson's disease

		Day													
ID	Dose	1	2	3	4	5	6	7	8	9	10	11	12	13	14
1	33.5	200	700	1000	800	1000	1000	900	900	800	900	1000	1000	1000	1000
2	67.0	100	300	400	500	700	700	700	700	700	700	700	700	700	700
3	0.0	0	150	150	150	150	150	150	150	200	200	250	300	300	300
4	8.4	0	100	200	300	400	400	400	500	600	600	600	600	800	800
5	16.8	150	300	400	250	300	325	450	450	450	450	600	600	600	600
6	67.0	0	0	0	0	0	0	0	0	0	0	0	0	0	0
7	16.8	0	0	0	0	0	0	0	0	0	0	0	0	0	0
8	8.4	250	625	750	1450	1700	1700	1700	1700	1375	1375	1700	1700	1500	1950
9	33.5	0	0	300	450	500	500	650	650	650	650	650	650	650	700
10	0.0	0	0	0	0	0	0	0	0	0	0	0	0	0	0
11	8.4	200	500	500	500	500	500	600	600	600	600	600	600	600	600
12	33.5	50	150	150	150	150	150	150	150	150	150	150	150	200	200
13	0.0	125	375	375	375	375	375	375	625	625	625	625	625	625	625
14	67.0	175	325	400	425	475	400	350	325	400	325	350	367	300	.
15	33.5	300	250	350	400	350	300	300	200	200	150	0	0	0	150
16	8.4	400	400	800	800	800	800	800	1000	1000	1000	800	1000	1000	1000
17	16.8	0	300	300	300	300	300	300	300	300	300	300	300	300	600
18	0.0	400	1200	1200	1700	1700	1700	1700	1700	1700	1650	1650	1800	1750	1750
19	67.0	0	0	0	0	100	150	150	150	150	150	150	300	200	200
20	67.0	300	500	500	600	800	600	600	700	700	700	700	700	700	700
21	33.5	250	750	625	875	1125	1000	1125	1125	1000	1125	1125	1125	1125	1125
22	16.8	125	0	300	300	300	200	400	400	500	500	500	500	600	500
23	8.4	200	0	150	150	150	150	200	200	200	350	350	350	350	600
24	0.0	100	200	150	150	150	150	150	150	300	300	300	300	300	300
25	16.8	200	450	500	500	600	500	500	600	550	550	550	600	600	600

(b) Repeat part (a) using the covariance structure incorporating only a random intercept at day 4 for each subject.

6.9 Crépeau et al. (1985) describe a study of the effect of halothane on responses to irreversible myocardial ischemia and subsequent infarction. The experiment consisted of inducing a heart attack in rats exposed to different concentrations of halothane (group 1: 0%, group 2: 0.25%, group 3: 0.5%, group 4: 1%). Table 6.11 displays blood pressure measurements (mm Hg) at up to nine time points ranging from one minute to 240 minutes after heart attack induction. Investigate the effect of halothane dose on blood pressure using an appropriate linear model, and justify your choice of covariance structure.

6.10 Section 5.4.2 discusses data from an experiment comparing dissolution times of a certain type of pill under four different storage conditions (Crowder, 1996). Table 5.4 displays the logarithms of the times, in seconds, for each pill to reach fractions remaining of 0.9, 0.7, 0.5, 0.3, 0.25, and 0.10.

TABLE 6.11. Blood pressure measurements (mm Hg) following heart attack induction in 43 rats

		Minutes after Ligation								
Grp	ID	1	5	10	15	30	60	120	180	240
1	1	112.5	100.5	102.5	102.5	107.5	107.5	95.0	102.5	100.5
	2	92.5	102.5	105.0	100.0	110.0	117.5	97.5	102.5	112.5
	3	132.5	125.0	115.0	112.5	110.0	110.0	127.5	.	.
	4	110.0	110.0	.	.	.	.	.	.	.
	5	122.5	127.5	.	.	.	.	.	.	.
	6	102.5	107.5	107.5	102.5	90.0	112.5	107.5	110.0	112.5
	7	42.5	42.5	.	.	.	.	.	.	.
	8	107.5	80.0	.	.	.	.	.	.	.
	9	110.0	130.0	115.0	105.0	112.5	110.0	115.0	102.5	92.5
	10	97.5	97.5	80.0	82.5	82.5	102.5	100.0	95.0	95.0
	11	90.0	70.0	85.0	85.0	92.5	97.5	107.5	97.5	90.0
2	1	115.0	115.0	107.5	107.5	112.5	107.5	112.5	107.5	107.5
	2	120.0	.	.	.	.	.	.	.	.
	3	125.0	125.0	120.0	120.0	117.5	125.0	122.5	120.0	120.0
	4	95.0	90.0	95.0	90.0	100.0	107.5	100.0	100.0	92.5
	5	97.5	70.0	.	.	.	.	.	.	.
	6	87.5	65.5	85.0	90.0	105.0	90.0	85.0	87.5	100.0
	7	90.0	87.5	97.5	95.0	100.0	95.0	102.5	.	.
	8	97.5	92.5	57.5	55.0	90.0	97.5	110.0	115.0	105.0
	9	107.5	107.5	145.0	110.0	105.0	105.0	112.5	.	.
	10	102.5	130.0	85.0	80.0	127.5	97.5	117.5	102.5	127.5
3	1	107.5	107.5	102.5	102.5	102.5	97.5	98.5	102.5	92.5
	2	67.5	20.0	.	.	.	.	.	.	.
	3	97.5	108.5	94.5	102.5	102.5	107.5	117.5	112.5	.
	4	105.0	105.0	.	.	.	.	.	.	.
	5	85.0	60.0	.	.	.	.	.	.	.
	6	100.0	105.0	105.0	105.0	110.0	110.0	115.0	107.5	105.0
	7	95.0	95.0	90.0	100.0	100.0	100.0	95.0	90.0	100.0
	8	85.0	92.5	92.5	92.5	90.0	110.0	100.0	102.5	87.5
	9	82.5	77.5	75.0	65.5	65.0	72.5	72.5	67.5	67.5
	10	92.5	75.0	40.0	35.0	.	.	.	.	.
	11	62.5	75.0	115.0	110.0	100.0	100.0	.	.	.
4	1	70.0	67.5	67.5	77.5	77.5	77.5	72.5	65.0	55.0
	2	45.0	37.5	45.0	45.0	47.5	45.0	50.0	45.0	50.0
	3	52.5	22.5	90.0	65.0	60.0	65.5	52.5	47.5	57.5
	4	100.0	100.0	100.0	100.0	97.5	92.5	.	.	.
	5	47.5	30.0	.	.	.	.	.	.	.
	6	102.5	90.0	.	.	.	.	.	.	.
	7	115.0	110.0	100.0	110.0	105.0	105.0	105.0	105.0	105.0
	8	97.5	97.5	97.5	105.0	95.0	92.5	92.5	92.5	92.5
	9	95.0	125.0	130.0	125.0	115.0	117.5	110.0	105.0	102.5
	10	72.5	87.5	65.0	57.5	92.5	82.5	57.5	50.0	50.0
	11	105.0	105.0	105.0	105.0	102.5	100.0	95.0	92.5	87.5

Based on the relevant kinetic considerations for diffusion of a small tablet in a large reservoir, Crowder considers the linear model

$$y = \beta_0 + \beta_1 x,$$

where $x = 1 - f^{2/3}$ and y is the time elapsed until fraction f of the pill remains. Note that Table 5.4 displays the values of $\log(y)$.

(a) Use REML estimation with a random intercept and slope for each tablet to fit Crowder's model to these data. Parameterize the model with a separate intercept and slope for each of the four groups.

(b) Test whether the rate of dissolution is the same for the four groups of tablets.

6.11 In a double-blind, placebo-controlled study, patients with postoperative pain were randomly assigned to one of three groups: treatment A, treatment B, or placebo. Subjects enrolled in the study received a single dose of their assigned treatment when they reported moderate to severe postoperative pain. The primary outcome variable was the quantity of rescue medication used; this was recorded at hourly intervals for 24 hours after dosing. Table 6.3 displays the data from the first ten subjects in each treatment group; Section 6.4.2 discusses the analysis of the repeated hourly measurements. The study protocol specified a secondary analysis to be carried out after combining the data over prespecified time intervals (0–3 hours, 4–6 hours, 7–12 hours, 13–24 hours). In this analysis, there are four repeated measurements, each computed as the average of the hourly measurements obtained during the interval.

(a) Using REML estimation to fit the model with a separate mean at each time point in each of the three groups, investigate the appropriateness of simplified covariance structures. In particular, test the adequacy of the banded, random intercept and slope, random intercept, first-order autoregressive, compound symmetry, and independence covariance structures versus the unstructured covariance model.

(b) Using the covariance model identified in part (a), determine an appropriate reduced model for the effect of treatment and time on rescue medication use.

(c) Summarize the results and conclusions of your analysis.

7 Weighted Least Squares Analysis of Repeated Categorical Outcomes

7.1 Introduction

The methods described in previous chapters are useful in the analysis of continuous, normally distributed outcome variables. This chapter introduces and discusses the use of weighted least squares methods for the analysis of repeated categorical outcomes.

The weighted least squares (WLS) methodology was the first general approach to the analysis of repeated measurements when the response variable is categorical. Grizzle et al. (1969) summarized previous research and provided the first systematic description of this general and versatile approach to the analysis of categorical data. Although Grizzle et al. (1969) considered two examples involving repeated measurements, Koch and Reinfurt (1971) and Koch et al. (1977) first discussed specifically the general use of this methodology in analyzing categorical repeated measurements.

The WLS approach makes no assumptions concerning the time dependence among the repeated measurements. This methodology is inherently nonparametric because it is based only on the multinomial sampling model for count data. Although this is a versatile approach, it is limited to situations in which the categorical response variable has only a few possible outcomes, all covariates are categorical, the number of measurement times is small, and the sample size is relatively large within each category of the cross-classification of response and time.

Section 7.2 presents the fundamental ideas of the WLS approach and its application to the analysis of categorical data. This material is not specific to the analysis of repeated measurements and can be omitted by readers who are already familiar with this background information. Section 7.3 then describes the basic application of the methodology to repeated measurements. Finally, Section 7.4 describes how the WLS approach can be used to accommodate missing data.

7.2 Background

7.2.1 The Multinomial Distribution

The WLS approach is based on the multinomial sampling model. Thus, the multinomial distribution is first defined, and some key results are presented. Johnson et al. (1997) provide an extensive discussion of this distribution.

Consider a sequence of n independent trials. On each trial, one of c mutually exclusive and exhaustive events $E_1, \ldots, E_c$ occurs. Let $\pi_i = \Pr(E_i)$ denote the probability that the event E_i occurs, where $0 < \pi_i < 1$ and $\sum_{i=1}^{c} \pi_i = 1$. The π_i values are assumed to remain constant across the n trials.

The probability that E_1 occurs x_1 times, ..., E_c occurs x_c times is given by

$$f(x_1, \ldots, x_c) = \frac{n!}{x_1!\, x_2! \cdots x_c!} \pi_1^{x_1} \pi_2^{x_2} \cdots \pi_c^{x_c},$$

where $x_i \geq 0$ and $\sum_{i=1}^{c} x_i = n$. The random vector $\boldsymbol{x} = (x_1, \ldots, x_c)'$ has the multinomial distribution with parameters n and $\boldsymbol{\pi} = (\pi_1, \ldots, \pi_c)'$; we write $\boldsymbol{x} \sim M_c(n, \boldsymbol{\pi})$. Note that the binomial distribution is the same as the $M_2(n, \boldsymbol{\pi})$ distribution.

The moments of the multinomial distribution are

$$\begin{aligned} \mathrm{E}(x_i) &= n\pi_i, \text{ for } i = 1, \ldots, c, \\ \mathrm{Var}(x_i) &= n\pi_i(1 - \pi_i), \text{ for } i = 1, \ldots, c, \\ \mathrm{Cov}(x_i, x_j) &= -n\pi_i\pi_j, \text{ for } i \neq j = 1, \ldots, c. \end{aligned}$$

The variance–covariance matrix of $\boldsymbol{x} = (x_1, \ldots, x_c)'$ is given by

$$\mathrm{Var}(\boldsymbol{x}) = \begin{pmatrix} n\pi_1(1-\pi_1) & -n\pi_1\pi_2 & \ldots & -n\pi_1\pi_c \\ -n\pi_1\pi_2 & n\pi_2(1-\pi_2) & \ldots & -n\pi_2\pi_c \\ \vdots & \vdots & \vdots & \vdots \\ -n\pi_1\pi_c & -n\pi_2\pi_c & \ldots & n\pi_c(1-\pi_c) \end{pmatrix}.$$

This variance–covariance matrix can be written as $n(\boldsymbol{D_\pi} - \boldsymbol{\pi}\boldsymbol{\pi}')$, where $\boldsymbol{D_\pi}$ is a diagonal matrix with the vector $\boldsymbol{\pi} = (\pi_1, \ldots, \pi_c)'$ on the main diagonal. Note that because the c components of $\boldsymbol{x}$ sum to one, $\mathrm{Var}(\boldsymbol{x})$ is a singular covariance matrix.

The maximum likelihood estimators of $\pi_1, \ldots, \pi_c$ are given by $p_i = x_i/n$ for $i = 1, \ldots, c$. Because $\mathrm{E}(p_i) = \pi_i$, the vector $\boldsymbol{p} = (p_1, \ldots, p_c)'$ is an unbiased estimator of $\boldsymbol{\pi} = (\pi_1, \ldots, \pi_c)'$. The variance–covariance matrix of $\boldsymbol{p}$ is

$$\begin{aligned}
\mathrm{Var}(\boldsymbol{p}) &= \frac{1}{n}\begin{pmatrix} \pi_1(1-\pi_1) & -\pi_1\pi_2 & \ldots & -\pi_1\pi_c \\ -\pi_1\pi_2 & \pi_2(1-\pi_2) & \ldots & -\pi_2\pi_c \\ \vdots & \vdots & \vdots & \vdots \\ -\pi_1\pi_c & -\pi_2\pi_c & \ldots & \pi_c(1-\pi_c) \end{pmatrix} \\
&= \frac{1}{n}(\boldsymbol{D_\pi} - \boldsymbol{\pi\pi}').
\end{aligned}$$

As $n \to \infty$, the asymptotic distribution of $\sqrt{n}(\boldsymbol{p}-\boldsymbol{\pi})$ is $N_c(\boldsymbol{0}_c, \boldsymbol{D_\pi}-\boldsymbol{\pi\pi}')$. A consistent estimator of $\mathrm{Var}(\boldsymbol{p})$ is

$$\begin{aligned}
\boldsymbol{V_p} &= \frac{1}{n}\begin{pmatrix} p_1(1-p_1) & -p_1p_2 & \ldots & -p_1p_c \\ -p_1p_2 & p_2(1-p_2) & \ldots & -p_2p_c \\ \vdots & \vdots & \vdots & \vdots \\ -p_1p_c & -p_2p_c & \ldots & p_c(1-p_c) \end{pmatrix} \\
&= \frac{1}{n}(\boldsymbol{D_p} - \boldsymbol{pp}').
\end{aligned}$$

The vector $\boldsymbol{p} = (p_1, \ldots, p_c)'$ has an approximate multivariate normal distribution with mean vector $\boldsymbol{\pi}$ and variance–covariance matrix $\boldsymbol{V_p}$. Note that this multivariate normal distribution is singular because the components of $\boldsymbol{p}$ sum to one.

7.2.2 Linear Models Using Weighted Least Squares

Because the covariance matrix of the vector of multinomial proportions has unequal diagonal elements and nonzero off-diagonal elements, the assumptions of ordinary least squares are not satisfied. This section describes weighted least squares, a generalization of ordinary least squares that permits observations to be correlated and have nonconstant variance.

Using the notation commonly used in discussions of linear models, let

$$\boldsymbol{y} = (y_1, \ldots, y_n)'$$

be an $n \times 1$ vector of observations. Suppose that

$$\boldsymbol{y} \sim N_n(\boldsymbol{X\beta}, \boldsymbol{V}),$$

where $\boldsymbol{X}$ is an $n \times p$ design (model) matrix with $p \leq n$, $\boldsymbol{\beta}$ is a $p \times 1$ vector of parameters, and $\boldsymbol{V}$ is the $n \times n$ variance–covariance matrix of $\boldsymbol{y}$. The linear model is

$$\boldsymbol{y} = \boldsymbol{X\beta} + \boldsymbol{\epsilon},$$

where $\boldsymbol{\epsilon} \sim N_n(\mathbf{0}_n, \boldsymbol{V})$.

The basic idea of weighted least squares is to transform the observations $\boldsymbol{y} = (y_1, \ldots, y_n)'$ to other variables $\boldsymbol{y}^*$ that satisfy the assumptions of the usual linear model with independent and identically distributed random errors; that is,

$$\boldsymbol{y}^* = \boldsymbol{X}^*\boldsymbol{\beta} + \boldsymbol{\epsilon}^*,$$

where $\boldsymbol{\epsilon}^* \sim N_n(\mathbf{0}_n, \boldsymbol{I}_n)$.

A unique nonsingular symmetric matrix $\boldsymbol{V}^{1/2}$ exists such that

$$\boldsymbol{V}^{1/2}\boldsymbol{V}^{1/2} = \boldsymbol{V}.$$

Multiplying both sides of the equation $\boldsymbol{y} = \boldsymbol{X\beta} + \boldsymbol{\epsilon}$ by $\boldsymbol{V}^{-1/2}$ yields

$$\boldsymbol{V}^{-1/2}\boldsymbol{y} = \boldsymbol{V}^{-1/2}\boldsymbol{X\beta} + \boldsymbol{V}^{-1/2}\boldsymbol{\epsilon}.$$

Thus, we have $\boldsymbol{y}^* = \boldsymbol{X}^*\boldsymbol{\beta} + \boldsymbol{\epsilon}^*$, where $\boldsymbol{y}^* = \boldsymbol{V}^{-1/2}\boldsymbol{y}$, $\boldsymbol{X}^* = \boldsymbol{V}^{-1/2}\boldsymbol{X}$, and $\boldsymbol{\epsilon}^* = \boldsymbol{V}^{-1/2}\boldsymbol{\epsilon}$.

In this case, $\mathrm{E}(\boldsymbol{\epsilon}^*) = \mathrm{E}(\boldsymbol{V}^{-1/2}\boldsymbol{\epsilon}) = \boldsymbol{V}^{-1/2}\mathrm{E}(\boldsymbol{\epsilon}) = \mathbf{0}_n$ and

$$\begin{aligned}
\mathrm{Var}(\boldsymbol{\epsilon}^*) &= \mathrm{Var}(\boldsymbol{V}^{-1/2}\boldsymbol{\epsilon}) \\
&= \boldsymbol{V}^{-1/2}\mathrm{Var}(\boldsymbol{\epsilon})\boldsymbol{V}^{-1/2'} \\
&= \boldsymbol{V}^{-1/2}\boldsymbol{V}\boldsymbol{V}^{-1/2} \\
&= \boldsymbol{V}^{-1/2}(\boldsymbol{V}^{1/2}\boldsymbol{V}^{1/2})\boldsymbol{V}^{-1/2} \\
&= \boldsymbol{I}_n.
\end{aligned}$$

Let $\boldsymbol{b} = \widehat{\boldsymbol{\beta}}$ denote the least squares estimator of $\boldsymbol{\beta}$. This estimator is found by minimizing the error sum of squares (SSE), which is given by

$$\begin{aligned}
\mathrm{SSE} &= \sum_{i=1}^{n} e_i^{*2} \\
&= (\boldsymbol{y}^* - \boldsymbol{X}^*\boldsymbol{b})'(\boldsymbol{y}^* - \boldsymbol{X}^*\boldsymbol{b}) \\
&= (\boldsymbol{V}^{-1/2}\boldsymbol{y} - \boldsymbol{V}^{-1/2}\boldsymbol{Xb})'(\boldsymbol{V}^{-1/2}\boldsymbol{y} - \boldsymbol{V}^{-1/2}\boldsymbol{Xb}) \\
&= [\boldsymbol{V}^{-1/2}(\boldsymbol{y} - \boldsymbol{Xb})]'[\boldsymbol{V}^{-1/2}(\boldsymbol{y} - \boldsymbol{Xb})] \\
&= (\boldsymbol{y} - \boldsymbol{Xb})'\boldsymbol{V}^{-1/2'}\boldsymbol{V}^{-1/2}(\boldsymbol{y} - \boldsymbol{Xb}) \\
&= (\boldsymbol{y} - \boldsymbol{Xb})'\boldsymbol{V}^{-1}(\boldsymbol{y} - \boldsymbol{Xb}) \\
&= (\boldsymbol{y}' - \boldsymbol{b}'\boldsymbol{X}')\boldsymbol{V}^{-1}(\boldsymbol{y} - \boldsymbol{Xb}) \\
&= \boldsymbol{y}'\boldsymbol{V}^{-1}\boldsymbol{y} - 2\boldsymbol{b}'\boldsymbol{X}'\boldsymbol{V}^{-1}\boldsymbol{y} + \boldsymbol{b}'\boldsymbol{X}'\boldsymbol{V}^{-1}\boldsymbol{Xb}.
\end{aligned}$$

The first derivative with respect to $\boldsymbol{b}$ is

$$\frac{\partial \mathrm{SSE}}{\partial \boldsymbol{b}} = -2\boldsymbol{X}'\boldsymbol{V}^{-1}\boldsymbol{y} + 2\boldsymbol{X}'\boldsymbol{V}^{-1}\boldsymbol{Xb}.$$

Setting this equal to zero gives

$$\boldsymbol{X}'\boldsymbol{V}^{-1}\boldsymbol{X}\boldsymbol{b} = \boldsymbol{X}'\boldsymbol{V}^{-1}\boldsymbol{y}.$$

If $\boldsymbol{X}$ is of full rank, $\boldsymbol{b} = (\boldsymbol{X}'\boldsymbol{V}^{-1}\boldsymbol{X})^{-1}(\boldsymbol{X}'\boldsymbol{V}^{-1}\boldsymbol{y})$.

Because $\boldsymbol{b}$ is a linear function of $\boldsymbol{y}$, $\boldsymbol{b}$ is normally distributed with mean

$$\mathrm{E}(\boldsymbol{b}) = (\boldsymbol{X}'\boldsymbol{V}^{-1}\boldsymbol{X})^{-1}\boldsymbol{X}'\boldsymbol{V}^{-1}\mathrm{E}(\boldsymbol{y}) = (\boldsymbol{X}'\boldsymbol{V}^{-1}\boldsymbol{X})^{-1}\boldsymbol{X}'\boldsymbol{V}^{-1}\boldsymbol{X}\boldsymbol{\beta} = \boldsymbol{\beta}$$

and variance

$$\begin{aligned}
\mathrm{Var}(\boldsymbol{b}) &= \mathrm{Var}[(\boldsymbol{X}'\boldsymbol{V}^{-1}\boldsymbol{X})^{-1}\boldsymbol{X}'\boldsymbol{V}^{-1}\boldsymbol{y}] \\
&= (\boldsymbol{X}'\boldsymbol{V}^{-1}\boldsymbol{X})^{-1}\boldsymbol{X}'\boldsymbol{V}^{-1}\mathrm{Var}(\boldsymbol{y})[(\boldsymbol{X}'\boldsymbol{V}^{-1}\boldsymbol{X})^{-1}\boldsymbol{X}'\boldsymbol{V}^{-1}]' \\
&= (\boldsymbol{X}'\boldsymbol{V}^{-1}\boldsymbol{X})^{-1}\boldsymbol{X}'\boldsymbol{V}^{-1}\boldsymbol{V}\boldsymbol{V}^{-1}\boldsymbol{X}(\boldsymbol{X}'\boldsymbol{V}^{-1}\boldsymbol{X})^{-1} \\
&= (\boldsymbol{X}'\boldsymbol{V}^{-1}\boldsymbol{X})^{-1}(\boldsymbol{X}'\boldsymbol{V}^{-1}\boldsymbol{X})(\boldsymbol{X}'\boldsymbol{V}^{-1}\boldsymbol{X})^{-1} \\
&= (\boldsymbol{X}'\boldsymbol{V}^{-1}\boldsymbol{X})^{-1}.
\end{aligned}$$

The total sum of squares (SST) is given by

$$\mathrm{SST} = \boldsymbol{y}^{*\prime}\boldsymbol{y}^{*} = (\boldsymbol{V}^{-1/2}\boldsymbol{y})'\boldsymbol{V}^{-1/2}\boldsymbol{y} = \boldsymbol{y}'\boldsymbol{V}^{-1/2}\boldsymbol{V}^{-1/2}\boldsymbol{y} = \boldsymbol{y}'\boldsymbol{V}^{-1}\boldsymbol{y}.$$

The SSE is given by

$$\begin{aligned}
\mathrm{SSE} &= \boldsymbol{y}'\boldsymbol{V}^{-1}\boldsymbol{y} - 2\boldsymbol{b}'\boldsymbol{X}'\boldsymbol{V}^{-1}\boldsymbol{y} + \boldsymbol{b}'\boldsymbol{X}'\boldsymbol{V}^{-1}\boldsymbol{X}\boldsymbol{b} \\
&= \boldsymbol{y}'\boldsymbol{V}^{-1}\boldsymbol{y} - \boldsymbol{b}'\boldsymbol{X}'\boldsymbol{V}^{-1}\boldsymbol{y} - \boldsymbol{b}'\boldsymbol{X}'\boldsymbol{V}^{-1}\boldsymbol{y} + \boldsymbol{b}'\boldsymbol{X}'\boldsymbol{V}^{-1}\boldsymbol{X}\boldsymbol{b} \\
&= \boldsymbol{y}'\boldsymbol{V}^{-1}\boldsymbol{y} - \boldsymbol{b}'\boldsymbol{X}'\boldsymbol{V}^{-1}\boldsymbol{y} - \boldsymbol{b}'(\boldsymbol{X}'\boldsymbol{V}^{-1}\boldsymbol{y} - \boldsymbol{X}'\boldsymbol{V}^{-1}\boldsymbol{X}\boldsymbol{b}) \\
&= \boldsymbol{y}'\boldsymbol{V}^{-1}\boldsymbol{y} - \boldsymbol{b}'\boldsymbol{X}'\boldsymbol{V}^{-1}\boldsymbol{y} \\
&\quad -\boldsymbol{b}'(\boldsymbol{X}'\boldsymbol{V}^{-1}\boldsymbol{y} - \boldsymbol{X}'\boldsymbol{V}^{-1}\boldsymbol{X}(\boldsymbol{X}'\boldsymbol{V}^{-1}\boldsymbol{X})^{-1}\boldsymbol{X}'\boldsymbol{V}^{-1}\boldsymbol{y}) \\
&= \boldsymbol{y}'\boldsymbol{V}^{-1}\boldsymbol{y} - \boldsymbol{b}'\boldsymbol{X}'\boldsymbol{V}^{-1}\boldsymbol{y} - \boldsymbol{b}'(\boldsymbol{X}'\boldsymbol{V}^{-1}\boldsymbol{y} - \boldsymbol{X}'\boldsymbol{V}^{-1}\boldsymbol{y}) \\
&= \boldsymbol{y}'\boldsymbol{V}^{-1}\boldsymbol{y} - \boldsymbol{b}'\boldsymbol{X}'\boldsymbol{V}^{-1}\boldsymbol{y}.
\end{aligned}$$

Because $\boldsymbol{X}'\boldsymbol{V}^{-1}\boldsymbol{y} = \boldsymbol{X}'\boldsymbol{V}^{-1}\boldsymbol{X}\boldsymbol{b}$,

$$\begin{aligned}
\mathrm{SSE} &= \boldsymbol{y}'\boldsymbol{V}^{-1}\boldsymbol{y} - \boldsymbol{b}'\boldsymbol{X}'\boldsymbol{V}^{-1}\boldsymbol{X}\boldsymbol{b} = \boldsymbol{y}'\boldsymbol{V}^{-1}\boldsymbol{y} - (\boldsymbol{X}\boldsymbol{b})'\boldsymbol{V}^{-1}\boldsymbol{X}\boldsymbol{b} \\
&= \mathrm{SST} - \mathrm{SSR},
\end{aligned}$$

where SSR is the regression sum of squares.

For theoretical purposes, it is useful to express SSE as a quadratic form in $\boldsymbol{y}$:

$$\begin{aligned}
\mathrm{SSE} &= \boldsymbol{y}'\boldsymbol{V}^{-1}\boldsymbol{y} - \boldsymbol{b}'\boldsymbol{X}'\boldsymbol{V}^{-1}\boldsymbol{y} \\
&= \boldsymbol{y}'\boldsymbol{V}^{-1}\boldsymbol{y} - [(\boldsymbol{X}'\boldsymbol{V}^{-1}\boldsymbol{X})^{-1}(\boldsymbol{X}'\boldsymbol{V}^{-1}\boldsymbol{y})]'\boldsymbol{X}'\boldsymbol{V}^{-1}\boldsymbol{y} \\
&= \boldsymbol{y}'\boldsymbol{V}^{-1}\boldsymbol{y} - \boldsymbol{y}'\boldsymbol{V}^{-1}\boldsymbol{X}(\boldsymbol{X}'\boldsymbol{V}^{-1}\boldsymbol{X})^{-1}\boldsymbol{X}'\boldsymbol{V}^{-1}\boldsymbol{y} \\
&= \boldsymbol{y}'\boldsymbol{L}\boldsymbol{y},
\end{aligned}$$

where $\boldsymbol{L} = \boldsymbol{V}^{-1} - \boldsymbol{V}^{-1}\boldsymbol{X}(\boldsymbol{X}'\boldsymbol{V}^{-1}\boldsymbol{X})^{-1}\boldsymbol{X}'\boldsymbol{V}^{-1}$. It can be shown that the rank of $\boldsymbol{L}$ is $n-p$, provided that $\boldsymbol{V}$ is of full rank n and that $\boldsymbol{X}$ is of full rank p.

The fit of the model can be tested using the minimum value of SSE

$$W = \min \text{SSE} = \boldsymbol{y}'\boldsymbol{V}^{-1}\boldsymbol{y} - (\boldsymbol{X}\boldsymbol{b})'\boldsymbol{b}\boldsymbol{V}^{-1}\boldsymbol{X}\boldsymbol{b}.$$

If the model fits, then W has a chi-square distribution with $n-p$ degrees of freedom (χ^2_{n-p}).

If the model fits, additional hypotheses of the form $H_0\colon \boldsymbol{C\beta} = \boldsymbol{0}_c$ may be tested, where $\boldsymbol{C}$ is a $c \times p$ coefficient matrix. Because

$$\boldsymbol{b} \sim N_p(\boldsymbol{\beta}, (\boldsymbol{X}'\boldsymbol{V}^{-1}\boldsymbol{X})^{-1}),$$

it follows that

$$\boldsymbol{Cb} \sim N_c(\boldsymbol{C\beta}, \boldsymbol{C}(\boldsymbol{X}'\boldsymbol{V}^{-1}\boldsymbol{X})^{-1}\boldsymbol{C}').$$

The Wald statistic

$$W_{\boldsymbol{C}} = (\boldsymbol{Cb})'[\boldsymbol{C}(\boldsymbol{X}'\boldsymbol{V}^{-1}\boldsymbol{X})^{-1}\boldsymbol{C}']^{-1}\boldsymbol{Cb}$$

has a χ^2_c distribution if H_0 is true.

The estimated parameter vector $\boldsymbol{b}$ yields predicted (smoothed) observations $\widehat{y}_i$. The vector $\widehat{\boldsymbol{y}} = (\widehat{y}_1, \ldots, \widehat{y}_n)'$ is given by

$$\widehat{\boldsymbol{y}} = \boldsymbol{Xb} = \boldsymbol{X}(\boldsymbol{X}'\boldsymbol{V}^{-1}\boldsymbol{X})^{-1}\boldsymbol{X}'\boldsymbol{V}^{-1}\boldsymbol{y}.$$

The mean and variance of $\widehat{\boldsymbol{y}}$ are

$$\begin{aligned}
\text{E}(\widehat{\boldsymbol{y}}) &= \text{E}(\boldsymbol{Xb}) = \boldsymbol{X\beta}, \\
\text{Var}(\widehat{\boldsymbol{y}}) &= \text{Var}(\boldsymbol{Xb}) = \boldsymbol{X}\text{Var}(\boldsymbol{b})\boldsymbol{X}' = \boldsymbol{X}(\boldsymbol{X}'\boldsymbol{V}^{-1}\boldsymbol{X})^{-1}\boldsymbol{X}'.
\end{aligned}$$

The fit of the model can also be examined by studying the residuals $r_i = y_i - \widehat{y}_i$. The residual vector $\boldsymbol{r} = (r_1, \ldots, r_n)'$ is given by

$$\boldsymbol{r} = \boldsymbol{y} - \widehat{\boldsymbol{y}} = \boldsymbol{y} - \boldsymbol{X}(\boldsymbol{X}'\boldsymbol{V}^{-1}\boldsymbol{X})^{-1}\boldsymbol{X}'\boldsymbol{V}^{-1}\boldsymbol{y}.$$

The mean of $\boldsymbol{r}$ is

$$\text{E}(\boldsymbol{r}) = \text{E}(\boldsymbol{y} - \widehat{\boldsymbol{y}}) = \boldsymbol{X\beta} - \boldsymbol{X\beta} = \boldsymbol{0}_n,$$

and the variance of $\boldsymbol{r}$ is

$$\begin{aligned}
\text{Var}(\boldsymbol{r}) &= \text{Var}[(\boldsymbol{I}_n - \boldsymbol{X}(\boldsymbol{X}'\boldsymbol{V}^{-1}\boldsymbol{X})^{-1}\boldsymbol{X}'\boldsymbol{V}^{-1})\boldsymbol{y}] \\
&= (\boldsymbol{I}_n - \boldsymbol{X}(\boldsymbol{X}'\boldsymbol{V}^{-1}\boldsymbol{X})^{-1}\boldsymbol{X}'\boldsymbol{V}^{-1})\boldsymbol{V} \times \\
&\qquad (\boldsymbol{I}_n - \boldsymbol{V}^{-1}\boldsymbol{X}(\boldsymbol{X}'\boldsymbol{V}^{-1}\boldsymbol{X})^{-1}\boldsymbol{X}') \\
&= (\boldsymbol{V} - \boldsymbol{X}(\boldsymbol{X}'\boldsymbol{V}^{-1}\boldsymbol{X})^{-1}\boldsymbol{X}')(\boldsymbol{I}_n - \boldsymbol{V}^{-1}\boldsymbol{X}(\boldsymbol{X}'\boldsymbol{V}^{-1}\boldsymbol{X})^{-1}\boldsymbol{X}') \\
&= \boldsymbol{V} - \boldsymbol{X}(\boldsymbol{X}'\boldsymbol{V}^{-1}\boldsymbol{X})^{-1}\boldsymbol{X}'.
\end{aligned}$$

7.2.3 Analysis of Categorical Data Using Weighted Least Squares

We now describe the use of weighted least squares to model a univariate categorical outcome variable. Grizzle et al. (1969) and Agresti (1990, pp. 458–462) provide a more detailed discussion of the application of the WLS approach to the analysis of a univariate response.

The general framework is as follows. In any experiment or study, two types of data are collected from each subject or experimental unit:

1. a description of the subpopulation or configuration of experimental conditions to which each experimental unit belongs;
2. a description of the outcome(s) for each experimental unit.

Variables of the first type are often called independent variables or factors, and variables of the second type are called dependent variables or response variables.

The underlying idea of the WLS approach to the analysis of categorical data is to structure the data as a two-way contingency table, where the rows of the table represent the subpopulations defined by the cross-classification of the factors (independent variables) and the columns represent the response variable (or, if there is more than one response, the cross-classification of the response variables). Using this *factor-response* framework, the data in any multidimensional contingency table can be regarded as the frequencies with which units belonging to the same subpopulation are classified into the same combination of response categories. Table 7.1 displays the cell counts n_{ij}, the underlying unknown probabilities π_{ij}, and the observed proportions $p_{ij} = n_{ij}/n_{i+}$, where $n_{i+} = \sum_{j=1}^{r} n_{ij}$.

The vector of responses $\boldsymbol{n}_i' = (n_{i1}, \ldots, n_{ir})$ for the ith subpopulation has the $M_r(n_{i+}, \boldsymbol{\pi}_i)$ distribution, where $\boldsymbol{\pi}_i = (\pi_{i1}, \ldots, \pi_{ir})'$. Because the rows of Table 7.1 are independent, the $sr \times 1$ vector $\boldsymbol{n}' = (\boldsymbol{n}_1', \ldots, \boldsymbol{n}_s')$ has the product-multinomial distribution with likelihood function

$$\Pr(\boldsymbol{n}) = \prod_{i=1}^{s} n_{i+}! \prod_{j=1}^{r} \pi_{ij}^{n_{ij}} / n_{ij}!.$$

Let $\boldsymbol{p}_i = (p_{i1}, \ldots, p_{ir})'$ denote the $r \times 1$ vector of observed proportions from the ith subpopulation, where $p_{ij} = n_{ij}/n_{i+}$. Using the results of Section 7.2.1, $\mathrm{E}(\boldsymbol{p}_i) = \boldsymbol{\pi}_i$ and

$$\mathrm{Cov}(\boldsymbol{p}_i) = \boldsymbol{V}_i = [\boldsymbol{D}_{\boldsymbol{\pi}_i} - \boldsymbol{\pi}_i \boldsymbol{\pi}_i'] / n_{i+},$$

where $\boldsymbol{D}_{\boldsymbol{\pi}_i}$ is a diagonal matrix with the elements of $\boldsymbol{\pi}_i$ on the main diagonal. In addition, the asymptotic distribution of $\sqrt{n}_{i+}(\boldsymbol{p}_i - \boldsymbol{\pi}_i)$ is $N_r(\boldsymbol{0}_r, n_{i+}\boldsymbol{V}_i)$. The matrix $\boldsymbol{V}_i$ can be consistently estimated by

$$\widehat{\boldsymbol{V}}_i = [\boldsymbol{D}_{\boldsymbol{p}_i} - \boldsymbol{p}_i \boldsymbol{p}_i'] / n_{i+}.$$

TABLE 7.1. Notation for the WLS approach to categorical data analysis

Observed Frequencies

Subpopulation	Response Category 1	$\cdots$	r	Total
1	n_{11}	$\cdots$	n_{1r}	n_{1+}
$\vdots$	$\vdots$		$\vdots$	$\vdots$
s	n_{s1}	$\cdots$	n_{sr}	n_{s+}

Underlying Probabilities

Subpopulation	Response Category 1	$\cdots$	r	Total
1	π_{11}	$\cdots$	π_{1r}	1
$\vdots$	$\vdots$		$\vdots$	$\vdots$
s	π_{s1}	$\cdots$	π_{sr}	1

Observed Proportions

Subpopulation	Response Category 1	$\cdots$	r	Total
1	p_{11}	$\cdots$	p_{1r}	1
$\vdots$	$\vdots$		$\vdots$	$\vdots$
s	p_{s1}	$\cdots$	p_{sr}	1

Now, let $\boldsymbol{p} = (\boldsymbol{p}_1', \ldots, \boldsymbol{p}_s')'$ denote the $sr \times 1$ vector of observed proportions from all s subpopulations. The mean of $\boldsymbol{p}$ is $\mathrm{E}(\boldsymbol{p}) = \boldsymbol{\pi}$, where $\boldsymbol{\pi} = (\boldsymbol{\pi}_1', \ldots, \boldsymbol{\pi}_s')'$ and the covariance matrix of $\boldsymbol{p}$ is the $sr \times sr$ matrix

$$\boldsymbol{V} = \begin{pmatrix} \boldsymbol{V}_1 & \boldsymbol{0}_{(r\times r)} & \cdots & \boldsymbol{0}_{(r\times r)} \\ \boldsymbol{0}_{(r\times r)} & \boldsymbol{V}_2 & & \boldsymbol{0}_{(r\times r)} \\ \vdots & & \ddots & \\ \boldsymbol{0}_{(r\times r)} & \boldsymbol{0}_{(r\times r)} & & \boldsymbol{V}_s \end{pmatrix}.$$

Let $n_{++} = \sum_{i=1}^{s} n_{i+}$. If $n_{++} \to \infty$ and $n_{i+}/n_{++} \to c_i > 0$, then the asymptotic distribution of $\sqrt{n_{++}}(\boldsymbol{p} - \boldsymbol{\pi})$ is multivariate normal with mean vector $\boldsymbol{0}_{sr}$ and covariance matrix $n_{++}\boldsymbol{V}$.

The vector $\boldsymbol{p}$ then has an approximate multivariate normal distribution with mean vector $\boldsymbol{\pi}$ and covariance matrix $\boldsymbol{V}$. Because $\boldsymbol{V}$ depends on the unknown true probabilities π_{ij}, we will replace it by the consistent estimator

$$\widehat{\boldsymbol{V}} = \begin{pmatrix} \widehat{\boldsymbol{V}}_1 & \boldsymbol{0}_{(r\times r)} & \cdots & \boldsymbol{0}_{(r\times r)} \\ \boldsymbol{0}_{(r\times r)} & \widehat{\boldsymbol{V}}_2 & & \boldsymbol{0}_{(r\times r)} \\ \vdots & & \ddots & \\ \boldsymbol{0}_{(r\times r)} & \boldsymbol{0}_{(r\times r)} & & \widehat{\boldsymbol{V}}_s \end{pmatrix}.$$

Thus, the vector $\boldsymbol{p}$ is approximately distributed as $N_{sr}(\boldsymbol{\pi}, \widehat{\boldsymbol{V}})$.

Now, let $\boldsymbol{F}(\boldsymbol{\pi}) = (F_1(\boldsymbol{\pi}), \ldots, F_u(\boldsymbol{\pi}))'$ be a vector of u linearly independent response functions of interest, where $u \leq s(r-1)$. Each of the functions is required to have continuous partial derivatives through order 2. Let

$$\boldsymbol{F}(\boldsymbol{p}) = (F_1(\boldsymbol{p}), \ldots, F_u(\boldsymbol{p}))'$$

denote the corresponding sample response functions, and let $\boldsymbol{Q} = (\partial \boldsymbol{F}/\partial \boldsymbol{\pi})$ denote the $u \times sr$ matrix of partial derivatives evaluated at the sample proportions $\boldsymbol{p}$. Then, $\boldsymbol{F}(\boldsymbol{p})$ is approximately distributed as $N_u(\boldsymbol{F}(\boldsymbol{\pi}), \widehat{\boldsymbol{V}}_{\boldsymbol{F}})$, where $\widehat{\boldsymbol{V}}_{\boldsymbol{F}} = \boldsymbol{Q}\widehat{\boldsymbol{V}}\boldsymbol{Q}'$. Although $\widehat{\boldsymbol{V}}$ is singular, $\widehat{\boldsymbol{V}}_{\boldsymbol{F}}$ is a nonsingular covariance matrix.

Although a wide variety of functions $\boldsymbol{F}(\boldsymbol{p})$ can be considered, a few types of functions are commonly used. In particular, $\boldsymbol{F}(\boldsymbol{\pi}) = \boldsymbol{A}\boldsymbol{\pi}$, where $\boldsymbol{A}$ is a matrix of known constants, is appropriate when the response functions are linear functions of the underlying probabilities. In this case, $\widehat{\boldsymbol{V}}_{\boldsymbol{F}} = \boldsymbol{A}\widehat{\boldsymbol{V}}\boldsymbol{A}'$. Many other useful functions can be generated as a sequence of linear, logarithmic, and exponential operators on the vector $\boldsymbol{\pi}$. The advantage of specifying the functions of interest in this way is that $\widehat{\boldsymbol{V}}_{\boldsymbol{F}}$ can then be estimated using the chain rule (Grizzle et al., 1969). This topic is described further in Section 7.2.4.

We can now use weighted least squares to fit models of the form

$$\boldsymbol{F}(\boldsymbol{\pi}) = \boldsymbol{X}\boldsymbol{\beta},$$

where $\boldsymbol{X}$ is a $u \times t$ full-rank matrix of known constants ($t \leq u$) and $\boldsymbol{\beta}$ is a $t \times 1$ vector of unknown parameters.

The procedure can be summarized as follows.

1. Lay out the data in the factor-response framework, as shown in Table 7.1.

2. Determine the number of response functions you wish to analyze from each subpopulation. (Note that there are at most $r-1$ linearly independent response functions per subpopulation.)

3. Determine the type of response function(s) you wish to analyze from each subpopulation (e.g., proportions, mean scores, logits, cumulative logits).

4. Specify the response functions $\boldsymbol{F}(\boldsymbol{p})$.

5. Specify a linear model relating the response functions to the independent variables: $\boldsymbol{F}(\boldsymbol{\pi}) = \boldsymbol{X}\boldsymbol{\beta}$.

6. Estimate the parameters using WLS.

7. Evaluate the goodness-of-fit of the model.

8. Test hypotheses of interest concerning model parameters.

9. Interpret the results of the fitted model.

7.2.4 Taylor Series Variance Approximations for Nonlinear Response Functions

When the response functions of interest are nonlinear functions of the vector of underlying multinomial proportions, the approximate variances and covariances of the response functions are computed using Taylor series approximations. This section discusses Taylor series approximations for a function of a scalar random variable, then for a scalar function of a random vector, and finally for a vector of functions of a random vector. The results for linear, logarithmic, and exponential functions are then summarized, followed by a description of the use of the chain rule for approximating variances of functions that can be defined using a sequence of linear, logarithmic, and exponential functions.

Univariate Taylor Series Approximations

Let X be a random variable with known mean and variance:

$$\mathrm{E}(X) = \mu, \qquad \mathrm{Var}(X) = \mathrm{E}[(X-\mu)^2] = \sigma^2.$$

Let $Y = g(X)$, where the continuous function $g(x)$ has first and second derivatives. Suppose that exact calculation of $\mathrm{E}(Y)$ and $\mathrm{Var}(Y)$ is difficult. One approach is to expand $g(X)$ in a Taylor series about μ and use this series representation to approximate $\mathrm{E}(Y)$ and $\mathrm{Var}(Y)$.

The first three terms of this expansion are

$$g(X) = g(\mu) + g'(\mu)(X - \mu) + \frac{1}{2} g''(\mu)(X - \mu)^2.$$

The approximation for the mean of Y is

$$\mathrm{E}(Y) \doteq \mathrm{E}\left[g(\mu) + g'(\mu)(X - \mu) + \frac{1}{2} g''(\mu)(X - \mu)^2\right] = g(\mu) + \frac{1}{2} g''(\mu)\mathrm{Var}(X).$$

Using the linear term only, $\mathrm{E}(Y) \doteq g(\mu)$. Similarly, the approximation for the variance of Y is

$$\begin{aligned}
\mathrm{Var}(Y) &= \mathrm{E}\left[\left(g(X) - \mathrm{E}[g(X)]\right)^2\right] \\
&\doteq \mathrm{E}\left[\left(g(\mu) + g'(\mu)(X - \mu) - g(\mu)\right)^2\right] \\
&= \mathrm{E}\left[\left(g'(\mu)(X - \mu)\right)^2\right] \\
&= \left(g'(\mu)\right)^2 \mathrm{E}\left[(X - \mu)^2\right] \\
&= \left(g'(\mu)\right)^2 \mathrm{Var}(X).
\end{aligned}$$

Multivariate Taylor Series Approximations

Now, let $\boldsymbol{X} = (X_1, \ldots, X_n)'$ be a random vector with known mean vector $\boldsymbol{\mu}$ and covariance matrix $\boldsymbol{\Sigma}$. Let $Y = g(X_1, \ldots, X_n)$, where $g(x_1, \ldots, x_n)$ is a continuous function with first and second partial derivatives. Expanding $g(\boldsymbol{X})$ in a Taylor series about $\boldsymbol{\mu}$ yields

$$g(\boldsymbol{X}) = g(\boldsymbol{\mu}) + \sum_{i=1}^{n} \frac{\partial g}{\partial \mu_i}(X_i - \mu_i) + \frac{1}{2} \sum_{i=1}^{n} \sum_{j=1}^{n} \frac{\partial^2 g}{\partial \mu_i \partial \mu_j}(X_i - \mu_i)(X_j - \mu_j),$$

where

$$\frac{\partial g}{\partial \mu_i} = \left.\frac{\partial g}{\partial X_i}\right|_{\boldsymbol{X}=\boldsymbol{\mu}}, \qquad \frac{\partial^2 g}{\partial \mu_i \partial \mu_j} = \left.\frac{\partial^2 g}{\partial X_i \partial X_j}\right|_{\boldsymbol{X}=\boldsymbol{\mu}}.$$

Let

$$g^{(1)}(\boldsymbol{\mu}) = \left(\frac{\partial g}{\partial \mu_1}, \ldots, \frac{\partial g}{\partial \mu_n}\right)$$

be the row vector of first partial derivatives. Then,

$$Y = g(X_1, \ldots, X_n) \doteq g(\boldsymbol{\mu}) + \left(g^{(1)}(\boldsymbol{\mu})\right)(\boldsymbol{X} - \boldsymbol{\mu}).$$

The approximate mean and variance of Y are

$$\mathrm{E}(Y) \doteq \mathrm{E}[g(\boldsymbol{\mu})] + \left(g^{(1)}(\boldsymbol{\mu})\right)\mathrm{E}(\boldsymbol{X} - \boldsymbol{\mu}) = g(\boldsymbol{\mu})$$

and

$$\begin{aligned}
\mathrm{Var}(Y) &= \mathrm{E}\left[\left(g(\boldsymbol{X}) - \mathrm{E}[g(\boldsymbol{X})]\right)^2\right] \\
&\doteq \mathrm{E}\left[\left(g(\boldsymbol{\mu}) + (g^{(1)}(\boldsymbol{\mu}))(\boldsymbol{X}-\boldsymbol{\mu}) - g(\boldsymbol{\mu})\right)^2\right] \\
&= \mathrm{E}\left[\left(g^{(1)}(\boldsymbol{\mu})(\boldsymbol{X}-\boldsymbol{\mu})\right)^2\right] \\
&= \mathrm{E}\left[(g^{(1)}(\boldsymbol{\mu}))(\boldsymbol{X}-\boldsymbol{\mu})(\boldsymbol{X}-\boldsymbol{\mu})'(g^{(1)}(\boldsymbol{\mu}))'\right] \\
&= (g^{(1)}(\boldsymbol{\mu}))\mathrm{E}[(\boldsymbol{X}-\boldsymbol{\mu})(\boldsymbol{X}-\boldsymbol{\mu})'](g^{(1)}(\boldsymbol{\mu}))' \\
&= (g^{(1)}(\boldsymbol{\mu}))\Sigma(g^{(1)}(\boldsymbol{\mu}))'.
\end{aligned}$$

Taylor Series Approximations for Multiple Functions of a Random Vector

Let $\boldsymbol{X} = (X_1, \ldots, X_n)'$ be a random vector with known mean vector $\boldsymbol{\mu}$ and covariance matrix $\boldsymbol{\Sigma}$. Let $\boldsymbol{Y} = (Y_1, \ldots, Y_m)'$, where $Y_i = g_i(X_1, \ldots, X_n)$, for $i = 1, \ldots, m$. From the results for a univariate function of a random vector,

$$\begin{aligned}
\mathrm{E}(Y_i) &\doteq g_i(\boldsymbol{\mu}), \\
\mathrm{Var}(Y_i) &\doteq (g_i^{(1)}(\boldsymbol{\mu}))\boldsymbol{\Sigma}(g_i^{(1)}(\boldsymbol{\mu}))'.
\end{aligned}$$

The covariance between Y_i and Y_j is approximated as follows:

$$\begin{aligned}
\mathrm{Cov}(Y_i, Y_j) &= \mathrm{E}[(Y_i - \mathrm{E}(Y_i))(Y_j - \mathrm{E}(Y_j))] \\
&\doteq \mathrm{E}\left[[g_i^{(1)}(\boldsymbol{\mu})](\boldsymbol{X}-\boldsymbol{\mu})[g_j^{(1)}(\boldsymbol{\mu})](\boldsymbol{X}-\boldsymbol{\mu})\right] \\
&= \mathrm{E}\left[[g_i^{(1)}(\boldsymbol{\mu})](\boldsymbol{X}-\boldsymbol{\mu})(\boldsymbol{X}-\boldsymbol{\mu})'[g_j^{(1)}(\boldsymbol{\mu})]'\right] \\
&= \left[g_i^{(1)}(\boldsymbol{\mu})\right]\mathrm{E}[(\boldsymbol{X}-\boldsymbol{\mu})(\boldsymbol{X}-\boldsymbol{\mu})']\left[g_j^{(1)}(\mu)\right]' \\
&= \left[g_i^{(1)}(\boldsymbol{\mu})\right]\boldsymbol{\Sigma}\left[g_j^{(1)}(\boldsymbol{\mu})\right]'.
\end{aligned}$$

Now, let $\left(\frac{\partial \boldsymbol{g}}{\partial \boldsymbol{\mu}}\right)$ denote the $m \times n$ matrix whose ith row is $g_i^{(1)}(\mu)$. The (i,j) element of $\left(\frac{\partial \boldsymbol{g}}{\partial \boldsymbol{\mu}}\right)$ is $\left.\frac{\partial g_i}{\partial X_j}\right|_{\boldsymbol{X}=\boldsymbol{\mu}}$. The approximate mean and covariance matrix of $\boldsymbol{Y}$ are

$$\begin{aligned}
\mathrm{E}(\boldsymbol{Y}) &\doteq \boldsymbol{g}(\boldsymbol{\mu}), \\
\mathrm{Var}(\boldsymbol{Y}) &\doteq \left(\frac{\partial \boldsymbol{g}}{\partial \boldsymbol{\mu}}\right)\boldsymbol{\Sigma}\left(\frac{\partial \boldsymbol{g}}{\partial \boldsymbol{\mu}}\right)'.
\end{aligned}$$

Variance Approximations for Special Classes of Functions

Let $\boldsymbol{X} = (X_1, \ldots, X_n)$ be a random vector with mean vector $\boldsymbol{\mu}$ and covariance matrix $\boldsymbol{\Sigma}$.

First, although Taylor series approximations are not necessary in this case, consider the class of linear functions of $\boldsymbol{X}$. Let $\boldsymbol{A}$ be an $m \times n$ matrix of constants, and let $\boldsymbol{Y} = \boldsymbol{AX}$ be an $m \times 1$ vector of functions of $\boldsymbol{X}$ defined by

$$\begin{aligned} \boldsymbol{Y} &= \boldsymbol{F}(\boldsymbol{X}) = \boldsymbol{AX} \\ &= \begin{pmatrix} a_{11} & \cdots & a_{1n} \\ \vdots & & \vdots \\ a_{m1} & \cdots & a_{mn} \end{pmatrix} \begin{pmatrix} X_1 \\ \vdots \\ X_n \end{pmatrix} \\ &= \begin{pmatrix} \sum_{j=1}^n a_{1j}X_j \\ \vdots \\ \sum_{j=1}^n a_{mj}X_j \end{pmatrix} = \begin{pmatrix} F_1(\boldsymbol{X}) \\ \vdots \\ F_m(\boldsymbol{X}) \end{pmatrix}. \end{aligned}$$

The partial derivatives are given by

$$\frac{\partial F_i}{\partial \boldsymbol{X}} = (a_{i1}, \ldots, a_{in})$$

for $i = 1, \ldots, m$ and

$$\left(\frac{\partial \boldsymbol{F}}{\partial \boldsymbol{X}}\right) = \begin{pmatrix} \dfrac{\partial F_1}{\partial \boldsymbol{X}} \\ \vdots \\ \dfrac{\partial F_m}{\partial \boldsymbol{X}} \end{pmatrix} = \boldsymbol{A}.$$

Therefore,

$$\mathrm{Var}(\boldsymbol{Y}) = \left(\frac{\partial \boldsymbol{F}}{\partial \boldsymbol{X}}\right) \boldsymbol{\Sigma} \left(\frac{\partial \boldsymbol{F}}{\partial \boldsymbol{X}}\right)' = \boldsymbol{A\Sigma A}'.$$

Now, consider the $n \times 1$ function vector $\boldsymbol{Y}$ of componentwise natural logarithms of $\boldsymbol{X}$. We write $\boldsymbol{Y} = \log(\boldsymbol{X})$, where $y_i = F_i(x_i) = \log(x_i)$, for $i = 1, \ldots, n$. The partial derivatives are given by

$$\begin{aligned} \frac{\partial F_1}{\partial \boldsymbol{X}} &= (1/X_1, 0, \ldots, 0) \\ \frac{\partial F_2}{\partial \boldsymbol{X}} &= (0, 1/X_2, 0, \ldots, 0) \\ &\vdots \\ \frac{\partial F_n}{\partial \boldsymbol{X}} &= (0, \ldots, 0, 1/X_n). \end{aligned}$$

Therefore,

$$\frac{\partial \boldsymbol{F}}{\partial \boldsymbol{X}} = \begin{pmatrix} \frac{\partial F_1}{\partial \boldsymbol{X}} \\ \frac{\partial F_2}{\partial \boldsymbol{X}} \\ \vdots \\ \frac{\partial F_n}{\partial \boldsymbol{X}} \end{pmatrix} = \begin{pmatrix} 1/X_1 & 0 & \cdots & 0 \\ 0 & 1/X_2 & \cdots & 0 \\ \vdots & \vdots & \ddots & 0 \\ 0 & 0 & \cdots & 1/X_n \end{pmatrix}.$$

Evaluated at $\boldsymbol{X} = \boldsymbol{\mu}$, we have

$$\left.\frac{\partial \boldsymbol{F}}{\partial \boldsymbol{X}}\right|_{\boldsymbol{X}=\boldsymbol{\mu}} = \begin{pmatrix} 1/\mu_1 & 0 & \cdots & 0 \\ 0 & 1/\mu_2 & \cdots & 0 \\ \vdots & \vdots & \ddots & 0 \\ 0 & 0 & \cdots & 1/\mu_n \end{pmatrix} = \boldsymbol{D}_{\boldsymbol{\mu}}^{-1},$$

where $\boldsymbol{D}_{\boldsymbol{\mu}}$ is a diagonal matrix with elements equal to $\mu_1, \ldots, \mu_n$. Then,

$$\text{Var}(\boldsymbol{Y}) \doteq \left(\left.\frac{\partial \boldsymbol{F}}{\partial \boldsymbol{X}}\right|_{\boldsymbol{X}=\boldsymbol{\mu}}\right) \boldsymbol{\Sigma} \left(\left.\frac{\partial \boldsymbol{F}}{\partial \boldsymbol{X}}\right|_{\boldsymbol{X}=\boldsymbol{\mu}}\right)' = \boldsymbol{D}_{\boldsymbol{\mu}}^{-1} \boldsymbol{\Sigma} \boldsymbol{D}_{\boldsymbol{\mu}}^{-1}.$$

Now, consider the $n \times 1$ vector $\boldsymbol{Y}$ of componentwise exponential functions of $\boldsymbol{X}$. We write $\boldsymbol{Y} = \exp(\boldsymbol{X})$, where $y_i = F_i(x_i) = \exp(x_i)$, for $i = 1, \ldots, n$. The partial derivatives are given by

$$\begin{aligned} \frac{\partial F_1}{\partial \boldsymbol{X}} &= (e^{X_1}, 0, \ldots, 0) \\ \frac{\partial F_2}{\partial \boldsymbol{X}} &= (0, e^{X_2}, 0, \ldots, 0) \\ &\vdots \\ \frac{\partial F_n}{\partial \boldsymbol{X}} &= (0, \ldots, 0, e^{X_n}). \end{aligned}$$

Therefore,

$$\frac{\partial \boldsymbol{F}}{\partial \boldsymbol{X}} = \begin{pmatrix} \frac{\partial F_1}{\partial \boldsymbol{X}} \\ \frac{\partial F_2}{\partial \boldsymbol{X}} \\ \vdots \\ \frac{\partial F_n}{\partial \boldsymbol{X}} \end{pmatrix} = \begin{pmatrix} e^{X_1} & 0 & \cdots & 0 \\ 0 & e^{X_2} & \cdots & 0 \\ \vdots & \vdots & \ddots & 0 \\ 0 & 0 & \cdots & e^{X_n} \end{pmatrix}.$$

Evaluated at $\boldsymbol{X} = \boldsymbol{\mu}$,

$$\left.\frac{\partial \boldsymbol{F}}{\partial \boldsymbol{X}}\right|_{\boldsymbol{X}=\boldsymbol{\mu}} = \begin{pmatrix} e^{\mu_1} & 0 & \cdots & 0 \\ 0 & e^{\mu_2} & \cdots & 0 \\ \vdots & \vdots & \ddots & 0 \\ 0 & 0 & \cdots & e^{\mu_n} \end{pmatrix} = \boldsymbol{D}_{e^{\mu}},$$

where $\boldsymbol{D}_{e^{\mu}}$ is a diagonal matrix with elements equal to $e^{\mu_1}, \ldots, e^{\mu_n}$. Therefore,

$$\mathrm{Var}(\boldsymbol{Y}) \doteq \left(\frac{\partial \boldsymbol{F}}{\partial \boldsymbol{X}}\bigg|_{\boldsymbol{X}=\boldsymbol{\mu}}\right)\boldsymbol{\Sigma}\left(\frac{\partial \boldsymbol{F}}{\partial \boldsymbol{X}}\bigg|_{\boldsymbol{X}=\boldsymbol{\mu}}\right)' = \boldsymbol{D}_{e^{\mu}}\boldsymbol{\Sigma}\boldsymbol{D}_{e^{\mu}}.$$

The preceding results for variances of linear, logarithmic, and exponential functions can be combined to approximate the variances and covariances of compound functions. Two types of compound functions are commonly used:

$$\begin{aligned}\boldsymbol{F}(\boldsymbol{X}) &= \boldsymbol{A}_2 \log(\boldsymbol{A}_1\boldsymbol{X}),\\ \boldsymbol{G}(\boldsymbol{X}) &= \exp(\boldsymbol{A}_2 \log(\boldsymbol{A}_1\boldsymbol{X})) = \exp(\boldsymbol{F}(\boldsymbol{X})).\end{aligned}$$

In this case, we wish to approximate $\boldsymbol{V}_{\boldsymbol{F}} = \mathrm{Var}(\boldsymbol{F}(\boldsymbol{X}))$ and $\boldsymbol{V}_{\boldsymbol{G}} = \mathrm{Var}(\boldsymbol{G}(\boldsymbol{X}))$.

First, let $\boldsymbol{F}_1(\boldsymbol{X}) = \boldsymbol{A}_1\boldsymbol{X}$. The variance of $\boldsymbol{F}_1(\boldsymbol{X})$ is

$$\boldsymbol{V}_{\boldsymbol{F}_1} = \mathrm{Var}(\boldsymbol{F}_1(\boldsymbol{X})) = \boldsymbol{A}_1\boldsymbol{\Sigma}\boldsymbol{A}_1'.$$

Now, let $\boldsymbol{F}_2(\boldsymbol{X}) = \log(\boldsymbol{F}_1(\boldsymbol{X})) = \log(\boldsymbol{A}_1\boldsymbol{X})$. The variance approximation for $\boldsymbol{F}_2(\boldsymbol{X})$ is

$$\begin{aligned}\boldsymbol{V}_{\boldsymbol{F}_2} &= \mathrm{Var}(\boldsymbol{F}_2(\boldsymbol{X})) = \mathrm{Var}(\log(\boldsymbol{F}_1(\boldsymbol{X})))\\ &\doteq \boldsymbol{D}_{\boldsymbol{F}_1}^{-1}\boldsymbol{V}_{\boldsymbol{F}_1}\boldsymbol{D}_{\boldsymbol{F}_1}^{-1} = \boldsymbol{D}_{\boldsymbol{F}_1}^{-1}\boldsymbol{A}_1\boldsymbol{\Sigma}\boldsymbol{A}_1'\boldsymbol{D}_{\boldsymbol{F}_1}^{-1}.\end{aligned}$$

Finally, let $\boldsymbol{F}(\boldsymbol{X}) = \boldsymbol{A}_2\boldsymbol{F}_2(\boldsymbol{X}) = \boldsymbol{A}_2\log(\boldsymbol{A}_1\boldsymbol{X})$. The variance approximation for $\boldsymbol{F}(\boldsymbol{X})$ is

$$\begin{aligned}\boldsymbol{V}_{\boldsymbol{F}} &= \mathrm{Var}(\boldsymbol{F}(\boldsymbol{X}))\\ &= \mathrm{Var}(\boldsymbol{A}_2\boldsymbol{F}_2(\boldsymbol{X}))\\ &= \boldsymbol{A}_2\boldsymbol{V}_{\boldsymbol{F}_2}\boldsymbol{A}_2'\\ &\doteq \boldsymbol{A}_2\boldsymbol{D}_{\boldsymbol{F}_1}^{-1}\boldsymbol{A}_1\boldsymbol{\Sigma}\boldsymbol{A}_1'\boldsymbol{D}_{\boldsymbol{F}_1}^{-1}\boldsymbol{A}_2'.\end{aligned}$$

Now, consider the function $\boldsymbol{G}(\boldsymbol{X}) = \exp(\boldsymbol{A}_2\log(\boldsymbol{A}_1\boldsymbol{X})) = \exp(\boldsymbol{F}(\boldsymbol{X}))$. The variance approximation for $\boldsymbol{G}(\boldsymbol{X})$ is

$$\begin{aligned}\boldsymbol{V}_{\boldsymbol{G}} &= \mathrm{Var}(\boldsymbol{G}(\boldsymbol{X}))\\ &= \mathrm{Var}(\exp(\boldsymbol{F}(\boldsymbol{X})))\\ &\doteq \boldsymbol{D}_{e^{\boldsymbol{F}}}\boldsymbol{V}_{\boldsymbol{F}}\boldsymbol{D}_{e^{\boldsymbol{F}}}\\ &= \boldsymbol{D}_{e^{\boldsymbol{F}}}\boldsymbol{A}_2\boldsymbol{D}_{\boldsymbol{F}_1}^{-1}\boldsymbol{A}_1\boldsymbol{\Sigma}\boldsymbol{A}_1'\boldsymbol{D}_{\boldsymbol{F}_1}^{-1}\boldsymbol{A}_2'\boldsymbol{D}_{e^{\boldsymbol{F}}}.\end{aligned}$$

This approach can be used for other types of compound response functions that can be expressed as combinations of linear, logarithmic, and exponential transformations.

7.3 Application to Repeated Measurements

7.3.1 Overview

The description of the WLS approach in Section 7.2.3 is applicable when there is a univariate response variable with r levels. The approach is equally applicable when there are multiple response variables for each experimental unit. In this case, r represents the number of levels defined by the cross-classification of the levels of the response variables.

In repeated measures applications, there are multiple response functions per subpopulation, and the correlation structure induced by the repeated measurements from each subject must be taken into consideration. In the general situation in which a c-category outcome variable is measured at t time points, the cross-classification of the possible outcomes results in $r = c^t$ response profiles. The response functions of interest could then be the $t(c-1)$ correlated marginal proportions, generalized logits, or cumulative logits. Alternatively, if the response variable is ordinal, the analysis of t correlated mean scores might be of interest.

Provided that the appropriate covariance matrix is computed for these correlated response functions, the WLS computations are no different from those described in Section 7.2. Koch and Reinfurt (1971) and Koch et al. (1977) first described the application of WLS to repeated measures categorical data. Stanish et al. (1978), Stanish and Koch (1984), Woolson and Clarke (1984), Stanish (1986), Agresti (1988, 1989), Landis et al. (1988), Stanek and Diehl (1988), Davis (1992), and Park and Davis (1993) further developed this methodology and illustrated various aspects of the use of the WLS approach in analyzing categorical repeated measures.

The basic ideas will be introduced by way of several examples.

7.3.2 One Population, Dichotomous Response, Repeated Measurements Factor Is Unordered

Grizzle et al. (1969) analyze data in which 46 subjects were treated with each of three drugs (A, B, and C). The response to each drug was recorded as favorable (F) or unfavorable (U). The null hypothesis of interest is that the marginal probability of a favorable response is the same for all three drugs. Because the same 46 subjects were used in testing each of the three drugs, the estimates of the three marginal probabilities are correlated. Table 7.2 displays the responses to each of the three drugs for each subject.

In terms of the factor-response framework discussed in Section 7.2.3, there is a single population ($s = 1$). Because there are $c = 2$ possible outcomes at each of $t = 3$ time points, there are

$$r = c^t = 2^3 = 8$$

TABLE 7.2. Favorable and unfavorable drug responses from 46 subjects

Subject	Drug A	Drug B	Drug C	Subject	Drug A	Drug B	Drug C
1	F	F	U	24	U	F	U
2	U	U	U	25	F	F	U
3	U	U	F	26	U	U	U
4	F	F	U	27	F	U	U
5	U	U	U	28	U	U	F
6	F	F	U	29	U	U	U
7	F	F	F	30	F	F	U
8	F	F	U	31	F	F	F
9	F	U	U	32	F	U	F
10	U	U	F	33	F	F	U
11	F	F	U	34	U	F	F
12	U	F	U	35	U	F	U
13	F	F	F	36	F	F	U
14	F	F	U	37	F	F	U
15	U	F	F	38	F	F	F
16	F	U	F	39	F	U	U
17	U	U	U	40	U	U	F
18	F	F	U	41	F	F	U
19	F	U	U	42	U	U	U
20	U	U	F	43	U	U	F
21	F	F	F	44	F	F	U
22	F	F	U	45	F	F	F
23	F	F	U	46	U	F	U

TABLE 7.3. Drug response data displayed in the WLS framework

	Response Profile (Drugs A, B, C)								
	F	F	F	F	U	U	U	U	
	F	F	U	U	F	F	U	U	
	F	U	F	U	F	U	F	U	Total
Number of subjects	6	16	2	4	2	4	6	6	46

potential response profiles. Table 7.3 displays the same data as Table 7.2 but this time in the general WLS framework.

Let p_i denote the observed proportion of subjects in the ith response profile (ordered from left to right as displayed in Table 7.3), and let

$$\boldsymbol{p} = (p_1, \ldots, p_8)'.$$

Similarly, let $\boldsymbol{\pi} = (\pi_1, \ldots, \pi_8)'$ denote the vector of population probabilities estimated by $\boldsymbol{p}$. For example, $\pi_1 = \Pr(\text{FFF})$ is the probability of a favorable response to all three drugs. Now, let p_A, p_B, and p_C denote the marginal proportions with a favorable response to drugs A, B, and C, respectively, and let π_A, π_B, and π_C denote the corresponding marginal probabilities. For example,

$$\pi_A = \Pr(\text{FFF or FFU or FUF or FUU}).$$

Note that $p_1, \ldots, p_8$ are the underlying multinomial proportions from the cross-classification of the values of the response variable at the three occasions, and p_A, p_B, and p_C are the marginal proportions. Similarly, $\pi_1, \ldots, \pi_8$ are the underlying multinomial probabilities, and π_A, π_B, and π_C are marginal probabilities. Although the same symbol is used for both types of proportions (probabilities), the differing types of subscripts are sufficient to distinguish these in this example. The vectors $\boldsymbol{p}$ and $\boldsymbol{\pi}$, however, refer to the underlying multinomial proportions and probabilities, respectively.

The vector of response functions $\boldsymbol{F}(\boldsymbol{p}) = (p_A, p_B, p_C)'$ can be computed by the linear transformation $\boldsymbol{F}(\boldsymbol{p}) = \boldsymbol{A}\boldsymbol{p}$, where

$$\boldsymbol{A} = \begin{pmatrix} 1 & 1 & 1 & 1 & 0 & 0 & 0 & 0 \\ 1 & 1 & 0 & 0 & 1 & 1 & 0 & 0 \\ 1 & 0 & 1 & 0 & 1 & 0 & 1 & 0 \end{pmatrix}.$$

The first row of $\boldsymbol{A}$ sums p_1, p_2, p_3, and p_4 to compute the proportion of subjects with a favorable response to drug A. Similarly, the second row of $\boldsymbol{A}$ sums p_1, p_2, p_5, and p_6 to yield the proportion with a favorable response to drug B. Finally, the corresponding proportion for drug C is computed by summing p_1, p_3, p_5, and p_7. The resulting vector of response functions is

$$\boldsymbol{F}(\boldsymbol{p}) = \begin{pmatrix} 0.60870 \\ 0.60870 \\ 0.34783 \end{pmatrix}.$$

The hypothesis of marginal homogeneity specifies that the marginal probabilities of a favorable response to drugs A, B, and C are equal. This hypothesis can be tested by fitting a model of the form $\boldsymbol{F}(\boldsymbol{\pi}) = \boldsymbol{X}\boldsymbol{\beta}$, where $\boldsymbol{X}$ is a known model matrix and $\boldsymbol{\beta}$ is a vector of unknown parameters. The most straightforward approach might be to fit the model

$$\boldsymbol{F}(\boldsymbol{\pi}) = \begin{pmatrix} 1 \\ 1 \\ 1 \end{pmatrix} \beta.$$

Because there are three response functions and one parameter, the lack-of-fit statistic W has $3 - 1 = 2$ degrees of freedom (df). With this choice of model matrix $\boldsymbol{X}$, the statistic W tests marginal homogeneity.

Using the model matrix $\boldsymbol{X} = (1, 1, 1)'$, the value of W is 6.58. With reference to the χ^2_2 distribution, $p = 0.037$. Therefore, the hypothesis of marginal homogeneity is rejected.

Another approach to this problem would be to fit a saturated model with

$$\boldsymbol{X} = \begin{pmatrix} 1 & 1 & 0 \\ 1 & 0 & 1 \\ 1 & -1 & -1 \end{pmatrix}, \qquad \boldsymbol{\beta} = \begin{pmatrix} \mu \\ \alpha_1 \\ \alpha_2 \end{pmatrix}.$$

This model includes an overall intercept and two parameters for the drug effect, which is parameterized using a "sum-to-zero" parameterization. Because this model is saturated, there are 0 df for lack of fit. In this case, the hypothesis of marginal homogeneity is specified as $H_0\colon \boldsymbol{C}\boldsymbol{\beta} = 0$, where

$$\boldsymbol{C} = \begin{pmatrix} 0 & 1 & 0 \\ 0 & 0 & 1 \end{pmatrix}.$$

The vector of estimated parameters is $\boldsymbol{b} = (0.5217, 0.0870, 0.0870)'$, and the test of marginal homogeneity is

$$W_C = (\boldsymbol{C}\boldsymbol{b})'[\boldsymbol{C}(\boldsymbol{X}'\boldsymbol{V}^{-1}\boldsymbol{X})^{-1}\boldsymbol{C}']^{-1}\boldsymbol{C}\boldsymbol{b} = 6.58$$

with 2 df, as before.

7.3.3 *One Population, Dichotomous Response, Repeated Measurements Factor Is Ordered*

Table 7.4 displays data from a longitudinal study of the health effects of air pollution (Ware et al., 1988). Agresti (1990) reported data from one component of this study, in which 1019 children were examined annually at ages 9, 10, 11, and 12 years. At each examination, the response variable was the presence or absence of wheezing. The questions of interest include:

- Does the prevalence of wheezing change with age?

TABLE 7.4. Classification of 1019 children by wheezing status

Presence of Wheezing				Number of
Age 9	Age 10	Age 11	Age 12	Children
Yes	Yes	Yes	Yes	94
Yes	Yes	Yes	No	30
Yes	Yes	No	Yes	15
Yes	Yes	No	No	28
Yes	No	Yes	Yes	14
Yes	No	Yes	No	9
Yes	No	No	Yes	12
Yes	No	No	No	63
No	Yes	Yes	Yes	19
No	Yes	Yes	No	15
No	Yes	No	Yes	10
No	Yes	No	No	44
No	No	Yes	Yes	17
No	No	Yes	No	42
No	No	No	Yes	35
No	No	No	No	572
Number of subjects				1019

- Is there a quantifiable trend in the age-specific prevalence rates?

In this example, there are $c = 2$ values of the outcome variable at each time point, $t = 4$ time points, and $c^t = 2^4 = 16$ response profiles. Note that Table 7.4 displays the counts for each of the 16 response profiles rather than the individual responses at the four time points for each child.

Let $\boldsymbol{p}$ denote the 16×1 vector of proportions corresponding to the multiway cross-classification of response at the four ages (ordered as shown in Table 7.4), and let P_x denote the marginal prevalence of wheezing at age x for $x = 9, \ldots, 12$. The response functions of interest are given by

$$\boldsymbol{F}(\boldsymbol{p}) = (P_9, P_{10}, P_{11}, P_{12})' = \boldsymbol{A}\boldsymbol{p},$$

where $\boldsymbol{A}$ is the 4×16 matrix

$$\begin{pmatrix} 1 & 1 & 1 & 1 & 1 & 1 & 1 & 1 & 0 & 0 & 0 & 0 & 0 & 0 & 0 & 0 \\ 1 & 1 & 1 & 1 & 0 & 0 & 0 & 0 & 1 & 1 & 1 & 1 & 0 & 0 & 0 & 0 \\ 1 & 1 & 0 & 0 & 1 & 1 & 0 & 0 & 1 & 1 & 0 & 0 & 1 & 1 & 0 & 0 \\ 1 & 0 & 1 & 0 & 1 & 0 & 1 & 0 & 1 & 0 & 1 & 0 & 1 & 0 & 1 & 0 \end{pmatrix}.$$

Thus, we have

$$\boldsymbol{F}(\boldsymbol{p}) = \begin{pmatrix} P_9 \\ P_{10} \\ P_{11} \\ P_{12} \end{pmatrix} = \begin{pmatrix} 0.26006 \\ 0.25025 \\ 0.23553 \\ 0.21197 \end{pmatrix}.$$

The question of whether the prevalence of wheezing changes with age is addressed by testing marginal homogeneity—that is, by testing

$$H_0\colon \Pi_9 = \Pi_{10} = \Pi_{11} = \Pi_{12},$$

where Π_x denotes the marginal probability of wheezing at age x. Several possible models of the form $\boldsymbol{F}(\boldsymbol{\pi}) = \boldsymbol{X}\boldsymbol{\beta}$ can be used to test this hypothesis. For example, the test of H_0 is given by the lack-of-fit statistic W if the model matrix

$$\boldsymbol{X} = \begin{pmatrix} 1 \\ 1 \\ 1 \\ 1 \end{pmatrix}$$

is used. Alternatively, the saturated model could be fit using the model matrix

$$\boldsymbol{X} = \begin{pmatrix} 1 & 1 & 0 & 0 \\ 1 & 0 & 1 & 0 \\ 1 & 0 & 0 & 1 \\ 1 & -1 & -1 & -1 \end{pmatrix}.$$

In this case, the test of H_0 is the test that the last three components of $\boldsymbol{\beta}$ are jointly equal to zero.

A useful approach that facilitates further model reduction, however, is the model $\boldsymbol{F}(\boldsymbol{\pi}) = \boldsymbol{X}_1\boldsymbol{\beta}$, where

$$\boldsymbol{X}_1 = \begin{pmatrix} 1 & -3 & 1 & -1 \\ 1 & -1 & -1 & 3 \\ 1 & 1 & -1 & -3 \\ 1 & 3 & 1 & 1 \end{pmatrix}, \qquad \boldsymbol{\beta} = \begin{pmatrix} \beta_0 \\ \beta_1 \\ \beta_2 \\ \beta_3 \end{pmatrix}.$$

This model parameterizes the effect of age using orthogonal polynomial coefficients for equally spaced time points (Pearson and Hartley, 1972, Table 47). The hypothesis of marginal homogeneity is $H_0\colon \boldsymbol{C}\boldsymbol{\beta} = \boldsymbol{0}$, where

$$\boldsymbol{C} = \begin{pmatrix} 0 & 1 & 0 & 0 \\ 0 & 0 & 1 & 0 \\ 0 & 0 & 0 & 1 \end{pmatrix}.$$

Because $W_C = 12.85$ with 3 df, this hypothesis is rejected ($p = 0.005$). This model also permits testing of the linear ($H_0\colon \beta_1 = 0$) and nonlinear ($H_0\colon \beta_2 = \beta_3 = 0$) components of the age effect. Although the linear component is highly significant ($W_C = 11.88$ with 1 df, $p = 0.0006$), the test of nonlinearity is not significant ($W_C = 0.54$ with 2 df, $p = 0.76$).

The results of the saturated model motivate the reduced model

$$\boldsymbol{F}(\boldsymbol{\pi}) = \boldsymbol{X}_2\boldsymbol{\beta},$$

where

$$\boldsymbol{X}_2 = \begin{pmatrix} 1 & 0 \\ 1 & 1 \\ 1 & 2 \\ 1 & 3 \end{pmatrix}, \qquad \boldsymbol{\beta} = \begin{pmatrix} \beta_0 \\ \beta_1 \end{pmatrix}.$$

The lack-of-fit statistic W is 0.54 with 2 df, indicating that the model provides a good fit. In this model, the estimated parameters have substantive interpretations. The intercept, $\widehat{\beta}_0 = 0.263$, is the predicted probability of wheezing at age 9. The estimated standard error of $\widehat{\beta}_0$ is 0.013. Similarly, $\widehat{\beta}_1 = -0.016$ is the estimated annual decline in the marginal probability of wheezing. The estimated standard error of $\widehat{\beta}_1$ is 0.005, and the Wald statistic assessing the significance of this parameter is highly significant ($W_C = 12.3$ with 1 df, $p = 0.0005$). Predicted marginal probabilities of wheezing at each age can then be estimated along with their standard errors.

In the preceding model, the marginal probability of wheezing at age x was modeled as a linear function of age:

$$\Pi_x = \beta_0 + \beta_1(x - 9), \qquad x = 9, 10, 11, 12.$$

It may also be of interest to analyze these data on the logit scale using the response functions

$$L_x = \log\left(\frac{\Pi_x}{1 - \Pi_x}\right).$$

In this case, the effect of age is multiplicative (instead of additive), predicted marginal probabilities are constrained to be between 0 and 1, and the estimated parameters have odds-ratio interpretations.

The marginal logit response functions can be defined as

$$\boldsymbol{F}(\boldsymbol{p}) = \boldsymbol{A}_2 \log(\boldsymbol{A}_1 \boldsymbol{p}),$$

where $\boldsymbol{p}$ is the 16×1 vector of multinomial proportions corresponding to the ordering in Table 7.4, $\boldsymbol{A}_1$ is the 8×16 matrix

$$\begin{pmatrix} 1 & 1 & 1 & 1 & 1 & 1 & 1 & 1 & 0 & 0 & 0 & 0 & 0 & 0 & 0 & 0 \\ 0 & 0 & 0 & 0 & 0 & 0 & 0 & 0 & 1 & 1 & 1 & 1 & 1 & 1 & 1 & 1 \\ 1 & 1 & 1 & 1 & 0 & 0 & 0 & 0 & 1 & 1 & 1 & 1 & 0 & 0 & 0 & 0 \\ 0 & 0 & 0 & 0 & 1 & 1 & 1 & 1 & 0 & 0 & 0 & 0 & 1 & 1 & 1 & 1 \\ 1 & 1 & 0 & 0 & 1 & 1 & 0 & 0 & 1 & 1 & 0 & 0 & 1 & 1 & 0 & 0 \\ 0 & 0 & 1 & 1 & 0 & 0 & 1 & 1 & 0 & 0 & 1 & 1 & 0 & 0 & 1 & 1 \\ 1 & 0 & 1 & 0 & 1 & 0 & 1 & 0 & 1 & 0 & 1 & 0 & 1 & 0 & 1 & 0 \\ 0 & 1 & 0 & 1 & 0 & 1 & 0 & 1 & 0 & 1 & 0 & 1 & 0 & 1 & 0 & 1 \end{pmatrix},$$

and $\boldsymbol{A}_2$ is the 4×8 matrix

$$\begin{pmatrix} 1 & -1 & 0 & 0 & 0 & 0 & 0 & 0 \\ 0 & 0 & 1 & -1 & 0 & 0 & 0 & 0 \\ 0 & 0 & 0 & 0 & 1 & -1 & 0 & 0 \\ 0 & 0 & 0 & 0 & 0 & 0 & 1 & -1 \end{pmatrix}.$$

Observe that rows 1, 3, 5, and 7 of $\boldsymbol{A}_1$ calculate the marginal proportions with wheezing present at ages 9–12, respectively, whereas rows 2, 4, 6, and 8 calculate the corresponding marginal proportions with wheezing absent. The four rows of $\boldsymbol{A}_2$ then compute the marginal logits at ages 9 12, respectively. $\boldsymbol{F}(\boldsymbol{p})$ is then the 4×1 vector of observed marginal logits

$$\begin{pmatrix} \widehat{L}_9 \\ \widehat{L}_{10} \\ \widehat{L}_{11} \\ \widehat{L}_{12} \end{pmatrix} = \begin{pmatrix} -1.046 \\ -1.097 \\ -1.177 \\ -1.313 \end{pmatrix}.$$

We can now use the model matrix

$$\boldsymbol{X}_2 = \begin{pmatrix} 1 & 0 \\ 1 & 1 \\ 1 & 2 \\ 1 & 3 \end{pmatrix}$$

to fit the same model $\boldsymbol{F}(\boldsymbol{\pi}) = \boldsymbol{X}_2\boldsymbol{\beta}$ as was fit on the proportion scale. This model also provides a good fit to the observed data ($W = 0.67$ with 2 df, $p = 0.72$), indicating that the nonlinear effects of age are nonsignificant. In addition, the linear effect of age is highly significant ($W_{\boldsymbol{C}} = 11.77$ with 1 df, $p < 0.001$). The results of these tests are similar to those from the linear model on the proportion scale.

The predicted model is

$$\widehat{L}_x = -1.028 - 0.088x.$$

Thus, we estimate that the log-odds in favor of wheezing decrease by 0.088 per year. Therefore, the estimated odds of wheezing are $e^{-0.088} = 0.92$ times as great at age x than at age $x-1$. Equivalently, we can state that the estimated odds against wheezing are 1.09 (= 1/0.92) times as high at age x than at age $x-1$.

In this example, the model hypothesizing a linear relationship between the response variable and age provided a good fit to the data both on the probability scale and also on the logit scale. Both models provide the same general conclusion—namely, that the probability of wheezing decreases as age increases. In general, the choice between an additive model on the probability scale and a multiplicative model on the logit scale might be based on subject matter considerations or on considerations related to model fit.

7.3.4 One Population, Polytomous Response

When the response is dichotomous, there is one response function per time point. Therefore, if there are t time points, the test of marginal homogeneity has $t-1$ df. If the response variable y_{ij} has c possible outcomes, then there are at most $c-1$ linearly independent response functions per time point. In this case, the test of marginal homogeneity has $(c-1)(t-1)$ df.

As an example, Table 7.5 displays data from the Iowa 65+ Rural Health Study (Cornoni-Huntley et al., 1986). In this example, 1926 elderly individuals were followed over a six-year period. Each individual was surveyed at years 0, 3, and 6. One of the variables of interest was the number of friends reported by each respondent. This was an ordered categorical variable with possible values 0 friends, 1–2 friends, and 3 or more friends. Table 7.5 displays the cross-classification of the responses at years 0, 3, and 6 for these 1926 individuals. The goal is to determine whether the distribution of the number of reported friends is changing over time.

In this example, there are $c = 3$ values of the outcome variable at each time point, $t = 3$ time points, and $c^t = 3^3 = 27$ response profiles. Note that Table 7.5 displays the counts for each of the 27 response profiles rather than the individual responses at the three time points for each subject.

Let $\boldsymbol{p}$ denote the 27×1 vector of proportions corresponding to the multiway cross-classification of response at the three survey years (ordered as shown in Table 7.5). Also, let p_{ij} denote the marginal proportion of subjects at year i in response category j for $i = 0, 3, 6$ and $j = 0, 1, 3$. Note that the index 1 for j represents the category of 1–2 friends, and the index 3 represents the category 3+ friends. As in Section 7.3.2, the subscripts are sufficient to distinguish marginal proportions from underlying multinomial proportions.

One choice for the vector of linearly independent response functions is to select the first two marginal proportions at each time point. In this case,

$$\boldsymbol{F}(\boldsymbol{p}) = (p_{00}, p_{01}, p_{30}, p_{31}, p_{60}, p_{61})' = \boldsymbol{A}\boldsymbol{p},$$

where $\boldsymbol{A}$ is the 6×27 matrix

$$\begin{pmatrix} 1&1&1&1&1&1&1&1&1&0&0&0&0&0&0&0&0&0&0&0&0&0&0&0&0&0&0 \\ 0&0&0&0&0&0&0&0&0&1&1&1&1&1&1&1&1&1&0&0&0&0&0&0&0&0&0 \\ 1&1&1&0&0&0&0&0&0&1&1&1&0&0&0&0&0&0&1&1&1&0&0&0&0&0&0 \\ 0&0&0&1&1&1&0&0&0&0&0&0&1&1&1&0&0&0&0&0&0&1&1&1&0&0&0 \\ 1&0&0&1&0&0&1&0&0&1&0&0&1&0&0&1&0&0&1&0&0&1&0&0&1&0&0 \\ 0&1&0&0&1&0&0&1&0&0&1&0&0&1&0&0&1&0&0&1&0&0&1&0&0&1&0 \end{pmatrix}.$$

The resulting vector of response functions is

$$\boldsymbol{F}(\boldsymbol{p}) = \begin{pmatrix} 0.196 \\ 0.238 \\ 0.122 \\ 0.229 \\ 0.084 \\ 0.181 \end{pmatrix}.$$

The question of whether the distribution of the number of friends changes over the three survey years is addressed by testing marginal homogeneity—

TABLE 7.5. Classification of 1926 Iowa 65+ Study participants by number of friends

Year 0	Year 3	Year 6	Number of Subjects
0	0	0	31
0	0	1–2	22
0	0	3+	54
0	1–2	0	15
0	1–2	1–2	25
0	1–2	3+	50
0	3+	0	22
0	3+	1–2	20
0	3+	3+	139
1–2	0	0	11
1–2	0	1–2	13
1–2	0	3+	30
1–2	1–2	0	12
1–2	1–2	1–2	64
1–2	1–2	3+	82
1–2	3+	0	13
1–2	3+	1–2	44
1–2	3+	3+	189
3+	0	0	9
3+	0	1–2	21
3+	0	3+	44
3+	1–2	0	18
3+	1–2	1–2	55
3+	1–2	3+	121
3+	3+	0	31
3+	3+	1–2	85
3+	3+	3+	706
Total number of subjects			1926

that is, by testing

$$H_0: \pi_{00} = \pi_{30} = \pi_{60}, \pi_{01} = \pi_{31} = \pi_{61},$$

where π_{ij} denotes the marginal probability of being in response category j at year i for $i = 0, 3, 6$ and $j = 0, 1, 3$. This hypothesis can be tested by fitting the model $\boldsymbol{F}(\boldsymbol{\pi}) = \boldsymbol{X\beta}$, where

$$\boldsymbol{X} = \begin{pmatrix} 1 & 0 \\ 0 & 1 \\ 1 & 0 \\ 0 & 1 \\ 1 & 0 \\ 0 & 1 \end{pmatrix}, \qquad \boldsymbol{\beta} = \begin{pmatrix} \beta_0 \\ \beta_1 \end{pmatrix}.$$

In this parameterization, β_0 is the probability of having 0 friends, and β_1 is the probability of having 1–2 friends; both of these probabilities are assumed to be common across the three surveys. The test of H_0 is given by the lack-of-fit statistic W. In this example, $W = 184.23$ with $6 - 2 = 4$ df, indicating a highly significant departure from marginal homogeneity ($p < 0.001$).

For nominal response variables, the natural linear response functions are marginal proportions. For ordinal response variables, other types of linear response functions that can be considered include cumulative marginal proportions and mean scores.

Provided that meaningful scores can be assigned to the levels of an ordered categorical response variable, one can analyze the change in the mean score over time (rather than the change in the entire distribution). We now have a single response function per time point and the hypothesis of homogeneity of means over time has $t - 1$ df (instead of $(c - 1)(t - 1)$ df).

In the general situation, consider an ordinal or discrete numeric response variable with c categories measured at each of t time points. Let a_j denote the score assigned to the jth level of the response for $j = 1, \ldots, c$. Let $\boldsymbol{F}_1(\boldsymbol{p}) = \boldsymbol{A}_1\boldsymbol{p}$ denote the $ct \times 1$ vector of marginal proportions, where $\boldsymbol{p}$ is the $c^t \times 1$ vector of underlying multinomial proportions and $\boldsymbol{A}_1$ is a $ct \times c^t$ matrix. The $t \times 1$ vector of marginal mean scores is given by

$$\boldsymbol{F}_2(\boldsymbol{p}) = \boldsymbol{A}_2\big(\boldsymbol{F}_1(\boldsymbol{p})\big),$$

where $\boldsymbol{A}_2$ is the $t \times ct$ matrix

$$\begin{pmatrix} a_1 \cdots a_c & 0 \cdots 0 & \cdots & 0 \cdots 0 \\ 0 \cdots 0 & a_1 \cdots a_c & \vdots & \vdots \\ \cdots\cdots & \cdots\cdots & \cdots & \cdots\cdots \\ 0 \cdots 0 & 0 \cdots 0 & \cdots & a_1 \cdots a_c \end{pmatrix}.$$

In this example, one possible choice of scores for the response categories 0, 1–2, 3+ is $a_1 = 0$, $a_2 = 1.5$, $a_3 = 4$. The 3×1 vector of marginal mean scores can be computed as

$$F(p) = A_2(A_1(p)),$$

where

$$A_1 = \begin{pmatrix}
1&1&1&1&1&1&1&1&1&0&0&0&0&0&0&0&0&0&0&0&0&0&0&0&0&0&0\\
0&0&0&0&0&0&0&0&0&1&1&1&1&1&1&1&1&1&0&0&0&0&0&0&0&0&0\\
0&0&0&0&0&0&0&0&0&0&0&0&0&0&0&0&0&0&1&1&1&1&1&1&1&1&1\\
1&1&1&0&0&0&0&0&0&1&1&1&0&0&0&0&0&0&1&1&1&0&0&0&0&0&0\\
0&0&0&1&1&1&0&0&0&0&0&0&1&1&1&0&0&0&0&0&0&1&1&1&0&0&0\\
0&0&0&0&0&0&1&1&1&0&0&0&0&0&0&1&1&1&0&0&0&0&0&0&1&1&1\\
1&0&0&1&0&0&1&0&0&1&0&0&1&0&0&1&0&0&1&0&0&1&0&0&1&0&0\\
0&1&0&0&1&0&0&1&0&0&1&0&0&1&0&0&1&0&0&1&0&0&1&0&0&1&0\\
0&0&1&0&0&1&0&0&1&0&0&1&0&0&1&0&0&1&0&0&1&0&0&1&0&0&1
\end{pmatrix}$$

and

$$A_2 = \begin{pmatrix}
0 & 1.5 & 4 & 0 & 0 & 0 & 0 & 0 & 0\\
0 & 0 & 0 & 0 & 1.5 & 4 & 0 & 0 & 0\\
0 & 0 & 0 & 0 & 0 & 0 & 0 & 1.5 & 4
\end{pmatrix}.$$

Of course, because the score for the first category is 0, the definition of the mean-score response functions can be simplified by omitting the first, fourth, and seventh rows of A_1 and the first, fourth, and seventh columns of A_2. In this case, we have

$$A_1 = \begin{pmatrix}
0&0&0&0&0&0&0&0&0&1&1&1&1&1&1&1&1&1&0&0&0&0&0&0&0&0&0\\
0&0&0&0&0&0&0&0&0&0&0&0&0&0&0&0&0&0&1&1&1&1&1&1&1&1&1\\
0&0&0&1&1&1&0&0&0&0&0&0&1&1&1&0&0&0&0&0&0&1&1&1&0&0&0\\
0&0&0&0&0&0&1&1&1&0&0&0&0&0&0&1&1&1&0&0&0&0&0&0&1&1&1\\
0&1&0&0&1&0&0&1&0&0&1&0&0&1&0&0&1&0&0&1&0&0&1&0&0&1&0\\
0&0&1&0&0&1&0&0&1&0&0&1&0&0&1&0&0&1&0&0&1&0&0&1&0&0&1
\end{pmatrix}$$

and

$$A_2 = \begin{pmatrix}
1.5 & 4 & 0 & 0 & 0 & 0\\
0 & 0 & 1.5 & 4 & 0 & 0\\
0 & 0 & 0 & 0 & 1.5 & 4
\end{pmatrix}.$$

With either choice of matrices A_1 and A_2, $F(p)$ is the 3×1 vector of correlated marginal mean scores

$$\begin{pmatrix} \widehat{m}_0 \\ \widehat{m}_3 \\ \widehat{m}_6 \end{pmatrix} = \begin{pmatrix} 2.62 \\ 2.94 \\ 3.21 \end{pmatrix}.$$

If we fit the model $F(\pi) = X\beta$, where $X' = (1, 1, 1)$, the hypothesis of marginal homogeneity of mean scores is tested using the lack-of-fit statistic W. The value of this statistic is 178.5 with $3-2=1$ df, indicating a highly significant departure from marginal homogeneity ($p < 0.001$).

One could also fit the model $\boldsymbol{F}(\boldsymbol{\pi}) = \boldsymbol{X}\beta$, where

$$\boldsymbol{X} = \begin{pmatrix} 1 & 0 \\ 1 & 3 \\ 1 & 6 \end{pmatrix}, \qquad \boldsymbol{\beta} = \begin{pmatrix} \beta_0 \\ \beta_1 \end{pmatrix}.$$

This model assumes that there is a linear trend in the marginal mean scores over time. The lack-of-fit statistic $W = 0.42$ with 1 df tests the hypothesis that the nonlinear component of the relationship between the mean score and time is equal to zero ($p = 0.52$). The estimated intercept is $\widehat{\beta}_0 = 2.629$ with an estimated standard error of 0.035. The estimated slope from this model is $\widehat{\beta}_1 = 0.098$ with an estimated standard error of 0.007. The test of $H_0\colon \beta_1 = 0$ indicates that the linear effect of survey year is highly significant ($W_C = 178.0$ with 1 df, $p < 0.001$). The resulting model is

$$\widehat{m}_j = 2.629 + 0.098j, \qquad j = 0, 3, 6.$$

Under the assumption that the marginal mean score represents the mean number of friends, this model indicates that the mean number of friends is estimated to increase by 0.098 per year.

7.3.5 Multiple Populations, Dichotomous Response

The previous examples involved the analysis of correlated response functions from a single population. This section extends the methodology to situations in which there are multiple groups of subjects.

The Iowa 65+ Rural Health Study (Cornoni-Huntley et al., 1986) followed a cohort of elderly males and females over a six-year period. At each of three surveys, the response to one of the variables of interest, church attendance, was classified as "yes" if the subject attends church regularly, or "no" if the subject does not attend church regularly. Table 7.6 displays the data from the 1311 females and 662 males who responded to all three surveys. Interest focuses on determining whether church attendance rates are changing over time, whether the attendance rates differ between females and males, and whether the observed patterns of change over time are the same for females and males.

When you obtain repeated measures data from multiple populations, you are interested not only in the effect of the repeated measures factor but also in the effect of the explanatory variables defining the multiple populations. In fact, when there are explanatory variables (factors) in a study involving repeated measures, there are three different types of variation:

- main effects and interactions of the repeated measurement factors (within-subjects variation);
- main effects and interactions of the explanatory variables (between-subjects variation);

TABLE 7.6. Classification of 1973 Iowa 65+ Study participants by regular church attendance

	Regularly Attended Church at			
Sex	Year 0	Year 3	Year 6	Count
Female	Yes	Yes	Yes	904
	Yes	Yes	No	88
	Yes	No	Yes	25
	Yes	No	No	51
	No	Yes	Yes	33
	No	Yes	No	22
	No	No	Yes	30
	No	No	No	158
Male	Yes	Yes	Yes	391
	Yes	Yes	No	36
	Yes	No	Yes	12
	Yes	No	No	26
	No	Yes	Yes	15
	No	Yes	No	21
	No	No	Yes	18
	No	No	No	143

- interactions between the explanatory variables and the repeated measurement factors.

In this example, there are two populations (females, males). Because a dichotomous response variable is measured at each of three time points (the repeated measurement factor), there are $r = 2^3 = 8$ response profiles. The between-subjects variation is due to differences between females and males, and the within-subjects variation is due to differences among time points. The analysis investigates both sources of variation as well as the variation due to their interaction.

Let $\boldsymbol{p}_h$ denote the underlying 8×1 multinomial proportion vector in subpopulation h, where $h = 1$ for females and $h = 2$ for males. The components of $\boldsymbol{p}_h$ are ordered as shown in Table 7.6. Suppose that the response functions of interest in this example are the marginal proportions p_{hj} of subjects from population h who regularly attend church at year j for $h = 1, 2$ and $j = 0, 3, 6$. In each subpopulation, let $\boldsymbol{F}(\boldsymbol{p}_h)$ denote the 3×1 vector of marginal proportions:

$$\boldsymbol{F}(\boldsymbol{p}_h) = (p_{h0}, p_{h3}, p_{h6})'.$$

In the case of multiple populations, the response functions are defined for each subpopulation. In population h, $\boldsymbol{F}(\boldsymbol{p}_h) = \boldsymbol{A}\boldsymbol{p}_h$, where

$$\boldsymbol{A} = \begin{pmatrix} 1 & 1 & 1 & 1 & 0 & 0 & 0 & 0 \\ 1 & 1 & 0 & 0 & 1 & 1 & 0 & 0 \\ 1 & 0 & 1 & 0 & 1 & 0 & 1 & 0 \end{pmatrix}.$$

In this example,

$$\boldsymbol{F}(\boldsymbol{p}_1) = \begin{pmatrix} 0.815 \\ 0.799 \\ 0.757 \end{pmatrix}, \quad \boldsymbol{F}(\boldsymbol{p}_2) = \begin{pmatrix} 0.702 \\ 0.699 \\ 0.659 \end{pmatrix}, \quad \boldsymbol{F}(\boldsymbol{p}) = \begin{pmatrix} \boldsymbol{F}(\boldsymbol{p}_1) \\ \boldsymbol{F}(\boldsymbol{p}_2) \end{pmatrix}.$$

The estimated covariance matrix of $\boldsymbol{F}(\boldsymbol{p})$ is the 6×6 matrix

$$\widehat{\boldsymbol{V}}_{\boldsymbol{F}} = \begin{pmatrix} \widehat{\boldsymbol{V}}_{\boldsymbol{F}_1} & \boldsymbol{0}_{(3\times 3)} \\ \boldsymbol{0}_{(3\times 3)} & \widehat{\boldsymbol{V}}_{\boldsymbol{F}_2} \end{pmatrix},$$

where $\widehat{\boldsymbol{V}}_{\boldsymbol{F}_h}$ is the estimated covariance matrix of $\boldsymbol{F}(\boldsymbol{p}_h)$.

One approach to the analysis of these data is first to fit a saturated model with separate parameters for females and males. Consider the model $\boldsymbol{F}(\boldsymbol{\pi}) = \boldsymbol{X}_1\boldsymbol{\beta}$, where

$$\boldsymbol{X}_1 = \begin{pmatrix} 1 & -1 & 1 & 0 & 0 & 0 \\ 1 & 0 & -2 & 0 & 0 & 0 \\ 1 & 1 & 1 & 0 & 0 & 0 \\ 0 & 0 & 0 & 1 & -1 & 1 \\ 0 & 0 & 0 & 1 & 0 & -2 \\ 0 & 0 & 0 & 1 & 1 & 1 \end{pmatrix}, \quad \boldsymbol{\beta} = \begin{pmatrix} \beta_{10} \\ \beta_{11} \\ \beta_{12} \\ \beta_{20} \\ \beta_{21} \\ \beta_{22} \end{pmatrix}.$$

In this parameterization, β_{h0}, β_{h1}, and β_{h2} are the intercept, linear time effect, and quadratic time effect for subpopulation h. Because the surveys were equally spaced, orthogonal polynomial coefficients are used for the time effects. Based on the results of hypothesis tests of interest concerning the parameters of the saturated model, we will then fit an appropriate reduced model.

Table 7.7 displays the coefficient matrices $\boldsymbol{C}$ for testing several hypotheses of the form $H_0: \boldsymbol{C}\boldsymbol{\beta} = 0$ along with the corresponding test statistics $W_{\boldsymbol{C}}$, degrees of freedom, and p-values. The effect of survey year is highly significant in both sexes combined as well as in females and males separately. In addition, the linear effect of survey year is significant in females, in males, and jointly. The joint test of nonlinearity in females and males is nearly significant, as are the separate tests of nonlinearity in females and in males. Finally, whereas the intercepts for females and males differ significantly, both the linear and quadratic survey-year effects do not differ significantly between females and males.

TABLE 7.7. Results of hypothesis tests from the saturated marginal probability model for the church attendance data

Hypothesis	C						W_C	df	p-value
No year effect	0	1	0	0	0	0	41.45	4	< 0.001
	0	0	1	0	0	0			
	0	0	0	0	1	0			
	0	0	0	0	0	1			
No year effect in females	0	1	0	0	0	0	30.46	2	< 0.001
	0	0	1	0	0	0			
No year effect in males	0	0	0	0	1	0	11.00	2	0.004
	0	0	0	0	0	1			
No linear year effect	0	1	0	0	0	0	38.20	2	< 0.001
	0	0	0	0	1	0			
No linear year effect in females	0	1	0	0	0	0	29.23	1	< 0.001
No linear year effect in males	0	0	0	0	1	0	8.97	1	0.003
No quadratic year effect	0	0	1	0	0	0	5.74	2	0.057
	0	0	0	0	0	1			
No quadratic year effect in females	0	0	1	0	0	0	2.97	1	0.085
No quadratic year effect in males	0	0	0	0	0	1	2.76	1	0.096
Equality of intercepts	1	0	0	−1	0	0	30.04	1	< 0.001
Equality of linear year effects	0	1	0	0	−1	0	0.61	1	0.435
Equality of quadratic year effects	0	0	1	0	0	−1	0.19	1	0.664

TABLE 7.8. Results of hypothesis tests from the reduced marginal probability model for the church attendance data

Hypothesis	$\boldsymbol{C}$	$W_{\boldsymbol{C}}$	df	p-value
No linear year effect	0 0 1 0	37.67	1	< 0.001
No quadratic year effect	0 0 0 1	5.47	1	0.019
Equality of intercepts	1 −1 0 0	30.63	1	< 0.001

A reasonable reduced model is $\boldsymbol{F}(\boldsymbol{\pi}) = \boldsymbol{X}_2\boldsymbol{\beta}$, where

$$\boldsymbol{X}_2 = \begin{pmatrix} 1 & 0 & -1 & 1 \\ 1 & 0 & 0 & -2 \\ 1 & 0 & 1 & 1 \\ 0 & 1 & -1 & 1 \\ 0 & 1 & 0 & -2 \\ 0 & 1 & 1 & 1 \end{pmatrix}, \qquad \boldsymbol{\beta} = \begin{pmatrix} \beta_{10} \\ \beta_{20} \\ \beta_1 \\ \beta_2 \end{pmatrix}.$$

In this parameterization, β_{10} and β_{20} are intercepts for females and males, respectively, and β_1 and β_2 are the common linear and quadratic effects of survey year. The lack-of-fit statistic W has 2 df and tests the hypothesis that the interaction between sex and survey year is equal to zero. Because $W = 0.87$ with 2 df, this model provides a good fit to the observed data.

Table 7.8 displays the coefficient matrices $\boldsymbol{C}$ for testing several hypotheses of the form $H_0\colon \boldsymbol{C\beta} = 0$ along with the corresponding test statistics $W_{\boldsymbol{C}}$, degrees of freedom, and p-values. Both the linear and quadratic survey-year effects are significantly different from zero. In addition, the intercepts for females and males are significantly different.

The parameter estimates are

$$\widehat{\beta}_{10} = 0.7905, \quad \widehat{\beta}_{20} = 0.6865, \quad \widehat{\beta}_1 = -0.0265, \quad \widehat{\beta}_2 = -0.00489.$$

Thus, the estimated probability of regular church attendance decreases over time. The rate of change is nonlinear; the decrease from year 0 to year 3 is less than the decrease from year 3 to year 6. At each time point, females are more likely than males to attend church regularly. The estimated difference in the probability of regular church attendance between females and males is $0.7905 - 0.6865 = 0.104$.

To produce parameter estimates that are more easily interpretable, this model will be refit on the natural time scale (years) instead of using orthogonal polynomial coefficients. The model is $\boldsymbol{F}(\boldsymbol{\pi}) = \boldsymbol{X}_3\boldsymbol{\beta}$, where

$$\boldsymbol{X}_3 = \begin{pmatrix} 1 & 0 & 0 & 0 \\ 1 & 0 & 3 & 9 \\ 1 & 0 & 6 & 36 \\ 0 & 1 & 0 & 0 \\ 0 & 1 & 3 & 9 \\ 0 & 1 & 6 & 36 \end{pmatrix}, \qquad \boldsymbol{\beta} = \begin{pmatrix} \beta_{10} \\ \beta_{20} \\ \beta_1 \\ \beta_2 \end{pmatrix}.$$

The lack-of-fit statistic W, the test of nonlinearity (H_0: $\beta_2 = 0$), and the test of equality of intercepts (H_0: $\beta_{10} = \beta_{20}$) are unchanged from the previous model. However, the test of H_0: $\beta_1 = 0$ yields $W_C = 0.05$ with 1 df ($p = 0.83$). This is because the linear and quadratic survey-year effects are highly correlated using this parameterization.

The parameter estimates are now

$$\widehat{\beta}_{10} = 0.8122, \quad \widehat{\beta}_{20} = 0.7081, \quad \widehat{\beta}_1 = 0.000932, \quad \widehat{\beta}_2 = -0.00163.$$

Using this parameterization, the intercepts $\widehat{\beta}_{10}$ and $\widehat{\beta}_{20}$ are the estimated probabilities of regular church attendance at year 0 for females and males, respectively. Although $\widehat{\beta}_1$ is positive, the magnitude of $\widehat{\beta}_2$ ensures that the results are identical with those from the model parameterized using orthogonal polynomial coefficients. Also note that the estimated difference in the probability of regular church attendance between females and males is $0.8122 - 0.7081 = 0.104$, the same as from the model $\boldsymbol{F}(\boldsymbol{\pi}) = \boldsymbol{X}_2\boldsymbol{\beta}$.

One might also choose to model these data on the logit scale using the response functions

$$\boldsymbol{F}(\boldsymbol{p}) = \begin{pmatrix} \boldsymbol{F}(\boldsymbol{p}_1) \\ \boldsymbol{F}(\boldsymbol{p}_2) \end{pmatrix},$$

where $\boldsymbol{F}(\boldsymbol{p}_h)$ is now the 3×1 vector of logits of marginal proportions:

$$\boldsymbol{F}(\boldsymbol{p}_h) = \begin{pmatrix} \log\left(\dfrac{p_{h0}}{1 - p_{h0}}\right) \\ \log\left(\dfrac{p_{h3}}{1 - p_{h3}}\right) \\ \log\left(\dfrac{p_{h6}}{1 - p_{h6}}\right) \end{pmatrix}.$$

In this case,

$$\boldsymbol{F}(\boldsymbol{p}_h) = \boldsymbol{A}_2 \log(\boldsymbol{A}_1 \boldsymbol{p}_h),$$

where

$$\boldsymbol{A}_1 = \begin{pmatrix} 1 & 1 & 1 & 1 & 0 & 0 & 0 & 0 \\ 0 & 0 & 0 & 0 & 1 & 1 & 1 & 1 \\ 1 & 1 & 0 & 0 & 1 & 1 & 0 & 0 \\ 0 & 0 & 1 & 1 & 0 & 0 & 1 & 1 \\ 1 & 0 & 1 & 0 & 1 & 0 & 1 & 0 \\ 0 & 1 & 0 & 1 & 0 & 1 & 0 & 1 \end{pmatrix}$$

and

$$\boldsymbol{A}_2 = \begin{pmatrix} 1 & -1 & 0 & 0 & 0 & 0 \\ 0 & 0 & 1 & -1 & 0 & 0 \\ 0 & 0 & 0 & 0 & 1 & -1 \end{pmatrix}.$$

The results of the saturated model $\boldsymbol{F}(\boldsymbol{\pi}) = \boldsymbol{X}_1\boldsymbol{\beta}$ are similar to those of the corresponding model on the probability scale. The reduced model

TABLE 7.9. Results of hypothesis tests from the reduced marginal logit model for the church attendance data

Hypothesis	C	W_C	df	p-value
No linear year effect	0 0 1 0	35.44	1	< 0.001
No quadratic year effect	0 0 0 1	4.98	1	0.026
Equality of intercepts	1 −1 0 0	31.45	1	< 0.001

$\boldsymbol{F}(\boldsymbol{\pi}) = \boldsymbol{X}_2\boldsymbol{\beta}$, where

$$\boldsymbol{X}_2 = \begin{pmatrix} 1 & 0 & -1 & 1 \\ 1 & 0 & 0 & -2 \\ 1 & 0 & 1 & 1 \\ 0 & 1 & -1 & 1 \\ 0 & 1 & 0 & -2 \\ 0 & 1 & 1 & 1 \end{pmatrix}, \quad \boldsymbol{\beta} = \begin{pmatrix} \beta_{10} \\ \beta_{20} \\ \beta_1 \\ \beta_2 \end{pmatrix},$$

also produces results similar to those of the model on the probability scale. The lack-of-fit statistic W has 2 df and tests the hypothesis that the interaction between sex and survey year is equal to zero. Because $W = 2.47$ with 2 df ($p = 0.29$), this model provides a good fit to the observed data.

Table 7.9 displays the coefficient matrices $\boldsymbol{C}$ for testing several hypotheses of the form $H_0\colon \boldsymbol{C\beta} = 0$ along with the corresponding test statistics $W_{\boldsymbol{C}}$, degrees of freedom, and p-values. Both the linear and quadratic survey-year effects are significantly different from zero. In addition, the intercepts for females and males are significantly different.

The parameter estimates are $\widehat{\beta}_{10} = 1.3241$, $\widehat{\beta}_{20} = 0.7911$, $\widehat{\beta}_1 = -0.1385$, and $\widehat{\beta}_2 = -0.0260$. Thus, the estimated logit of the probability of regular church attendance decreases over time. The rate of change is nonlinear; the decrease from year 0 to year 3 is less than the decrease from year 3 to year 6. At each time point, females are more likely than males to attend church regularly. The estimated difference in the logit of the probability of regular church attendance between females and males is $1.3241 - 0.7911 = 0.533$. At each time point, the odds of regularly attending church are estimated to be $e^{0.533} = 1.7$ times higher for females than for males.

Although both models provide a reasonable fit to the observed data, the fit of the marginal logit model is not quite as good as the fit of the corresponding model on the marginal probability scale (based on a comparison of the lack-of-fit statistics W). Figure 7.1 displays the observed marginal proportions and predicted marginal probabilities of regular church attendance from the two models. In this example, there is little to distinguish between the two models.

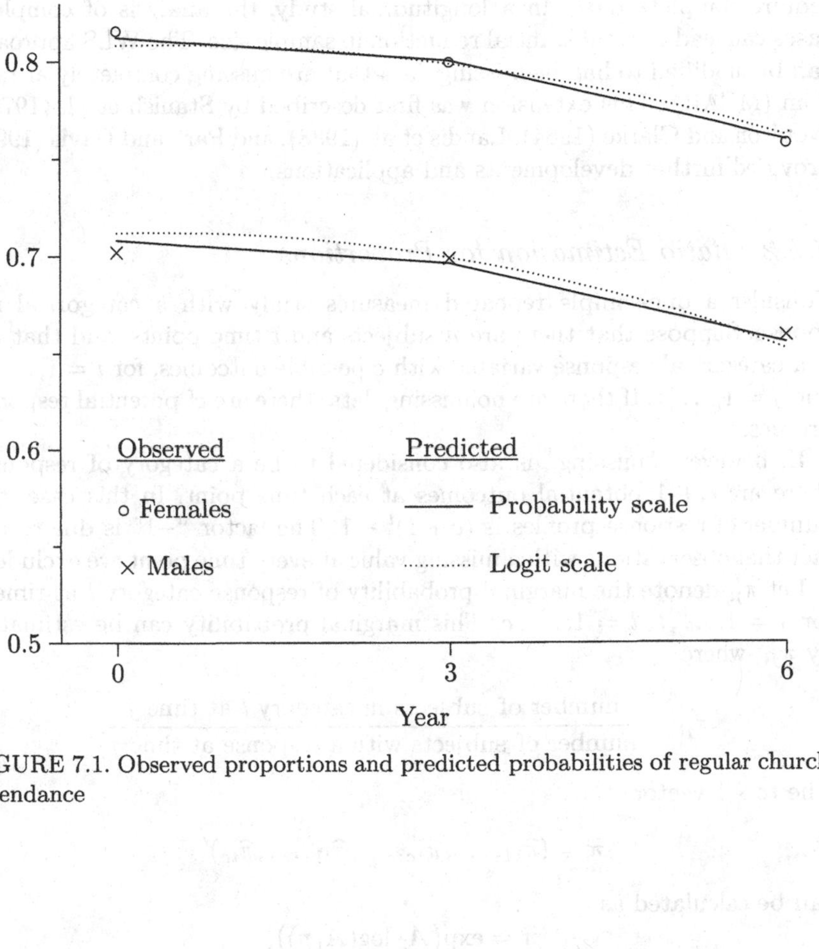

FIGURE 7.1. Observed proportions and predicted probabilities of regular church attendance

7.4 Accommodation of Missing Data

7.4.1 Overview

Data collected in longitudinal studies are often incomplete. Generally, some of the individuals who are intended to be followed over time will fail to provide information at one or more of the scheduled follow-up times. An observation may be missing by design, at random, or due to known or unknown characteristics of the subject.

Many of the standard methods for the analysis of repeated measurements require complete data. In a longitudinal study, the analysis of complete cases can lead to a substantial reduction in sample size. The WLS approach can be modified to handle missing data that are missing completely at random (MCAR). This extension was first described by Stanish et al. (1978). Woolson and Clarke (1984), Landis et al. (1988), and Park and Davis (1993) provided further developments and applications.

7.4.2 Ratio Estimation for Proportions

Consider a one-sample repeated measures study with a categorical response. Suppose that there are n subjects and t time points, and that y_{ij} is a categorical response variable with c possible outcomes, for $i = 1, \ldots, n$ and $j = 1, \ldots, t$. If there are no missing data, there are c^t potential response profiles.

If, however, "missing" is also considered to be a category of response, there are $c + 1$ potential outcomes at each time point. In this case, the number of response profiles is $(c+1)^t - 1$. The factor "-1" is due to the fact that observations with a missing value at every time point are excluded.

Let π_{jl} denote the marginal probability of response category l at time j for $j = 1, \ldots, t$, $l = 1, \ldots, c$. This marginal probability can be estimated by $\widehat{\pi}_{jl}$, where

$$\widehat{\pi}_{jl} = \frac{\text{number of subjects in category } l \text{ at time } j}{\text{number of subjects with a response at time } j}.$$

The $tc \times 1$ vector

$$\widehat{\boldsymbol{\pi}} = (\widehat{\pi}_{11}, \ldots, \widehat{\pi}_{1c}, \ldots, \widehat{\pi}_{t1}, \ldots, \widehat{\pi}_{tc})'$$

can be calculated as

$$\widehat{\boldsymbol{\pi}} = \exp\bigl(\boldsymbol{A}_2 \log(\boldsymbol{A}_1 \boldsymbol{p})\bigr),$$

where $\boldsymbol{p}$ is the $((c+1)^t - 1) \times 1$ vector of proportions corresponding to the multiway cross-classification of the response at the t time points.

The matrix $\boldsymbol{A}_1$ is a $t(c+1) \times ((c+1)^t - 1)$ matrix whose rows compute the proportions displayed in Table 7.10. The matrix $\boldsymbol{A}_2$ is the $tc \times t(c+1)$ matrix $\boldsymbol{I}_t \otimes [\boldsymbol{I}_c, -\boldsymbol{1}_c]$, where $\otimes$ denotes the direct (Kronecker) product

TABLE 7.10. Rows of matrix $\boldsymbol{A}_1$ for ratio estimation of proportions

Row	Proportion of Subjects with:
1	response category 1 at time 1
2	response category 2 at time 1
$\vdots$	$\vdots$
c	response category c at time 1
$c+1$	nonmissing response at time 1
$(t-1)(c+1)+1$	response category 1 at time t
$(t-1)(c+1)+2$	response category 2 at time t
$\vdots$	$\vdots$
$(t-1)(c+1)+c$	response category c at time t
$(t-1)(c+1)+c+1$ $[=t(c+1)]$	nonmissing response at time t

(Searle, 1982, p. 265). Because the elements of $\hat{\boldsymbol{\pi}}$ are linearly dependent, additional transformations can then be used to compute marginal proportions, marginal logits, marginal mean scores, or other types of response functions of interest. In practice, the matrices $\boldsymbol{A}_1$ and $\boldsymbol{A}_2$ can often be simplified to compute only the specific marginal proportions of interest.

This methodology is more clearly demonstrated by example.

7.4.3 One Population, Dichotomous Response

The Muscatine Coronary Risk Factor Study was a longitudinal study of coronary risk factors in school children. From 1971 to 1981, six biennial cross-sectional school screens were completed. In this study, children currently enrolled in school were eligible to participate, and about 70% of eligible children were screened. One variable of interest was obesity. Height and weight were measured on each participating child, from which relative weight was computed (the ratio of the child's weight to the median weight in the sex–age–height group).

Woolson and Clarke (1984) analyzed data on the prevalence of obesity in 1977, 1979, and 1981. In their analysis, children with relative weight greater than 110% of the median weight were classified as obese. Table 7.11 displays the cross-classification of the cohort of males who were 7–9 years old in 1977 by obesity status in 1977, 1979, and 1981. Of this group of 522 children, 356 participated in the 1977 survey, 375 participated in the 1979 survey, and 380 participated in the 1981 survey. However, only 225 children participated in all three surveys.

In this example, the response is dichotomous ($c = 2$) and there are $t = 3$ time points. Thus, the underlying multinomial vector of probabilities $\boldsymbol{\pi}$ has

$$(c+1)^t - 1 = 3^3 - 1 = 27 - 1 = 26$$

TABLE 7.11. Classification of 522 7–9 year old males from the Muscatine Coronary Risk Factor Study by obesity status

Classified as Obese in:			
1977	1979	1981	Number of Children
Yes	Yes	Yes	20
Yes	Yes	No	7
Yes	Yes	Missing	11
Yes	No	Yes	9
Yes	No	No	8
Yes	No	Missing	1
Yes	Missing	Yes	3
Yes	Missing	No	1
Yes	Missing	Missing	7
No	Yes	Yes	8
No	Yes	No	8
No	Yes	Missing	3
No	No	Yes	15
No	No	No	150
No	No	Missing	38
No	Missing	Yes	6
No	Missing	No	16
No	Missing	Missing	45
Missing	Yes	Yes	13
Missing	Yes	No	3
Missing	Yes	Missing	4
Missing	No	Yes	2
Missing	No	No	42
Missing	No	Missing	33
Missing	Missing	Yes	14
Missing	Missing	No	55
Total			522

components, ordered as shown in Table 7.11. Let π_{77}, π_{79}, and π_{81} denote the marginal probability of being classified as obese at year 1977, 1979, and 1981, respectively. Similarly, let p_{77}, p_{79}, and p_{81} denote the observed marginal proportions classified as obese at the three time points. These marginal proportions are estimated using all available data from each time point.

The response functions $\boldsymbol{F}(\boldsymbol{p}) = (p_{77}, p_{79}, p_{81})'$ can be computed as

$$\boldsymbol{F}(\boldsymbol{p}) = \exp\big(\boldsymbol{A}_2 \log(\boldsymbol{A}_1 \boldsymbol{p})\big),$$

where $\boldsymbol{A}_1$ is the 6×26 matrix

$$\begin{pmatrix} 1&1&1&1&1&1&1&1&1&0&0&0&0&0&0&0&0&0&0&0&0&0&0&0&0&0 \\ 1&1&1&1&1&1&1&1&1&1&1&1&1&1&1&1&1&1&0&0&0&0&0&0&0&0 \\ 1&1&1&0&0&0&0&0&0&1&1&1&0&0&0&0&0&0&1&1&1&0&0&0&0&0 \\ 1&1&1&1&1&1&0&0&0&1&1&1&1&1&1&0&0&0&1&1&1&1&1&1&0&0 \\ 1&0&0&1&0&0&1&0&0&1&0&0&1&0&0&1&0&0&1&0&0&1&0&0&1&0 \\ 1&1&0&1&1&0&1&1&0&1&1&0&1&1&0&1&1&0&1&1&0&1&1&0&1&1 \end{pmatrix},$$

and

$$\boldsymbol{A}_2 = \begin{pmatrix} 1 & -1 & 0 & 0 & 0 & 0 \\ 0 & 0 & 1 & -1 & 0 & 0 \\ 0 & 0 & 0 & 0 & 1 & -1 \end{pmatrix}.$$

The general approach of first computing the marginal proportions and then applying subsequent transformations, as described in Section 7.4.2, could have been followed. The computation of the response functions for this example was simplified, however, by first computing the proportions who were obese at years 1977, 1979, and 1981 (rows 1, 3, and 5 of $\boldsymbol{A}_1$) along with the proportions who had a nonmissing response at years 1977, 1979, and 1981 (rows 2, 4, and 6 of $\boldsymbol{A}_1$). The marginal proportions of interest are then the pairwise differences on the log scale (matrix $\boldsymbol{A}_2$).

The resulting vector of response functions is

$$\boldsymbol{F}(\boldsymbol{p}) = \begin{pmatrix} 0.188 \\ 0.205 \\ 0.237 \end{pmatrix}.$$

We will first fit the model $\boldsymbol{F}(\boldsymbol{\pi}) = \boldsymbol{X}\boldsymbol{\beta}$, where

$$\boldsymbol{X} = \begin{pmatrix} 1 & 0 \\ 1 & 2 \\ 1 & 4 \end{pmatrix}, \qquad \boldsymbol{\beta} = \begin{pmatrix} \beta_0 \\ \beta_1 \end{pmatrix}.$$

In this parameterization, β_0 is the probability of obesity in 1977 and β_1 is the linear effect of year. The lack-of-fit statistic W tests the null hypothesis that the nonlinear effect of year is equal to zero. In this example, $W = 0.15$

TABLE 7.12. Classification of 225 7–9 year old males from the Muscatine Coronary Risk Factor Study who participated in all three surveys

Classified as Obese in:			
1977	1979	1981	Number of Children
Yes	Yes	Yes	20
Yes	Yes	No	7
Yes	No	Yes	9
Yes	No	No	8
No	Yes	Yes	8
No	Yes	No	8
No	No	Yes	15
No	No	No	150
Total			225

with 3 − 2 = 1 df, indicating that the linear model provides a good fit ($p = 0.70$).

The parameter estimates are $\widehat{\beta}_1 = 0.186$ and $\widehat{\beta}_2 = 0.012$, with estimated standard errors of 0.020 and 0.006, respectively. The test of $H_0: \beta_1 = 0$ tests marginal homogeneity. Because $W_C = 3.83$ with 1 df, there is some evidence that the probability of obesity is not the same at the three surveys ($p = 0.05$). The resulting model is

$$\widehat{\pi}_x = 0.1863 + 0.0120(x - 77), \quad \text{for } x = 77, 79, 81.$$

Thus, we estimate that the probability of obesity is increasing by 0.012 per year.

Suppose that subjects with missing data had instead been excluded from the analysis. Table 7.12 displays the data from the subset of 225 children who participated in all three surveys. In this case, the response functions

$$\boldsymbol{F}(\boldsymbol{p}) = (p_{77}, p_{79}, p_{81})' = (0.19556, 0.19111, 0.23111)'$$

are computed as

$$\boldsymbol{F}(\boldsymbol{p}) = \boldsymbol{A}\boldsymbol{p},$$

where

$$\boldsymbol{A} = \begin{pmatrix} 1 & 1 & 1 & 1 & 0 & 0 & 0 & 0 \\ 1 & 1 & 0 & 0 & 1 & 1 & 0 & 0 \\ 1 & 0 & 1 & 0 & 1 & 0 & 1 & 0 \end{pmatrix}.$$

If we again fit the model

$$\boldsymbol{F}(\boldsymbol{\pi}) = \begin{pmatrix} 1 & 0 \\ 1 & 2 \\ 1 & 4 \end{pmatrix} \begin{pmatrix} \beta_0 \\ \beta_1 \end{pmatrix},$$

the lack-of-fit statistic is $W = 0.95$ with $3 - 2 = 1$ df, indicating that the linear model provides a good fit ($p = 0.33$). However, the test of $H_0\colon \beta_1 = 0$ is not significant ($W_C = 1.49$ with 1 df, $p = 0.22$).

One would then conclude that the model hypothesizing marginal homogeneity,

$$\boldsymbol{F}(\boldsymbol{\pi}) = \begin{pmatrix} 1 \\ 1 \\ 1 \end{pmatrix} \beta,$$

is appropriate. The lack-of-fit statistic is $W_C = 2.44$ with 2 df ($p = 0.30$). The conclusion from this model would be that the prevalence of obesity is not changing significantly across the three surveys. The estimated probability of obesity from this model is $\widehat{\beta} = 0.204$ with an estimated standard error of 0.022.

7.4.4 Multiple Populations, Dichotomous Response

As a second illustration of the use of the WLS methodology to accommodate missing data, we return to the "church attendance" example of Section 7.3.5. Table 7.6 displayed the data from the 1973 individuals (1311 females, 662 males) who responded to all three surveys. In fact, this study included 3085 subjects (1935 females, 1150 males). Whereas subjects with missing data were excluded from the analyses described in Section 7.3.5, we will now analyze the data displayed in Table 7.13. As indicated in Table 7.13, there were a substantial number of missing values. Most occur at the end of a sequence of nonmissing responses and were due largely to deaths or losses to follow-up.

As in Section 7.3.5, interest focuses on determining whether church attendance rates are changing over time, whether the attendance rates differ between females and males, and whether the observed patterns of change over time are the same for females and males. The exclusion of subjects with incomplete data resulted in a substantially reduced sample size (from 3085 subjects to 1973 subjects). We will now use all available data at each time point by estimating the marginal probabilities of regular church attendance using ratios of sums of underlying multinomial proportions.

In this example, a dichotomous response variable ($c = 2$) was scheduled to be measured at $t = 3$ time points. Including "missing" as a possible response gives

$$(c+1)^t - 1 = 3^3 - 1 = 26$$

potential response profiles. Table 7.13 shows, however, that only 23 of these potential response profiles were observed. (There were no occurrences of the profiles Missing–Missing–No, Missing–Missing–Yes, or Missing–Yes–No). Therefore, the underlying vector $\boldsymbol{p}_h$ of multinomial proportions in subpopulation h, where $h = 1$ for females and $h = 2$ for males, has 23 com-

TABLE 7.13. Classification of 3085 Iowa 65+ Study participants by regular church attendance

Attend Church Regularly at			Frequency		
Year 0	Year 3	Year 6	Female	Male	Total
Missing	No	Missing	3	2	5
Missing	No	No	1	3	4
Missing	No	Yes	1	1	2
Missing	Yes	Missing	2	2	4
Missing	Yes	Yes	2	0	2
No	Missing	Missing	101	122	223
No	Missing	No	11	5	16
No	Missing	Yes	3	2	5
No	No	Missing	71	86	157
No	No	No	158	143	301
No	No	Yes	30	18	48
No	Yes	Missing	14	5	19
No	Yes	No	22	21	43
No	Yes	Yes	33	15	48
Yes	Missing	Missing	195	125	320
Yes	Missing	No	4	0	4
Yes	Missing	Yes	18	9	27
Yes	No	Missing	28	16	44
Yes	No	No	51	26	77
Yes	No	Yes	25	12	37
Yes	Yes	Missing	170	110	280
Yes	Yes	No	88	36	124
Yes	Yes	Yes	904	391	1295
Total			1935	1150	3085

ponents. Similarly, $\boldsymbol{\pi}_h$, the vector of underlying multinomial probabilities, is also 23×1.

As in Section 7.3.5, the response functions of interest are the marginal proportions p_{hj} of subjects from population h who regularly attend church at year j for $h = 1, 2$ and $j = 0, 3, 6$. In each subpopulation,

$$\boldsymbol{F}(\boldsymbol{p}_h) = (p_{h0}, p_{h3}, p_{h6})'$$

is computed as $\boldsymbol{F}(\boldsymbol{p}_h) = \exp\big(\boldsymbol{A}_2 \log(\boldsymbol{A}_1 \boldsymbol{p}_h)\big)$, where $\boldsymbol{A}_1$ is

$$\begin{pmatrix} 0&0&0&0&0&0&0&0&0&0&0&0&0&0&1&1&1&1&1&1&1&1&1 \\ 0&0&0&0&0&1&1&1&1&1&1&1&1&1&1&1&1&1&1&1&1&1&1 \\ 0&0&0&1&1&0&0&0&0&0&0&1&1&1&0&0&0&0&0&0&1&1&1 \\ 1&1&1&1&1&0&0&0&1&1&1&1&1&1&0&0&0&1&1&1&1&1&1 \\ 0&0&1&0&1&0&0&1&0&0&1&0&0&1&0&0&1&0&0&1&0&0&1 \\ 0&1&1&0&1&0&1&1&0&1&1&0&1&1&0&1&1&0&1&1&0&1&1 \end{pmatrix}$$

and

$$\boldsymbol{A}_2 = \boldsymbol{I}_3 \otimes (1, -1) = \begin{pmatrix} 1 & -1 & 0 & 0 & 0 & 0 \\ 0 & 0 & 1 & -1 & 0 & 0 \\ 0 & 0 & 0 & 0 & 1 & -1 \end{pmatrix}.$$

In this example,

$$\boldsymbol{F}(\boldsymbol{p}_1) = \begin{pmatrix} 0.770 \\ 0.770 \\ 0.752 \end{pmatrix}, \quad \boldsymbol{F}(\boldsymbol{p}_2) = \begin{pmatrix} 0.635 \\ 0.654 \\ 0.657 \end{pmatrix}, \quad \boldsymbol{F}(\boldsymbol{p}) = \begin{pmatrix} \boldsymbol{F}(\boldsymbol{p}_1) \\ \boldsymbol{F}(\boldsymbol{p}_2) \end{pmatrix}.$$

We will first fit the same saturated model as was considered in Section 7.3.5. The model is $\boldsymbol{F}(\boldsymbol{\pi}) = \boldsymbol{X}_1 \boldsymbol{\beta}$, where

$$\boldsymbol{X}_1 = \begin{pmatrix} 1 & -1 & 1 & 0 & 0 & 0 \\ 1 & 0 & -2 & 0 & 0 & 0 \\ 1 & 1 & 1 & 0 & 0 & 0 \\ 0 & 0 & 0 & 1 & -1 & 1 \\ 0 & 0 & 0 & 1 & 0 & -2 \\ 0 & 0 & 0 & 1 & 1 & 1 \end{pmatrix}, \quad \boldsymbol{\beta} = \begin{pmatrix} \beta_{10} \\ \beta_{11} \\ \beta_{12} \\ \beta_{20} \\ \beta_{21} \\ \beta_{22} \end{pmatrix}.$$

In this parameterization, β_{h0}, β_{h1}, and β_{h2} are the intercept, linear time effect, and quadratic time effect for subpopulation h. Because the surveys were equally spaced, orthogonal polynomial coefficients are used for the time effects.

Table 7.14 displays the coefficient matrices $\boldsymbol{C}$ for testing several hypotheses of the form $H_0\colon \boldsymbol{C}\boldsymbol{\beta} = 0$ along with the corresponding test statistics $W_{\boldsymbol{C}}$, degrees of freedom, and p-values. In contrast to the results of the analysis of the complete data (Table 7.7), the 4-df test of the year effect is not significant in both sexes combined as well as in females and males separately. The tests of the linear and quadratic components of the survey-year effect are also not statistically significant.

TABLE 7.14. Results of hypothesis tests from the saturated marginal probability model for the church attendance data

Hypothesis	C	W_C	df	p-value
No year effect	0 1 0 0 0 0 0 0 1 0 0 0 0 0 0 0 1 0 0 0 0 0 0 1	6.00	4	0.199
No year effect in females	0 1 0 0 0 0 0 0 1 0 0 0	3.28	2	0.194
No year effect in males	0 0 0 0 1 0 0 0 0 0 0 1	2.73	2	0.256
No linear year effect	0 1 0 0 0 0 0 0 0 0 1 0	4.19	2	0.123
No linear year effect in females	0 1 0 0 0 0	2.44	1	0.118
No linear year effect in males	0 0 0 0 1 0	1.75	1	0.186
No quadratic year effect	0 0 1 0 0 0 0 0 0 0 0 1	1.83	2	0.401
No quadratic year effect in females	0 0 1 0 0 0	1.36	1	0.244
No quadratic year effect in males	0 0 0 0 0 1	0.47	1	0.493
Equality of intercepts	1 0 0 −1 0 0	50.81	1	< 0.001
Equality of linear year effects	0 1 0 0 −1 0	3.90	1	0.048
Equality of quadratic year effects	0 0 1 0 0 −1	0.01	1	0.922

These results suggest fitting a model with separate intercepts for females and males. The model $\boldsymbol{F}(\boldsymbol{\pi}) = \boldsymbol{X}_2\boldsymbol{\beta}$, where

$$\boldsymbol{X}_2 = \begin{pmatrix} 1 & 0 \\ 1 & 0 \\ 1 & 0 \\ 1 & 1 \\ 1 & 1 \\ 1 & 1 \end{pmatrix}, \qquad \boldsymbol{\beta} = \begin{pmatrix} \beta_1 \\ \beta_2 \end{pmatrix},$$

incorporates an intercept for females (β_1) and an incremental effect for males (β_2). This model provides an adequate fit to the observed data ($W = 6.00$ with 4 df, $p = 0.2$). The estimated probability of regular church attendance for females is $\widehat{\beta}_1 = 0.7660$ with an estimated standard error of 0.0086. Because $\widehat{\beta}_2 = -0.1225$, the probability of regular church attendance is estimated to be 0.1225 less for males than for females. The Wald test of $H_0\colon \beta_2 = 0$ is

$$\left(\frac{\widehat{\beta}_2}{\text{s.e.}(\widehat{\beta}_2)}\right)^2 = \left(\frac{-0.1225}{0.0158}\right)^2 = 60.12$$

with 1 df, indicating that the intercept difference is highly significant.

The analysis of all data results in a similar conclusion concerning the difference between females and males as does the analysis of the complete data (Section 7.3.5). The two analyses, however, give quite different conclusions concerning the effect of survey year.

As in Section 7.3.5, we might prefer to analyze the data on the logit scale rather than on the probability scale. Consider the response functions

$$\boldsymbol{F}(\boldsymbol{p}) = \begin{pmatrix} \boldsymbol{F}(\boldsymbol{p}_1) \\ \boldsymbol{F}(\boldsymbol{p}_2) \end{pmatrix},$$

where $\boldsymbol{F}(\boldsymbol{p}_h)$ is now the 3×1 vector of logits of marginal proportions:

$$\boldsymbol{F}(\boldsymbol{p}_h) = \begin{pmatrix} \log\left(\dfrac{p_{h0}}{1 - p_{h0}}\right) \\ \log\left(\dfrac{p_{h3}}{1 - p_{h3}}\right) \\ \log\left(\dfrac{p_{h6}}{1 - p_{h6}}\right) \end{pmatrix}.$$

These response functions are computed via the transformation

$$\boldsymbol{F}(\boldsymbol{p}_h) = \boldsymbol{A}_2 \log(\boldsymbol{A}_1 \boldsymbol{p}_h),$$

where

$$\boldsymbol{A}_1 = \begin{pmatrix} 0&0&0&0&0&0&0&0&0&0&0&0&0&0&1&1&1&1&1&1&1&1&1 \\ 0&0&0&0&0&1&1&1&1&1&1&1&1&1&0&0&0&0&0&0&0&0&0 \\ 0&0&0&1&1&0&0&0&0&0&0&1&1&1&0&0&0&0&0&0&1&1&1 \\ 1&1&1&0&0&0&0&0&1&1&1&0&0&0&0&0&0&1&1&1&0&0&0 \\ 0&0&1&0&1&0&0&1&0&0&1&0&0&1&0&0&1&0&0&1&0&0&1 \\ 0&1&0&0&0&0&1&0&0&1&0&0&1&0&0&1&0&0&1&0&0&1&0 \end{pmatrix}$$

and

$$A_2 = I_3 \otimes (1, -1) = \begin{pmatrix} 1 & -1 & 0 & 0 & 0 & 0 \\ 0 & 0 & 1 & -1 & 0 & 0 \\ 0 & 0 & 0 & 0 & 1 & -1 \end{pmatrix}.$$

Row 1 of $\boldsymbol{A}_1$ computes the proportion of subjects who regularly attend church at year 0; row 2 computes the proportion who do not regularly attend church at year 0. Rows 3–4 and 5–6 of $\boldsymbol{A}_1$ compute these proportions at year 3 and year 6, respectively. The rows of $\boldsymbol{A}_2$ then compute the logit response functions at years 0, 3, and 6.

The logit model with an intercept for females and an incremental effect for males ($\boldsymbol{F}(\boldsymbol{\pi}) = \boldsymbol{X}_2\boldsymbol{\beta}$) provides an adequate fit to the data ($W = 6.07$ with 4 df, $p = 0.19$). The estimated logit of the probability of regular church attendance for females is $\widehat{\beta}_1 = 1.181$ with an estimated standard error of 0.048. Because $\widehat{\beta}_2 = -0.594$, the logit of the probability of regular church attendance is estimated to be 0.594 less for males than for females. Hence, we estimate that the odds of regular church attendance are $e^{-0.594} = 0.55$ times as high for males as for females (or $e^{0.594} = 1.8$ times higher for females than for males). The Wald test of $H_0\colon \beta_2 = 0$ is

$$\left(\frac{\widehat{\beta}_2}{\text{s.e.}(\widehat{\beta}_2)}\right)^2 = \left(\frac{-0.594}{0.075}\right)^2 = 62.5$$

with 1 df, indicating that the intercept difference is highly significant.

7.4.5 *Assessing the Missing-Data Mechanism*

The example considered in Sections 7.3.5 and 7.4.4 illustrates the situation where the analysis of complete cases gives different conclusions than the analysis of all available data. Park and Davis (1993) describe a test of the missing-data mechanism for repeated categorical data. The basic idea is to fit a single model to two subgroups (subjects with complete data, subjects with incomplete data) and then to test whether the parameter estimates for the complete cases are significantly different (individually and jointly) from the parameter estimates for the incomplete cases. This methodology will be illustrated using the church attendance data displayed in Table 7.13.

If we again consider analyzing the data on the marginal proportion scale, let

$$\boldsymbol{F}(\boldsymbol{p}_h) = (p_{h0c}, p_{h3c}, p_{h6c}, p_{h0i}, p_{h3i}, p_{h6i})'$$

denote the 6×1 vector of response functions from population h for $h = 1, 2$, where $h = 1$ for females and $h = 2$ for males. In this case, the third subscript is "c" for subjects with complete data and "i" for subjects with one or more missing responses. Thus, the response function vector

$$\boldsymbol{F}(\boldsymbol{p}) = (\boldsymbol{F}(\boldsymbol{p}_1), \boldsymbol{F}(\boldsymbol{p}_2))'$$

now has 12 components. The response functions in population h are computed as

$$\boldsymbol{F}(\boldsymbol{p}_h) = \exp\big(\boldsymbol{A}_2 \log(\boldsymbol{A}_1 \boldsymbol{p}_h)\big),$$

where $\boldsymbol{A}_1$ is

$$\begin{pmatrix}
0&0&0&0&0&0&0&0&0&0&0&0&0&0&0&0&0&0&1&1&0&1&1\\
0&0&0&0&0&0&0&0&0&0&0&0&1&1&0&0&0&0&0&0&0&1&1\\
0&0&0&0&0&0&0&0&0&0&1&0&0&1&0&0&0&0&0&1&0&0&1\\
0&0&0&0&0&0&0&0&0&1&1&0&1&1&0&0&0&0&1&1&0&1&1\\
0&0&0&0&0&0&0&0&0&0&0&0&0&0&1&1&1&1&0&0&1&0&0\\
0&0&0&0&0&1&1&1&1&0&0&1&0&0&1&1&1&1&0&0&1&0&0\\
0&0&0&1&1&0&0&0&0&0&0&1&0&0&0&0&0&0&0&0&1&0&0\\
1&1&1&1&1&0&0&0&1&0&0&1&0&0&0&0&0&1&0&0&1&0&0\\
0&0&1&0&1&0&0&1&0&0&0&0&0&0&0&0&1&0&0&0&0&0&0\\
0&1&1&0&1&0&1&1&0&0&0&0&0&0&0&1&1&0&0&0&0&0&0
\end{pmatrix}$$

and

$$\boldsymbol{A}_2 = \begin{pmatrix}
1&0&0&-1&0&0&0&0&0&0\\
0&1&0&-1&0&0&0&0&0&0\\
0&0&1&-1&0&0&0&0&0&0\\
0&0&0&0&1&-1&0&0&0&0\\
0&0&0&0&0&0&1&-1&0&0\\
0&0&0&0&0&0&0&0&1&-1
\end{pmatrix}.$$

Rows 1–4 of $\boldsymbol{A}_1$ compute relevant proportions from the subgroup of subjects who responded to all three surveys. The first three rows of $\boldsymbol{A}_1$ compute the proportions who attended church regularly at years 0, 3, and 6, respectively, and row 4 of $\boldsymbol{A}_1$ computes the proportion who responded to all three surveys. Rows 5–10 of $\boldsymbol{A}_1$ compute relevant proportions from the subgroup of subjects who had at least one missing response. Rows 5–6 compute the numerator (proportion who attend church regularly) and denominator (proportion who responded) of the marginal proportion at year 0. Rows 7–8 and 9–10 compute the corresponding quantities for years 3 and 6, respectively.

Similarly, rows 1–3 of $\boldsymbol{A}_2$ pertain to subjects who responded to all three surveys; these rows compute the difference between the logarithm of the proportion who attended church regularly at year j and the logarithm of the proportion who responded to all three surveys, for $j = 0, 3, 6$, respectively. Rows 4–6 of $\boldsymbol{A}_2$ pertain to subjects who had at least one missing response and compute the difference between the logarithm of the proportion who attended church regularly at year j and the logarithm of the proportion who responded at year j, for $j = 0, 3, 6$, respectively.

The resulting response functions are

$$\boldsymbol{F}(\boldsymbol{p}_1) = \begin{pmatrix} p_{10c} \\ p_{13c} \\ p_{16c} \\ p_{10i} \\ p_{13i} \\ p_{16i} \end{pmatrix} = \begin{pmatrix} 0.815 \\ 0.799 \\ 0.757 \\ 0.675 \\ 0.644 \\ 0.600 \end{pmatrix}, \quad \boldsymbol{F}(\boldsymbol{p}_2) = \begin{pmatrix} p_{20c} \\ p_{23c} \\ p_{26c} \\ p_{20i} \\ p_{23i} \\ p_{26i} \end{pmatrix} = \begin{pmatrix} 0.702 \\ 0.699 \\ 0.659 \\ 0.542 \\ 0.520 \\ 0.600 \end{pmatrix}.$$

By referring to the observed counts displayed in Table 7.13, it is not difficult to check the computation of these response functions. For example, the observed proportion of males with incomplete data at year 0 or year 3 who regularly attended church at year 6 is

$$p_{26i} = \frac{1+0+2+9}{3+1+0+5+2+0+9} = \frac{12}{20} = 0.6.$$

Similarly, the observed proportion of females with incomplete data at year 0 or year 6 who regularly attended church at year 3 is

$$p_{13i} = \frac{2+2+14+170}{3+1+1+2+2+71+14+28+170} = \frac{188}{292} = 0.644.$$

As in Section 7.4.4, we will first fit a saturated model with separate intercepts, linear year effects, and quadratic year effects in each of the four subpopulations (complete females, complete males, incomplete females, incomplete males). The model is $\boldsymbol{F}(\boldsymbol{\pi}) = \boldsymbol{X}_1\boldsymbol{\beta}$, where

$$\boldsymbol{X}_1 = \begin{pmatrix} 1 & -1 & 1 & 0 & 0 & 0 & 0 & 0 & 0 & 0 & 0 & 0 \\ 1 & 0 & -2 & 0 & 0 & 0 & 0 & 0 & 0 & 0 & 0 & 0 \\ 1 & 1 & 1 & 0 & 0 & 0 & 0 & 0 & 0 & 0 & 0 & 0 \\ 0 & 0 & 0 & 0 & 0 & 0 & 1 & -1 & 1 & 0 & 0 & 0 \\ 0 & 0 & 0 & 0 & 0 & 0 & 1 & 0 & -2 & 0 & 0 & 0 \\ 0 & 0 & 0 & 0 & 0 & 0 & 1 & 1 & 1 & 0 & 0 & 0 \\ 0 & 0 & 0 & 1 & -1 & 1 & 0 & 0 & 0 & 0 & 0 & 0 \\ 0 & 0 & 0 & 1 & 0 & -2 & 0 & 0 & 0 & 0 & 0 & 0 \\ 0 & 0 & 0 & 1 & 1 & 1 & 0 & 0 & 0 & 0 & 0 & 0 \\ 0 & 0 & 0 & 0 & 0 & 0 & 0 & 0 & 0 & 1 & -1 & 1 \\ 0 & 0 & 0 & 0 & 0 & 0 & 0 & 0 & 0 & 1 & 0 & -2 \\ 0 & 0 & 0 & 0 & 0 & 0 & 0 & 0 & 0 & 1 & 1 & 1 \end{pmatrix}$$

and

$$\boldsymbol{\beta} = (\beta_{10c}, \beta_{11c}, \beta_{12c}, \beta_{20c}, \beta_{21c}, \beta_{22c}, \beta_{10i}, \beta_{11i}, \beta_{12i}, \beta_{20i}, \beta_{21i}, \beta_{22i})'.$$

The parameters β_{h0c}, β_{h1c}, and β_{h2c} are the intercept, linear, and quadratic effects among subjects with complete data from population h, and β_{h0i}, β_{h1i}, and β_{h2i} are the corresponding parameters from subjects with incomplete data.

We first test whether the parameters from subjects with complete data are equal to the corresponding parameters from subjects with incomplete data. The null hypothesis is

$$\beta_{10c} = \beta_{10i}, \beta_{11c} = \beta_{11i}, \beta_{12c} = \beta_{12i}, \beta_{20c} = \beta_{20i}, \beta_{21c} = \beta_{21i}, \beta_{22c} = \beta_{22i}.$$

In matrix notation, we wish to test $H_0: \boldsymbol{C\beta} = \mathbf{0}$, where

$$\boldsymbol{C} = \begin{pmatrix} 1 & 0 & 0 & 0 & 0 & 0 & -1 & 0 & 0 & 0 & 0 & 0 \\ 0 & 1 & 0 & 0 & 0 & 0 & 0 & -1 & 0 & 0 & 0 & 0 \\ 0 & 0 & 1 & 0 & 0 & 0 & 0 & 0 & -1 & 0 & 0 & 0 \\ 0 & 0 & 0 & 1 & 0 & 0 & 0 & 0 & 0 & -1 & 0 & 0 \\ 0 & 0 & 0 & 0 & 1 & 0 & 0 & 0 & 0 & 0 & -1 & 0 \\ 0 & 0 & 0 & 0 & 0 & 1 & 0 & 0 & 0 & 0 & 0 & -1 \end{pmatrix}.$$

Because $W_C = 82.7$ with 6 df, the difference between subjects with complete data and subjects with incomplete data is highly significant ($p < 0.001$).

To determine a parsimonious model for the data, one can also test additional hypotheses comparing complete and incomplete cases. For example, we can test whether the time effects in subjects with complete data are the same as those in subjects with incomplete data. The null hypothesis is $H_0: \beta_{11c} = \beta_{11i}, \beta_{12c} = \beta_{12i}, \beta_{21c} = \beta_{21i}, \beta_{22c} = \beta_{22i}$, or $H_0: \boldsymbol{C\beta} = \mathbf{0}$, where

$$\boldsymbol{C} = \begin{pmatrix} 0 & 1 & 0 & 0 & 0 & 0 & 0 & -1 & 0 & 0 & 0 & 0 \\ 0 & 0 & 1 & 0 & 0 & 0 & 0 & 0 & -1 & 0 & 0 & 0 \\ 0 & 0 & 0 & 0 & 1 & 0 & 0 & 0 & 0 & 0 & -1 & 0 \\ 0 & 0 & 0 & 0 & 0 & 1 & 0 & 0 & 0 & 0 & 0 & -1 \end{pmatrix}.$$

Because $W_C = 1.58$ with 4 df, this hypothesis is not rejected ($p = 0.81$).

These results motivate fitting a reduced model with separate intercepts for complete females, incomplete females, complete males, and incomplete males (four parameters) and common linear and quadratic time effects for females (two parameters) and for males (two parameters). The model is

$$\boldsymbol{F}(\boldsymbol{\pi}) = \boldsymbol{X}_2\boldsymbol{\beta},$$

where

$$\boldsymbol{X}_2 = \begin{pmatrix} 1 & 0 & -1 & 1 & 0 & 0 & 0 & 0 \\ 1 & 0 & 0 & -2 & 0 & 0 & 0 & 0 \\ 1 & 0 & 1 & 1 & 0 & 0 & 0 & 0 \\ 0 & 1 & -1 & 1 & 0 & 0 & 0 & 0 \\ 0 & 1 & 0 & -2 & 0 & 0 & 0 & 0 \\ 0 & 1 & 1 & 1 & 0 & 0 & 0 & 0 \\ 0 & 0 & 0 & 0 & 1 & 0 & -1 & 1 \\ 0 & 0 & 0 & 0 & 1 & 0 & 0 & -2 \\ 0 & 0 & 0 & 0 & 1 & 0 & 1 & 1 \\ 0 & 0 & 0 & 0 & 0 & 1 & -1 & 1 \\ 0 & 0 & 0 & 0 & 0 & 1 & 0 & -2 \\ 0 & 0 & 0 & 0 & 0 & 1 & 1 & 1 \end{pmatrix}, \quad \boldsymbol{\beta} = \begin{pmatrix} \beta_{10c} \\ \beta_{10i} \\ \beta_{11} \\ \beta_{12} \\ \beta_{20c} \\ \beta_{20i} \\ \beta_{21} \\ \beta_{22} \end{pmatrix}.$$

The parameters β_{h0c} and β_{h0i} are the intercepts for subjects with complete and incomplete data from population h, and β_{h1} and β_{h2} are the linear and quadratic time effects in population h.

This model provides a good fit to the data ($W_C = 1.58$ with 4 df, $p = 0.81$). One hypothesis of interest is equality of time effects for females and males; that is,

$$H_0: \beta_{11} = \beta_{21}, \beta_{12} = \beta_{22}$$

or, equivalently, $H_0: \boldsymbol{C\beta} = \boldsymbol{0}$, where

$$\boldsymbol{C} = \begin{pmatrix} 0 & 0 & 1 & 0 & 0 & 0 & -1 & 0 \\ 0 & 0 & 0 & 1 & 0 & 0 & 0 & -1 \end{pmatrix}.$$

Because $W_C = 1.01$ with 2 df, the time effects in males and females are not significantly different ($p = 0.60$).

This motivates a further reduced model with four intercepts (complete and incomplete females and males) and common linear and quadratic time effects (two parameters). The model is $\boldsymbol{F}(\boldsymbol{\pi}) = \boldsymbol{X}_3\boldsymbol{\beta}$, where

$$\boldsymbol{X}_3 = \begin{pmatrix} 1 & 0 & 0 & 0 & -1 & 1 \\ 1 & 0 & 0 & 0 & 0 & -2 \\ 1 & 0 & 0 & 0 & 1 & 1 \\ 0 & 1 & 0 & 0 & -1 & 1 \\ 0 & 1 & 0 & 0 & 0 & -2 \\ 0 & 1 & 0 & 0 & 1 & 1 \\ 0 & 0 & 1 & 0 & -1 & 1 \\ 0 & 0 & 1 & 0 & 0 & -2 \\ 0 & 0 & 1 & 0 & 1 & 1 \\ 0 & 0 & 0 & 1 & -1 & 1 \\ 0 & 0 & 0 & 1 & 0 & -2 \\ 0 & 0 & 0 & 1 & 1 & 1 \end{pmatrix}, \quad \boldsymbol{\beta} = \begin{pmatrix} \beta_{10c} \\ \beta_{10i} \\ \beta_{20c} \\ \beta_{20i} \\ \beta_1 \\ \beta_2 \end{pmatrix}.$$

The parameters β_1 and β_2 are the linear and quadratic time effects, assumed to be common across complete and incomplete females and males. This model provides a good fit to the data ($W_C = 2.58$ with 6 df, $p = 0.86$). In addition, both components of the effect of survey year are statistically significant (linear: $W_C = 40.7$ with 1 df, $p < 0.001$; quadratic: $W_C = 4.9$ with 1 df, $p = 0.03$).

To produce parameter estimates that are more easily interpretable, this model will be refit on the natural time scale (years) instead of using or-

TABLE 7.15. Parameter estimates from the final marginal probability model for the church attendance data

Parameter	Estimate	Standard Error
Complete female intercept	0.8128	0.0103
Incomplete female intercept	0.6710	0.0182
Complete male intercept	0.7089	0.0166
Incomplete male intercept	0.5426	0.0223
Linear year	−0.0001	0.0040
Quadratic year	−0.0015	0.0007

thogonal polynomial coefficients. The model is $\boldsymbol{F}(\boldsymbol{\pi}) = \boldsymbol{X}_4\boldsymbol{\beta}$, where

$$\boldsymbol{X}_4 = \begin{pmatrix} 1 & 0 & 0 & 0 & 0 & 0 \\ 1 & 0 & 0 & 0 & 3 & 9 \\ 1 & 0 & 0 & 0 & 6 & 36 \\ 0 & 1 & 0 & 0 & 0 & 0 \\ 0 & 1 & 0 & 0 & 3 & 9 \\ 0 & 1 & 0 & 0 & 6 & 36 \\ 0 & 0 & 1 & 0 & 0 & 0 \\ 0 & 0 & 1 & 0 & 3 & 9 \\ 0 & 0 & 1 & 0 & 6 & 36 \\ 0 & 0 & 0 & 1 & 0 & 0 \\ 0 & 0 & 0 & 1 & 3 & 9 \\ 0 & 0 & 0 & 1 & 6 & 36 \end{pmatrix}, \qquad \boldsymbol{\beta} = \begin{pmatrix} \beta_{10c} \\ \beta_{10i} \\ \beta_{20c} \\ \beta_{20i} \\ \beta_1 \\ \beta_2 \end{pmatrix}.$$

The lack-of-fit statistic W and the test of nonlinearity ($H_0\colon \beta_2 = 0$) are unchanged from the previous model. The test of $H_0\colon \beta_1 = 0$, however, yields $W_C = 0.00$ with 1 df ($p = 0.99$). This is because the linear and quadratic survey-year effects are highly correlated using this parameterization.

Table 7.15 displays the parameter estimates and their standard errors. Because the profiles over time are parallel across the four groups of subjects (complete females, incomplete females, complete males, incomplete males), the results of this model are easy to interpret. In each subpopulation, the estimated probability of regular church attendance decreases nonlinearly over time. The decrease from year 0 to year 3 is greater than the decrease from year 3 to year 6. In addition, the probability of regular church attendance is highest for females with complete data, followed by males with complete data, females with incomplete data, and males with incomplete data.

The test of equality of the four intercepts is highly significant ($W_C = 150.9$ with 3 df, $p < 0.001$). In addition, Table 7.16 displays the results of other joint and pairwise comparisons among intercepts. All of these tests are statistically significant.

TABLE 7.16. Results of hypothesis tests on intercepts from the final marginal probability model for the church attendance data

Comparison	Test	C	W_C	df	p-value
Females vs. males	Joint	1 0 −1 0 0 0 0 1 0 −1 0 0	50.5	2	< 0.001
	Complete	1 0 −1 0 0 0	30.6	1	< 0.001
	Incomplete	0 1 0 −1 0 0	20.0	1	< 0.001
Complete vs. incomplete	Joint	1 −1 0 0 0 0 0 0 1 −1 0 0	81.9	2	< 0.001
	Females	1 −1 0 0 0 0	46.9	1	< 0.001
	Males	0 0 1 −1 0 0	36.1	1	< 0.001

As was seen in the two other analyses of these data (complete cases only: Section 7.3.5; all data: Section 7.4.4), this analysis also leads to the conclusion that females are more likely to attend church regularly than are males. This analysis also shows that, within each sex, the subjects who responded to all three surveys are significantly more likely to attend regularly than are subjects with at least one missing response. Although the analysis of the complete cases only also revealed a statistically significant decrease in the estimated probability of regular church attendance over time, this was not identified in the analysis of all data that did not allow separate parameters for complete and incomplete cases (Section 7.4.4).

7.5 Problems

7.1 Suppose that a dichotomous response variable (coded as 0 or 1) is measured at two time points for each of n subjects. The proportion of subjects in each of the $2^2 = 4$ combinations of the cross-classification of time and response can be summarized in the vector $\boldsymbol{p} = (p_1, \ldots, p_4)'$, as shown in Table 7.17.

(a) State the matrix $\boldsymbol{A}$ for defining the vector of response functions

$$\boldsymbol{F}(\boldsymbol{p}) = \boldsymbol{A}\boldsymbol{p} = (P_1, P_2)',$$

where P_i is the marginal proportion with response = 1 at time i.

TABLE 7.17. Response proportions for a dichotomous outcome measured at two time points

Response		
Time 1	Time 2	Proportion
0	0	p_1
0	1	p_2
1	0	p_3
1	1	p_4

(b) Find $\boldsymbol{V_F} = \boldsymbol{AVA'}$, where $\boldsymbol{V} = \frac{1}{n}(\boldsymbol{D_p} - \boldsymbol{pp'})$ and $\boldsymbol{D_p}$ is a diagonal matrix with the vector $\boldsymbol{p}$ on the main diagonal.

(c) Consider the model $\boldsymbol{F}(\boldsymbol{p}) = \boldsymbol{X}\beta$, where β is a scalar and $\boldsymbol{X}' = (1, 1)$. Find and interpret the weighted least squares estimator of β.

7.2 Suppose that a dichotomous response variable (coded as 0 or 1) is measured at four equally spaced time points for each of n subjects. The proportion of subjects in each of the $2^4 = 16$ combinations of the cross-classification of time and response can be summarized in the vector $\boldsymbol{p} = (p_1, \ldots, p_{16})'$, as shown in Table 7.18.

(a) State the matrix $\boldsymbol{A}$ for defining the vector of response functions

$$\boldsymbol{F}(\boldsymbol{p}) = \boldsymbol{Ap} = (P_1, P_2, P_3, P_4)',$$

where P_i is the marginal proportion with response = 1 at time i.

(b) Consider the model $\boldsymbol{F}(\boldsymbol{p}) = \boldsymbol{X\beta}$, where $\boldsymbol{\beta}' = (\beta_1, \beta_2, \beta_3)$ and

$$\boldsymbol{X} = \begin{pmatrix} 1 & 0 & 0 \\ 1 & 1 & 0 \\ 1 & 1 & 1 \\ 1 & 1 & 1 \end{pmatrix}.$$

Interpret the parameters β_1, β_2, and β_3.

(c) With respect to the model from part (b), state the hypothesis that is tested by the lack-of-fit statistic.

(d) Suppose that the model from part (b) provides a good fit to the observed data. Specify the matrix $\boldsymbol{C}$ for testing $H_0\colon \boldsymbol{C\beta} = \boldsymbol{0}$ that the marginal probabilities of response = 1 at the four time points are equal.

TABLE 7.18. Response proportions for a dichotomous outcome measured at four time points

Response at Time:				
1	2	3	4	Proportion
0	0	0	0	p_1
0	0	0	1	p_2
0	0	1	0	p_3
0	0	1	1	p_4
0	1	0	0	p_5
0	1	0	1	p_6
0	1	1	0	p_7
0	1	1	1	p_8
1	0	0	0	p_9
1	0	0	1	p_{10}
1	0	1	0	p_{11}
1	0	1	1	p_{12}
1	1	0	0	p_{13}
1	1	0	1	p_{14}
1	1	1	0	p_{15}
1	1	1	1	p_{16}

7.3 Suppose that an ordered categorical response (coded as 0 = none, 1 = moderate, 2 = severe) is measured at months 0, 2, and 6 for each of n subjects. The proportion of subjects in each of the $3^3 = 27$ combinations of the cross-classification of month and response can be summarized in the vector $\boldsymbol{p} = (p_1, \ldots, p_{27})'$, as shown in Table 7.19. Let π_{jk} denote the marginal probability of response k at month j for $j = 0, 2, 6$ and $k = 0, 1, 2$. Suppose that you wish to analyze the cumulative logit response functions

$$L_{j1} = \log\left(\frac{\pi_{j0}}{\pi_{j1} + \pi_{j2}}\right), \qquad L_{j2} = \log\left(\frac{\pi_{j0} + \pi_{j1}}{\pi_{j2}}\right), \qquad \text{for } j = 0, 2, 6.$$

(a) Define this vector of response functions $\boldsymbol{F}(\boldsymbol{p})$ as a sequence of linear, logarithmic, and/or exponential transformations of $\boldsymbol{p}$.

(b) State the degrees of freedom for testing the hypothesis of marginal homogeneity using these response functions.

(c) Repeat parts (a) and (b) for analyzing the marginal mean scores at each of the three time points (using the scores 0, 1, and 2 for none, moderate, and severe, respectively.

7.4 Consider a study in which an ordered categorical response with three levels (0 = none, 1 = moderate, 2 = severe) is measured at three time

TABLE 7.19. Response proportions for an ordered categorical outcome measured at three time points

Response at Month:			
0	2	6	Proportion
0	0	0	p_1
		1	p_2
		2	p_3
	1	0	p_4
		1	p_5
		2	p_6
	2	0	p_7
		1	p_8
		2	p_9
1	0	0	p_{10}
		1	p_{11}
		2	p_{12}
	1	0	p_{13}
		1	p_{14}
		2	p_{15}
	2	0	p_{16}
		1	p_{17}
		2	p_{18}
2	0	0	p_{19}
		1	p_{20}
		2	p_{21}
	1	0	p_{22}
		1	p_{23}
		2	p_{24}
	2	0	p_{25}
		1	p_{26}
		2	p_{27}

points from a large number of subjects in each of two groups. Let

$$\boldsymbol{L} = (L_{111}, L_{112}, L_{121}, L_{122}, L_{131}, L_{132}, L_{211}, L_{212}, L_{221}, L_{222}, L_{231}, L_{232})'$$

denote the 12×1 vector of cumulative logit response functions, where L_{hjk} is the kth cumulative logit at time j in group h for $h = 1, 2$, $j = 1, 2, 3$, $k = 1, 2$. Thus, in group h at time j,

$$L_{hj1} = \log\left(\frac{\Pr(\text{response} = 0)}{\Pr(\text{response} = 1 \text{ or } 2)}\right), L_{hj2} = \log\left(\frac{\Pr(\text{response} = 0 \text{ or } 1)}{\Pr(\text{response} = 2)}\right).$$

Consider the model $\boldsymbol{L} = \boldsymbol{X\beta}$, where

$$\boldsymbol{X} = \begin{pmatrix} 1 & 0 & 1 & 0 & 1 & 0 \\ 0 & 1 & 0 & 1 & 0 & 1 \\ 1 & 0 & 1 & 0 & 2 & 0 \\ 0 & 1 & 0 & 1 & 0 & 2 \\ 1 & 0 & 1 & 0 & 3 & 0 \\ 0 & 1 & 0 & 1 & 0 & 3 \\ 1 & 0 & -1 & 0 & 1 & 0 \\ 0 & 1 & 0 & -1 & 0 & 1 \\ 1 & 0 & -1 & 0 & 2 & 0 \\ 0 & 1 & 0 & -1 & 0 & 2 \\ 1 & 0 & -1 & 0 & 3 & 0 \\ 0 & 1 & 0 & -1 & 0 & 3 \end{pmatrix}.$$

(a) If this model is fit using weighted least squares, state in words the hypothesis tested by the lack-of-fit statistic.

(b) Specify the coefficient matrix $\boldsymbol{C}$ for testing the hypothesis $H_0\colon \boldsymbol{C\beta} = \boldsymbol{0}$ of no group effect.

(c) Repeat part (b) for the hypothesis of no time effect.

7.5 Suppose that a dichotomous response with possible values 0 and 1 is measured at months 0, 2, and 5 for each of n subjects from a single population. Because the response may be missing at any of the three time points, the proportion of subjects in each of the $3^3 - 1 = 26$ combinations of the cross-classification of time and response can be summarized in the vector $\boldsymbol{p} = (p_1, \ldots, p_{26})'$, as shown in Table 7.20.

(a) Let $\boldsymbol{F}(\boldsymbol{p}) = (L_0, L_2, L_5)'$, where

$$L_j = \log\left(\frac{\Pr(\text{response 1 at time } j)}{\Pr(\text{response 0 at time } j)}\right)$$

denotes the log-odds of response $= 1$ at time j for $j = 0, 2, 5$. Define this vector of response functions $\boldsymbol{F}(\boldsymbol{p})$ as a sequence of linear, logarithmic, and/or exponential transformations of $\boldsymbol{p}$.

(b) Now, suppose that $\boldsymbol{F}(\boldsymbol{p}) = (P_0, P_2, P_5)'$, where P_j is the probability of response $= 1$ at time j for $j = 0, 2, 5$. Using all available data, define this vector of response functions $\boldsymbol{F}(\boldsymbol{p})$ as a sequence of linear, logarithmic, and/or exponential transformations of $\boldsymbol{p}$.

(c) If you wish to model these data using the weighted least squares approach to fit models of the form $\boldsymbol{F}(\boldsymbol{p}) = \boldsymbol{X\beta}$, discuss the factors you would consider in deciding whether to use the response functions L_j or P_j.

7.6 Two diagnostic procedures (standard and test) were evaluated on each of two occasions in 793 subjects (MacMillan et al., 1981). At each of the four treatment–time combinations, the response was categorized as negative or positive. Table 7.21 displays the cross-classification of the four results for each subject.

(a) Test the null hypothesis that the marginal probability of a negative result is the same across the four treatment–time combinations.

(b) Fit a model permitting separate tests of the effects of time, treatment, and time × treatment interaction.

(c) Fit a reduced model incorporating only those effects that are judged to be statistically significant.

(d) Summarize the results of your analysis.

7.7 In the Iowa 65+ Rural Health Study (Cornoni-Huntley et al., 1986), 1926 elderly individuals were followed over a six-year period. Each individual was surveyed at years 0, 3, and 6. One of the variables of interest was the number of friends reported by each respondent. This was an ordered categorical variable with possible values 0 friends, 1–2 friends, and 3 or more friends. Table 7.5 displays the cross-classification of the responses at years 0, 3, and 6 for these 1926 individuals; Section 7.3.4 illustrated the analysis of marginal proportions and marginal mean scores.

(a) Analyze the cumulative marginal proportions; that is, the two response functions at each time point are Pr(no friends) and Pr(less than three friends). Test the hypothesis of marginal homogeneity of the distributions across the three times and investigate whether linear time trends are sufficient to describe the results.

(b) Compare your results from part (a) with those obtained from the analysis of marginal proportions presented in Section 7.3.4.

7.8 In a randomized experiment designed to determine whether driver education reduces the number of collisions and violations among teenage

TABLE 7.20. Response proportions for a dichotomous outcome measured at three time points

Response at Month			
0	2	5	Proportion
0	0	0	p_1
		1	p_2
		Missing	p_3
	1	0	p_4
		1	p_5
		Missing	p_6
	Missing	0	p_7
		1	p_8
		Missing	p_9
1	0	0	p_{10}
		1	p_{11}
		Missing	p_{12}
	1	0	p_{13}
		1	p_{14}
		Missing	p_{15}
	Missing	0	p_{16}
		1	p_{17}
		Missing	p_{18}
Missing	0	0	p_{19}
		1	p_{20}
		Missing	p_{21}
	1	0	p_{22}
		1	p_{23}
		Missing	p_{24}
	Missing	0	p_{25}
		1	p_{26}

TABLE 7.21. Diagnostic test results from 793 subjects

Time 1		Time 2		
Standard	Test	Standard	Test	Count
Negative	Negative	Negative	Negative	509
Negative	Negative	Negative	Positive	4
Negative	Negative	Positive	Negative	17
Negative	Negative	Positive	Positive	3
Negative	Positive	Negative	Negative	13
Negative	Positive	Negative	Positive	8
Negative	Positive	Positive	Negative	0
Negative	Positive	Positive	Positive	8
Positive	Negative	Negative	Negative	14
Positive	Negative	Negative	Positive	1
Positive	Negative	Positive	Negative	17
Positive	Negative	Positive	Positive	9
Positive	Positive	Negative	Negative	7
Positive	Positive	Negative	Positive	4
Positive	Positive	Positive	Negative	9
Positive	Positive	Positive	Positive	170
Total				793

drivers (Stock et al., 1983), eligible students were randomized to one of three groups: (a) safe performance curriculum (SPC), (b) pre-driver licensing curriculum (PDL), (c) control. At the time of the study, the 70-hour SPC was considered to be the most advanced and thorough high school driver education program in the U.S. In contrast, the PDL was a 30-hour course containing only the minimum training required to pass a license test. Students assigned to the control group received no formal driver education coursework through the school system and were expected to be taught to drive by their parents and/or private driver-training schools. Follow-up data concerning the occurrence of collisions and moving violations were obtained using records from the state Department of Motor Vehicles.

Table 7.22 displays data from 2409 males who were randomized to the control group and followed for four years. During each year of follow-up, it was determined whether the subject had been cited for any traffic violations. The goal is to assess the relationship between the probability of having a traffic violation (more precisely, the probability of one or more violations) and year of follow-up.

(a) Test the null hypothesis that the probability of a traffic violation is the same at each of the four years. If the null hypothesis of equality of proportions is rejected, carry out separate pairwise comparisons between years.

TABLE 7.22. Traffic violation data from 2409 male subjects in the control group of the driver education study

Traffic Violation Status				
Year 1	Year 2	Year 3	Year 4	Count
No	No	No	No	731
No	No	No	Yes	310
No	No	Yes	No	256
No	No	Yes	Yes	196
No	Yes	No	No	156
No	Yes	No	Yes	121
No	Yes	Yes	No	114
No	Yes	Yes	Yes	152
Yes	No	No	No	61
Yes	No	No	Yes	40
Yes	No	Yes	No	45
Yes	No	Yes	Yes	39
Yes	Yes	No	No	47
Yes	Yes	No	Yes	42
Yes	Yes	Yes	No	46
Yes	Yes	Yes	Yes	53
Total				2409

(b) Test the null hypothesis that the relationship between the probability of a traffic violation and year of follow-up is linear.

(c) Fit a polynomial model for predicting the probability of a violation as a function of follow-up year. Report the goodness-of-fit of this model and plot observed and predicted probabilities.

7.9 In a longitudinal study of coronary risk factors in children (Woolson and Clarke, 1984), biennial cross-sectional school screens were conducted from 1971 to 1981. At each screening, height and weight were measured on participating children, from which relative weight was computed (the ratio of the child's weight to the median weight in the sex–age–height group). Children with relative weight greater than 110% of the median weight were classified as obese. Table 7.11 displays the results from the 1977, 1979, and 1981 surveys for the cohort of males who were 7–9 years old in 1977. Section 7.4.3 illustrated the fitting of models for the proportion classified as obese.

(a) Let $L_x = \log(\pi_x/(1-\pi_x))$, where π_x is the marginal probability of being classified as obese at year x for $x = 77, 79, 81$. Using all of the data, fit the model $L_x = \alpha + \beta(x - 77)$ via weighted least squares. Comment on the fit of the model and the statistical significance of

TABLE 7.23. Responses from 975 parents at three interviews concerning the problems of rearing children

Problem in the Previous Week			Years of Education	
Time1	Time2	Time3	11+	< 11
Yes	Yes	Yes	135	95
Yes	Yes	No	26	32
Yes	No	Yes	30	33
Yes	No	No	32	30
No	Yes	Yes	79	74
No	Yes	No	29	35
No	No	Yes	65	57
No	No	No	94	129

the resulting parameter estimates. Give an odds-ratio interpretation of the estimate of β.

(b) Repeat part (a) using the subgroup of 225 children who participated in all three surveys. Compare the results and interpretations of the two models.

7.10 Duncan (1985) describes a study in which parents participated in discussions concerning the problems of rearing children. At each of three interviews, subjects were asked to respond to the question, "In the past week, did any of your children come to you with a problem that was bothering them?" The first interview took place prior to the discussions, the second interview was conducted at the conclusion of the 6–8 week period in which the discussions took place, and the third interview occurred 6–8 weeks after the discussion period ended. Table 7.23 displays the responses from 485 subjects with fewer than 11 years of education and from 490 subjects with at least 11 years of education. Using the probability of a "yes" response as the outcome variable, fit one or more models to answer the following questions:

(a) Are the changes over the three interviews in the probability of a "yes" response the same for the two groups of subjects?

(b) Are there changes over time in the probability of a "yes" response?

(c) Are there differences between the two groups of subjects with respect to the overall probability of responding "yes"?

7.11 Mislevy (1985) gives counts of correct and incorrect responses for four items from the arithmetic reasoning test of the Armed Services Vocational Aptitude Battery from samples of white males, white females, black

TABLE 7.24. Correct (1) and incorrect (0) responses to four items from the Armed Services Vocational Aptitude Battery from samples of white males, white females, black males, and black females

Item				White	White	Black	Black
1	2	3	4	Males	Females	Males	Females
0	0	0	0	23	20	27	29
0	0	0	1	5	8	5	8
0	0	1	0	12	14	15	7
0	0	1	1	2	2	3	3
0	1	0	0	16	20	16	14
0	1	0	1	3	5	5	5
0	1	1	0	6	11	4	6
0	1	1	1	1	7	3	0
1	0	0	0	22	23	15	14
1	0	0	1	6	8	10	10
1	0	1	0	7	9	8	11
1	0	1	1	19	6	1	2
1	1	0	0	21	18	7	19
1	1	0	1	11	15	9	5
1	1	1	0	23	20	10	8
1	1	1	1	86	42	2	4

males, and black females. Table 7.24 displays the cross-classification of correct (1) and incorrect (0) responses for the four items in each of the four samples. In analyzing these data, note that there is no order to the four responses from each subject.

(a) Develop a model for predicting the logit of the probability of a correct response as a function of item number, sex, and race.

(b) Repeat part (a) using the probability of a correct response as the outcome variable.

7.12 Table 7.25 displays collision data from the first three years of the driver education experiment described in Problem 7.8 for 14,127 individuals with complete follow-up. The response variable is "Yes" if the individual was involved in one or more collisions during the year and "No" otherwise. We wish to determine whether randomization to one of the two driver education groups affects the probability of being involved in a collision and, if so, how long any effects persist.

(a) Using the logit of the probability of a collision as the response variable, fit a saturated model including effects for program, sex, time, and all interactions.

TABLE 7.25. Collision data from 14,127 participants in the driver education study

		Year 1 = No				Year 1 = Yes				
		Year 2 = No		Year 2 = Yes		Year 2 = No		Year 2 = Yes		
		Year 3		Year 3		Year 3		Year 3		
Program	Sex	No	Yes	No	Yes	No	Yes	No	Yes	Total
SPC	M	1467	295	305	79	190	68	60	19	2483
	F	1659	218	217	28	120	30	17	4	2293
PDL	M	1495	264	278	80	206	52	46	25	2446
	F	1618	228	191	24	122	12	17	3	2215
Control	M	1552	288	271	94	167	47	55	23	2497
	F	1640	217	185	24	96	13	16	2	2193

(b) After moving any nonsignificant interactions to the error space, fit a reduced factorial model involving the factors program, sex, follow-up year, and their interactions (again using named effects rather than an explicitly specified design matrix). Justify your choice of model by documenting the results of any preliminary models that you first fit to the data.

(c) Suppose that the investigator is interested in summarizing these data in terms of a model with separate program and sex effects for each of the three years of follow-up. Fit an equivalent model to part (b) with nested effects rather than factorial effects. Partition the two degrees of freedom (df) for differences among programs into two "meaningful" 1-df effects.

(d) Based on the results from part (c), fit a reduced model that adequately explains the variation in the observed data. Summarize your final model in terms of the estimated parameters and predicted odds ratios.

7.13 Table 7.26 displays the wheezing status (yes, no) of 537 children from Steubenville, Ohio at ages 7, 8, 9, and 10 years of age (Fitzmaurice and Laird, 1993). In 187 of these children, the child's mother was a regular smoker. Analyze these data to determine how the logit of the probability of wheezing is affected by maternal smoking, child's age, and the interaction between maternal smoking and child's age. Summarize your results.

7.14 Using the data from Problem 7.7 (as displayed in Table 7.5), let $p_{j,0}$, $p_{j,1-2}$, and $p_{j,3+}$ denote the marginal probabilities of each response category at time j, for $j = 0, 3, 6$, and consider the following three sets of response functions:

TABLE 7.26. Wheezing status of 537 children from Steubenville, Ohio

Maternal Smoking									
No					Yes				
Age 7	Age 8	Age 9	Age 10	No. of Children	Age 7	Age 8	Age 9	Age 10	No. of Children
No	No	No	No	237	No	No	No	No	118
			Yes	10				Yes	6
		Yes	No	15			Yes	No	8
			Yes	4				Yes	2
	Yes	No	No	16		Yes	No	No	11
			Yes	2				Yes	1
		Yes	No	7			Yes	No	6
			Yes	3				Yes	4
Yes	No	No	No	24	Yes	No	No	No	7
			Yes	3				Yes	3
		Yes	No	3			Yes	No	3
			Yes	2				Yes	1
	Yes	No	No	6		Yes	No	No	4
			Yes	2				Yes	2
		Yes	No	5			Yes	No	4
			Yes	11				Yes	7
Total				350					187

- logits:

$$L_{j1} = \ln(p_{j,1-2}/p_{j,0}), \quad L_{j2} = \ln(p_{j,3+}/p_{j,0});$$

- adjacent-category logits:

$$L_{j1} = \ln(p_{j,1-2}/p_{j,0}), \quad L_{j2} = \ln(p_{j,3+}/p_{j,1-2});$$

- cumulative logits:

$$L_{j1} = \ln\big((p_{j,1-2} + p_{j,3+})/p_{j,0}\big), \quad L_{j2} = \ln\big(p_{j,3+}/(p_{j,0} + p_{j,1-2})\big).$$

For each of these sets of response functions:

(a) Fit a saturated model incorporating linear and nonlinear time effects.

(b) Test whether the linear and quadratic time effects are significantly different from zero (for each response function as well as for both response functions simultaneously).

(c) Test whether the linear (quadratic) effects are the same for the two response functions.

(d) If warranted, fit a reduced model including only those time effects that are significantly different from zero and using common effects for the two response functions.

(e) Interpret the parameter estimates from your final model in terms of odds ratios.

Which of the three analyses leads to the simplest interpretation of the data?

7.15 Of the 15,541 students who participated in the driver education trial considered in Problems 7.8 and 7.12, nearly 95% (14,714) completed at least one year of follow-up. Table 7.27 displays collision data from the first three years of the study for these subjects. The response variable is "Yes" if the individual was involved in one or more collisions during the year, "No" if the individual was not involved in a collision, and "Unk" if follow-up information was not available.

(a) Using the probability of a collision as the response, fit a saturated model including effects for program, sex, time, and all interactions.

(b) After moving any nonsignificant interactions to the error space, fit a reduced factorial model involving the factors program, sex, follow-up year, and their interactions. Justify your choice of model by documenting the results of any preliminary models that you first fit to the data.

(c) Suppose that the investigator is specifically interested in summarizing these data in terms of a model involving separate effects for each year of follow-up. Fit an equivalent model to part (b) with nested effects rather than factorial effects. Partition the two df for differences among programs into two "meaningful" 1-df effects.

(d) Based on the results from part (c), fit a reduced model that adequately explains the variation in the observed data. Summarize your final model in terms of the estimated parameters and predicted probabilities.

7.16 In a placebo-controlled clinical trial of the efficacy of a new drug for treating a skin condition, patients were randomly assigned to one of two groups (drug, placebo). Prior to treatment, each patient was evaluated to determine the initial severity of the skin condition (moderate or severe). At three follow-up visits, patients were evaluated according to a five-point ordinal response scale defining extent of improvement (1 = rapidly improving, 2 = slowly improving, 3 = stable, 4 = slowly worsening, 5 = rapidly worsening). Table 7.28 displays the ordinal response scores at visits 1, 2, and 3 for the 88 patients in the active treatment group and the 84 patients in the placebo group (Stanish et al., 1978; Landis et al., 1988).

(a) Using all available data, determine a parsimonious factorial model for the mean improvement scores as a function of treatment, initial status, and visit. Justify your choice of model by documenting the results of any preliminary models that you first fit to the data.

(b) Reparameterize your factorial model from part (a) to have separate incremental effects from visit 1 to visit 2 and from visit 2 to visit 3 in each treatment group. Test the equality of the visit effects in the two groups.

(c) Based on the results of part (b), fit a reduced model that explains the variation in mean scores using as few parameters as possible. Interpret the results of your final model.

7.17 With reference to the longitudinal study of coronary risk factors in children described in Section 7.4.3 and Problem 7.9 (Woolson and Clarke, 1984), Table 7.29 displays the cross-classification of obesity outcomes in 1977, 1979, and 1981 for 4856 children from ten age–sex populations (five 2-year age intervals for males and females). There are many patterns of participation over the course of the study due to absences, children entering school, children leaving school, and other factors.

(a) Using all available data, model the marginal probability of obesity as a quadratic function of age (using the midpoints of the age intervals)

TABLE 7.27. Collision data from 14,714 participants in the driver education study

SPC					PDL					Control				
	Year					Year					Year			
Sex	1	2	3	n	Sex	1	2	3	n	Sex	1	2	3	n
M	No	Unk	Unk	41	M	No	Unk	Unk	33	M	No	Unk	Unk	31
	No	No	Unk	34		No	No	Unk	30		No	No	Unk	29
	No	No	No	1467		No	No	No	1495		No	No	No	1552
	No	No	Yes	295		No	No	Yes	264		No	No	Yes	288
	No	Yes	Unk	11		No	Yes	Unk	16		No	Yes	Unk	21
	No	Yes	No	305		No	Yes	No	278		No	Yes	No	271
	No	Yes	Yes	79		No	Yes	Yes	80		No	Yes	Yes	94
	Yes	Unk	Unk	11		Yes	Unk	Unk	8		Yes	Unk	Unk	8
	Yes	No	Unk	4		Yes	No	Unk	2		Yes	No	Unk	1
	Yes	No	No	190		Yes	No	No	206		Yes	No	No	167
	Yes	No	Yes	68		Yes	No	Yes	52		Yes	No	Yes	47
	Yes	Yes	Unk	3		Yes	Yes	Unk	4		Yes	Yes	Unk	2
	Yes	Yes	No	60		Yes	Yes	No	46		Yes	Yes	No	55
	Yes	Yes	Yes	19		Yes	Yes	Yes	25		Yes	Yes	Yes	23
F	No	Unk	Unk	34	F	No	Unk	Unk	45	F	No	Unk	Unk	48
	No	No	Unk	35		No	No	Unk	49		No	No	Unk	36
	No	No	No	1659		No	No	No	1618		No	No	No	1640
	No	No	Yes	218		No	No	Yes	228		No	No	Yes	217
	No	Yes	Unk	7		No	Yes	Unk	6		No	Yes	Unk	9
	No	Yes	No	217		No	Yes	No	191		No	Yes	No	185
	No	Yes	Yes	28		No	Yes	Yes	24		No	Yes	Yes	24
	Yes	Unk	Unk	9		Yes	Unk	Unk	8		Yes	Unk	Unk	4
	Yes	No	Unk	4		Yes	No	Unk	2		Yes	No	Unk	1
	Yes	No	No	120		Yes	No	No	122		Yes	No	No	96
	Yes	No	Yes	30		Yes	No	Yes	12		Yes	No	Yes	13
	Yes	Yes	Unk	1		Yes	Yes	Unk	0		Yes	Yes	Unk	0
	Yes	Yes	No	17		Yes	Yes	No	17		Yes	Yes	No	16
	Yes	Yes	Yes	4		Yes	Yes	Yes	3		Yes	Yes	Yes	2

TABLE 7.28. Improvement scores from 172 subjects in a randomized trial of a new drug for treating a skin condition

Active Treatment										Placebo Treatment									
	Initial	Visit				Initial	Visit				Initial	Visit				Initial	Visit		
ID	Status	1	2	3	ID	Status	1	2	3	ID	Status	1	2	3	ID	Status	1	2	3
1	Mod	3	.	3	45	Mod	1	1	1	1	Mod	4	3	3	45	Mod	3	.	5
2	Mod	3	2	2	46	Sev	3	3	4	2	Mod	4	4	4	46	Sev	4	3	4
3	Sev	3	2	2	47	Mod	2	2	1	3	Sev	4	5	4	47	Mod	2	3	3
4	Mod	2	2	1	48	Mod	2	1	1	4	Mod	4	4	5	48	Sev	3	3	3
5	Mod	3	2	2	49	Sev	2	1	1	5	Mod	4	4	4	49	Sev	3	3	3
6	Sev	2	1	3	50	Sev	2	2	2	6	Sev	4	4	4	50	Sev	4	3	3
7	Sev	1	1	1	51	Sev	3	2	1	7	Sev	4	.	.	51	Mod	3	3	3
8	Sev	1	1	1	52	Sev	2	1	1	8	Mod	4	4	.	52	Mod	4	4	4
9	Sev	5	.	.	53	Sev	2	2	1	9	Mod	2	2	.	53	Mod	1	1	1
10	Mod	1	1	1	54	Sev	2	2	1	10	Sev	3	3	4	54	Mod	2	2	.
11	Sev	4	4	4	55	Mod	1	1	1	11	Mod	4	4	4	55	Mod	2	2	2
12	Sev	3	1	1	56	Mod	1	1	1	12	Mod	4	4	.	56	Mod	4	4	.
13	Sev	1	1	1	57	Mod	2	2	1	13	Sev	4	4	.	57	Mod	1	1	2
14	Sev	3	3	3	58	Mod	2	2	1	14	Sev	4	5	.	58	Mod	2	3	3
15	Sev	1	1	1	59	Mod	1	1	1	15	Sev	4	4	.	59	Mod	4	3	3
16	Mod	1	1	.	60	Mod	3	2	1	16	Mod	4	.	.	60	Mod	3	3	3
17	Mod	4	4	4	61	Mod	2	2	2	17	Sev	1	1	.	61	Sev	3	3	4
18	Mod	3	.	.	62	Mod	1	1	1	18	Mod	4	4	4	62	Mod	3	3	4
19	Sev	.	1	.	63	Mod	3	1	1	19	Sev	3	3	3	63	Mod	3	3	3
20	Mod	3	3	3	64	Mod	2	2	2	20	Sev	4	4	4	64	Mod	5	.	.
21	Sev	2	2	2	65	Mod	3	2	2	21	Sev	2	2	2	65	Mod	2	2	1
22	Sev	3	2	2	66	Mod	3	3	2	22	Sev	4	4	.	66	Mod	4	4	4
23	Sev	4	.	.	67	Mod	1	1	1	23	Sev	2	2	2	67	Mod	4	3	3
24	Sev	2	2	2	68	Mod	1	1	1	24	Mod	3	3	.	68	Sev	2	2	1
25	Sev	2	2	1	69	Mod	3	3	3	25	Sev	4	4	.	69	Sev	4	4	4
26	Sev	3	3	3	70	Mod	1	1	1	26	Sev	4	3	3	70	Sev	4	4	4
27	Mod	1	1	1	71	Mod	2	2	2	27	Sev	5	.	.	71	Sev	4	3	4
28	Sev	3	1	1	72	Mod	2	2	1	28	Mod	1	.	1	72	Mod	4	4	.
29	Sev	2	2	1	73	Sev	2	1	1	29	Mod	4	2	4	73	Sev	4	3	3
30	Mod	2	.	1	74	Mod	4	3	3	30	Sev	5	.	.	74	Sev	2	2	2
31	Mod	3	4	4	75	Sev	3	.	.	31	Sev	4	5	.	75	Mod	4	4	.
32	Sev	2	2	2	76	Mod	2	1	1	32	Sev	4	4	3	76	Sev	4	3	3
33	Sev	2	1	1	77	Sev	.	3	2	33	Sev	3	4	4	77	Sev	4	3	3
34	Sev	3	4	4	78	Sev	3	.	.	34	Sev	4	3	3	78	Sev	3	3	3
35	Sev	1	1	1	79	Sev	2	2	2	35	Mod	1	1	2	79	Sev	2	2	1
36	Sev	1	1	1	80	Sev	2	2	2	36	Sev	2	2	3	80	Mod	4	3	3
37	Sev	.	4	4	81	Sev	2	2	1	37	Mod	2	2	3	81	Sev	4	4	4
38	Sev	3	2	1	82	Sev	2	1	1	38	Mod	3	5	5	82	Mod	4	4	3
39	Sev	1	.	1	83	Mod	1	1	.	39	Mod	2	2	2	83	Sev	4	3	3
40	Sev	1	1	1	84	Mod	2	1	1	40	Sev	3	3	3	84	Mod	4	3	3
41	Mod	2	1	.	85	Mod	3	2	2	41	Mod	3	3	3					.
42	Sev	2	1	1	86	Sev	2	2	1	42	Sev	4	3	3					.
43	Mod	1	1	1	87	Sev	1	1	1	43	Sev	4	4	5					.
44	Sev	2	2	2	88	Sev	2	1	1	44	Sev	4	.	.					.

with separate intercepts and linear and quadratic age parameters for males and females. Does this model provide an adequate fit to the observed data?

(b) Test hypotheses regarding the equality of the constant, linear, and quadratic parameters for males and females. Use the results to fit a reduced model.

(c) Consider "completeness" to be an additional stratification variable, and refit the model from part (a) with separate parameters for complete and incomplete cases. Test the hypothesis that the corresponding parameter estimates for complete and incomplete cases are equal.

(d) Using the results of part (c), fit one or more reduced models that combine parameters for complete and incomplete cases, as appropriate.

(e) Compare the results from parts (b) and (d); comment on any differences in the conclusions of the two models.

TABLE 7.29. Classification of 4856 children from the Muscatine Coronary Risk Factor Study by obesity status

N=not obese O=obese M=missing			Males					Females				
			Age in 1977 (yrs.)					Age in 1977 (yrs.)				
1977	1979	1981	5–7	7–9	9–11	11–13	13–15	5–7	7–9	9–11	11–13	13–15
N	N	N	90	150	152	119	101	75	154	148	129	91
N	N	0	9	15	11	7	4	8	14	6	8	9
N	O	N	3	8	8	8	2	2	13	10	7	5
N	O	0	7	8	10	3	7	4	19	8	9	3
O	N	N	0	8	7	13	8	2	2	12	6	6
O	N	0	1	9	7	4	0	2	6	0	2	0
O	O	N	1	7	9	11	6	1	6	8	7	6
O	O	0	8	20	25	16	15	8	21	27	14	15
N	N	M	16	38	48	42	82	20	25	36	36	83
N	O	M	5	3	6	4	9	0	3	0	9	15
O	N	M	0	1	2	4	8	0	1	7	4	6
O	O	M	0	11	14	13	12	4	11	17	13	23
N	M	N	9	16	13	14	6	7	16	8	31	5
N	M	O	3	6	5	2	1	2	3	1	4	0
O	M	N	0	1	0	1	0	0	0	1	2	0
O	M	O	0	3	3	4	1	1	4	4	6	1
M	N	N	129	42	36	18	13	109	47	39	19	11
M	N	O	18	2	5	3	1	22	4	6	1	1
M	O	N	6	3	4	3	2	7	1	7	2	2
M	O	O	13	13	3	1	2	24	8	13	2	3
N	M	M	32	45	59	82	95	23	47	53	58	89
O	M	M	5	7	17	24	23	5	7	16	37	32
M	N	M	33	33	31	23	34	27	23	25	21	43
M	O	M	11	4	9	6	12	5	5	9	1	15
M	M	N	70	55	40	37	15	65	39	23	23	14
M	M	O	24	14	9	14	3	19	13	8	10	5

8 Randomization Model Methods for One-Sample Repeated Measurements

8.1 Introduction

In many settings in which the response variable is categorical, the WLS approach described in Chapter 7 cannot be used. For example, the sample size may be too small, the number of time points may be too large, and/or the response variable may have too many possible values. In addition, the methods described in Chapters 3–6 for analyzing continuous response variables are also often inapplicable. For example, the distribution of the outcome variable may be markedly nonnormal. This chapter describes an alternative methodology based on the randomization model and the multiple hypergeometric distribution.

The randomization model approach is useful for assessing the strength of association between a response variable and a repeated measurements factor in a relatively assumption-free context. This methodology applies to both categorical and continuous outcomes. The basic idea is that the data from each subject or experimental unit are structured as a two-way table of counts. The levels of the repeated measurements factor define the rows of this table, and the values of the outcome variable define the columns. One then carries out a stratified analysis of multiple two-way tables, where each subject (experimental unit) defines a stratum. This approach does not require random sampling of subjects from some underlying probabilistic framework.

The randomization model test statistics are valid when sample sizes are too small to warrant the use of other large-sample methods. This is because the sample size requirements for validity of asymptotic tests apply to across-strata (across-subject) totals rather than to within-strata totals. The methodology also easily accommodates missing data (provided that the missing-data mechanism is MCAR, as described in Section 1.4).

There are, however, several limitations of the randomization model approach to the analysis of repeated measurements. The major limitation is that the use of this methodology is restricted to one-sample problems. Thus, although it is possible to test the strength of association between the response variable and the repeated measurements factor, one cannot assess the influence of additional covariates. In addition, this approach provides hypothesis testing procedures only; estimation of parameters and their standard errors, as well as construction of confidence intervals, is not generally possible. Another shortcoming is that the scope of inference is restricted to the actual subjects under study rather than to some broad population that the subjects might conceptually represent. Finally, the randomization model test statistics are insensitive to alternatives in which associations vary in direction across strata (subjects).

The randomization model approach is based on the use of Cochran–Mantel–Haenszel (CMH) test statistics. Landis et al. (1978) give a general overview of the three types of CMH statistics. Landis et al. (1988) and Crowder and Hand (1990, Section 8.6) describe the use of these procedures in analyzing repeated measurements.

We first introduce the special case where a binary response variable is measured at two time points for each experimental unit. Section 8.2 provides background material on the hypergeometric distribution, and Section 8.3 applies these results to the analysis of repeated measurements. We then consider the more general case where a response variable with c levels is measured at t time points for $c > 2$ and $t > 2$. Section 8.4 describes the multiple hypergeometric distribution, and Section 8.5 applies the results to the repeated measurements setting. Section 8.6 describes the use of the randomization model approach when there are missing data, and Section 8.7 discusses the use of this methodology when the response variable is continuous rather than categorical.

8.2 The Hypergeometric Distribution and Large-Sample Tests of Randomness for 2 × 2 Tables

8.2.1 The Hypergeometric Distribution

Consider a population of n objects, of which $n_{.1}$ are of type 1 and $n - n_{.1}$ are of type 2. Suppose that a random sample of size $n_{1.}$ is selected from this population (without replacement). Let the random variable X denote

TABLE 8.1. Hypergeometric sampling model

Sampled	Type 1	Type 2	Total
Yes	X	$n_{1.} - X$	$n_{1.}$
No	$n_{.1} - X$	$n - n_{1.} - n_{.1} + X$	$n - n_{1.}$
Total	$n_{.1}$	$n - n_{.1}$	n

the number of type 1 objects in the sample. Table 8.1 displays the data from such an experiment in a 2×2 contingency table.

The probability function of the random variable X is

$$\begin{aligned} \Pr(X = x) &= \binom{n_{.1}}{x}\binom{n - n_{.1}}{n_{1.} - x} \Big/ \binom{n}{n_{1.}} \\ &= \frac{\dfrac{n_{.1}!}{x!(n_{.1} - x)!}\,\dfrac{(n - n_{.1})!}{(n_{1.} - x)!(n - n_{.1} - n_{1.} + x)!}}{\dfrac{n!}{n_{1.}!(n - n_{1.})!}} \\ &= \frac{n_{.1}!\,(n - n_{.1})!\,n_{1.}!\,(n - n_{1.})!}{n!\,x!(n_{.1} - x)!(n_{1.} - x)!(n - n_{.1} - n_{1.} + x)!} \end{aligned} \tag{8.1}$$

for $\max(0, n_{1.} + n_{.1} - n) \leq x \leq \min(n_{1.}, n_{.1})$. The random variable X has the hypergeometric distribution with parameters n, $n_{1.}$, and $n_{.1}$; we write this as $X \sim H(n, n_{1.}, n_{.1})$.

The hypergeometric distribution has mean and variance given by

$$\mathrm{E}(X) = \frac{n_{1.}n_{.1}}{n}, \tag{8.2}$$

$$\mathrm{Var}(X) = \frac{n_{1.}(n - n_{1.})n_{.1}(n - n_{.1})}{n^2(n-1)}. \tag{8.3}$$

Note that $n_{.1}/n$ is the proportion of objects of type 1, and $n_{1.}$ is the sample size. Thus, $\mathrm{E}(X)$ is equivalent to the mean of the binomial distribution with sample size $n = n_{1.}$ and success probability $\pi = n_{.1}/n$, and $\mathrm{Var}(X)$ is then

$$n\pi(1-\pi) \times \frac{n - n_{1.}}{n - 1}.$$

When n is much larger than $n_{1.}$, the hypergeometric variance is only slightly smaller than the corresponding binomial variance.

8.2.2 Test of Randomness for a 2×2 Contingency Table

Consider a sample of n observations classified with respect to two dichotomous variables. Table 8.2 displays the resulting frequencies as a 2×2 contingency table. If the row and column marginal totals are fixed (either by

TABLE 8.2. Cell frequencies for a 2 × 2 contingency table

Row	Column Variable		
Variable	Level 1	Level 2	Total
Level 1	n_{11}	n_{12}	$n_{1.}$
Level 2	n_{21}	n_{22}	$n_{2.}$
Total	$n_{.1}$	$n_{.2}$	n

design or by conditioning), then the distribution of n_{11}, the count in the (1,1) cell of Table 8.2, is $H(n, n_{1.}, n_{.1})$.

Under the null hypothesis of randomness, the probability function of n_{11} is

$$f(n_{11}) = \frac{n_{1.}!\, n_{2.}!\, n_{.1}!\, n_{.2}!}{n!\, n_{11}!\, n_{12}!\, n_{21}!\, n_{22}!}$$

for $\max(0, n_{1.} + n_{.1} - n) \leq n_{11} \leq \min(n_{1.}, n_{.1})$. Using Equations (8.2) and (8.3) for the mean and variance of a hypergeometric random variable,

$$\mathrm{E}(n_{11}) = \frac{n_{1.} n_{.1}}{n}, \tag{8.4}$$

$$\mathrm{Var}(n_{11}) = \frac{n_{1.} n_{2.} n_{.1} n_{.2}}{n^2(n-1)}. \tag{8.5}$$

A large-sample test of randomness is based on the statistic

$$Q = \frac{\left(n_{11} - \mathrm{E}(n_{11})\right)^2}{\mathrm{Var}(n_{11})},$$

which has an asymptotic χ_1^2 distribution. This statistic differs slightly from the usual Pearson chi-square statistic

$$X^2 = \sum_{i=1}^{2} \sum_{j=1}^{2} \frac{(n_{ij} - \widehat{m}_{ij})^2}{\widehat{m}_{ij}},$$

where $\widehat{m}_{ij} = n_{i.} n_{.j}/n$. One can show that

$$Q = \frac{n-1}{n} X^2.$$

8.2.3 Test of Randomness for s 2 × 2 Contingency Tables

Consider a set of s independent 2×2 tables with the counts in the hth table denoted as shown in Table 8.3. The null hypothesis of interest in this situation is:

H_0: no association between the row and column variables in any of the s tables.

TABLE 8.3. Cell frequencies for table h

Row	Column Variable		
Variable	Level 1	Level 2	Total
Level 1	n_{h11}	n_{h12}	$n_{h1.}$
Level 2	n_{h21}	n_{h22}	$n_{h2.}$
Total	$n_{h.1}$	$n_{h.2}$	n_h

If the row and column marginal totals in each table are fixed, the n_{h11} counts are independent hypergeometric random variables with

$$n_{h11} \sim H(n_h, n_{h1.}, n_{h.1}).$$

If H_0 is true,

$$\begin{aligned} \mathrm{E}(n_{h11}) &= \frac{n_{h1.}n_{h.1}}{n_h}, \\ \mathrm{Var}(n_{h11}) &= \frac{n_{h1.}n_{h2.}n_{h.1}n_{h.2}}{n_h^2(n_h - 1)}. \end{aligned}$$

Now, let $X = \sum_{h=1}^{s} n_{h11}$. This random variable has mean and variance given by

$$\begin{aligned} \mathrm{E}(X) &= \sum_{h=1}^{s} \mathrm{E}(n_{h11}) = \sum_{h=1}^{s} \frac{n_{h1.}n_{h.1}}{n_h}, \\ \mathrm{Var}(X) &= \sum_{h=1}^{s} \mathrm{Var}(n_{h11}) = \sum_{h=1}^{s} \frac{n_{h1.}n_{h2.}n_{h.1}n_{h.2}}{n_h^2(n_h - 1)}. \end{aligned}$$

H_0 can then be tested using the statistic

$$Q = \frac{(X - \mathrm{E}(X))^2}{\mathrm{Var}(X)}, \tag{8.6}$$

which has an asymptotic null χ_1^2 distribution.

The statistic Q is the Mantel–Haenszel statistic (Mantel and Haenszel, 1959), one of the most widely used tools in the analysis of epidemiologic and medical data. The asymptotic null distribution of Q is valid when s is small, provided that the stratum-specific totals $\{n_h\}$ are large. The statistic Q also has an asymptotic χ_1^2 distribution when s is large, even if the counts $\{n_h\}$ are small.

The value of Q will be large when $n_{h11} - \mathrm{E}(n_{h11})$ is consistently positive or consistently negative across strata. If the direction of the association changes dramatically across strata, that is, if $n_{h11} - \mathrm{E}(n_{h11})$ is positive in some strata and negative in others, the Mantel–Haenszel test will have low power for detecting an overall association.

TABLE 8.4. Contingency table layout for data from the ith subject

Row	Response Category		
Time	+	−	Total
1	n_{i11}	n_{i12}	1
2	n_{i21}	n_{i22}	1
Total	$n_{i.1}$	$n_{i.2}$	2

8.3 Application to Repeated Measurements: Binary Response, Two Time Points

Suppose that a dichotomous outcome (coded as "+" or "−") is measured at $t = 2$ time points for each of n subjects. Let y_{ij} denote the response of the ith subject at time j for $j = 1, 2$ and $i = 1, \ldots, n$. The data from subject i can be displayed in a 2×2 contingency table, as shown in Table 8.4. Note that in each row of Table 8.4 one of the n_{ijk} values will be equal to 0 and one will be equal to 1.

Table 8.5 displays the four possible 2×2 tables. Using Equations (8.4) and (8.5) from Section 8.2.2, the expected value and variance of the (1, 1) cell for each of the four table types are also displayed. Let a, b, c, and d denote the number of subjects from each of the four types; note that

$$n = a + b + c + d.$$

The statistic Q [Equation (8.6) from Section 8.2.3] is computed as follows:

$$\begin{aligned} X &= \sum_{i=1}^{n} n_{i11} \\ &= (a \times 1) + (b \times 1) + (c \times 0) + (d \times 0) \\ &= a + b, \end{aligned}$$

$$\begin{aligned} \mathrm{E}(X) &= \sum_{i=1}^{n} \mathrm{E}(n_{i11}) \\ &= \left(a \times 1\right) + \left(b \times \frac{1}{2}\right) + \left(c \times \frac{1}{2}\right) + \left(d \times 0\right) \\ &= a + \frac{b+c}{2}, \end{aligned}$$

$$\begin{aligned} \mathrm{Var}(X) &= \sum_{i=1}^{n} \mathrm{Var}(n_{i11}) \\ &= \left(a \times 0\right) + \left(b \times \frac{1}{4}\right) + \left(c \times \frac{1}{4}\right) + \left(d \times 0\right) \\ &= \frac{b+c}{4}. \end{aligned}$$

TABLE 8.5. Four possible tables for the case of a binary response measured at two time points

Type of Table				No. of Subjects	E(n_{i11})	Var(n_{i11})
	Response					
Time	+	−	Total			
1	1	0	1	*a*	1	0
2	1	0	1			
Total	2	0	2			
	Response					
Time	+	−	Total			
1	1	0	1	*b*	1/2	1/4
2	0	1	1			
Total	1	1	2			
	Response					
Time	+	−	Total			
1	0	1	1	*c*	1/2	1/4
2	1	0	1			
Total	1	1	2			
	Response					
Time	+	−	Total			
1	0	1	1	*d*	0	0
2	0	1	1			
Total	0	2	2			

TABLE 8.6. Summary 2 × 2 table

Time 1	Time 2: +	Time 2: −	Total
+	a	b	$a+b$
−	c	d	$c+d$
Total	$a+c$	$b+d$	n

Finally, we have

$$\begin{aligned} Q &= \frac{\left(X - \mathrm{E}(X)\right)^2}{\mathrm{Var}(X)} \\ &= \frac{\left(a + b - \left(a + \dfrac{b+c}{2}\right)\right)^2}{\dfrac{b+c}{4}} \\ &= \frac{(b-c)^2}{b+c}. \end{aligned}$$

If we display the data in a summary 2 × 2 table as shown in Table 8.6, the test based on the Mantel–Haenszel statistic Q is shown to be equivalent to McNemar's (1947) test.

With respect to the sample size required for the use of this test, Mantel and Fleiss (1980) proposed a validity criterion for Q for the general case of s 2 × 2 tables. Their discussion was in terms of the minimum (L_i) and maximum (U_i) possible values of n_{i11}, the (1, 1) cell count for the ith table. Using the layout of Table 8.4,

$$L_i = \max(0, n_{i11} - n_{i22}), \qquad U_i = \min(n_{i1.}, n_{i.1}).$$

Provided that each of the two quantities

$$\sum_{i=1}^{n} \mathrm{E}(n_{i11}) - \sum_{i=1}^{n} L_i, \qquad \sum_{i=1}^{n} U_i - \sum_{i=1}^{n} \mathrm{E}(n_{i11})$$

exceeds 5, the χ_1^2 distribution should adequately approximate the exact distribution of Q. In the repeated measures setting, this requirement simplifies to $b + c \geq 10$.

8.4 The Multiple Hypergeometric Distribution and Large-Sample Tests of Randomness for $r \times c$ Tables

The multiple hypergeometric distribution extends this methodology for the analysis of one-sample repeated measurements to situations where there are more than two time points or when the response variable has more than two possible outcomes.

8.4.1 The Multiple Hypergeometric Distribution

Consider a population of n objects, of which $n_{.1}$ are of type 1, ..., $n_{.t}$ are of type t; note that $n = \sum_{j=1}^{t} n_{.j}$. Suppose that s successive random samples of size $n_{1.}, \ldots, n_{s.}$ are selected from this population without replacement. Let X_{ij} denote the number of elements of type j in sample i for $i = 1, \ldots, s, j = 1, \ldots, t$. The probability that the ith sample contains x_{ij} elements of type j is given by

$$f(\{x_{ij}\}) = \frac{\prod_{i=1}^{s} n_{i.}! \prod_{j=1}^{t} n_{.j}!}{n! \prod_{i=1}^{s} \prod_{j=1}^{t} x_{ij}!}.$$

The random vector $\boldsymbol{X} = (X_{11}, \ldots, X_{st})'$ has the multiple hypergeometric distribution with parameters n, $\{n_{i.}\}$, and $\{n_{.j}\}$; we denote this by

$$\boldsymbol{X} \sim H(n, \{n_{i.}\}, \{n_{.j}\}).$$

This distribution simplifies to the hypergeometric distribution [Equation (8.1)] if $s = t = 2$. To avoid confusion with similar distributions, it should be noted that this is not the same as the multivariate hypergeometric distribution discussed in Bishop et al. (1975, p. 450). It is also not the same as the multiple hypergeometric distribution discussed by Lehmann (1998, p. 381). It is, however, equivalent to the generalized multiple hypergeometric distribution discussed in Lehmann (1998, pp. 382–383).

The expected values, variances, and covariances of the components of the random vector $\boldsymbol{X}$ are as follows:

$$\begin{aligned}
\mathrm{E}(X_{ij}) &= \frac{n_{i.} n_{.j}}{n}, \\
\mathrm{Var}(X_{ij}) &= \frac{n_{i.}(n - n_{i.}) n_{.j}(n - n_{.j})}{n^2(n-1)}, \\
\mathrm{Cov}(X_{ij}, X_{ij'}) &= \frac{-n_{i.}(n - n_{i.}) n_{.j} n_{.j'}}{n^2(n-1)}, \\
\mathrm{Cov}(X_{ij}, X_{i'j}) &= \frac{-n_{i.} n_{i'.} n_{.j}(n - n_{.j})}{n^2(n-1)}, \\
\mathrm{Cov}(X_{ij}, X_{i'j'}) &= \frac{n_{i.} n_{i'.} n_{.j} n_{.j'}}{n^2(n-1)}.
\end{aligned}$$

A general expression for the variances and covariances is

$$\mathrm{Cov}(X_{ij}, X_{i'j'}) = \frac{n_{i.}(\delta_{ii'} n - n_{i'.}) n_{.j}(\delta_{jj'} n - n_{.j'})}{n^2(n-1)},$$

TABLE 8.7. Cell frequencies for an $r \times c$ table

Row	Column Variable					Total
Variable	1	$\cdots$	j	$\cdots$	c	Total
1	n_{11}	$\cdots$	n_{1j}	$\cdots$	n_{1c}	$n_{1.}$
$\vdots$	$\vdots$		$\vdots$		$\vdots$	$\vdots$
i	n_{i1}	$\cdots$	n_{ij}	$\cdots$	n_{ic}	$n_{i.}$
$\vdots$	$\vdots$		$\vdots$		$\vdots$	$\vdots$
r	n_{r1}	$\cdots$	n_{rj}	$\cdots$	n_{rc}	$n_{r.}$
Total	$n_{.1}$	$\cdots$	$n_{.j}$	$\cdots$	$n_{.c}$	N

where $\delta_{ij} = 1$ if $i = j$ and 0 otherwise.

8.4.2 Test of Randomness for an $r \times c$ Contingency Table

Consider a sample of N observations classified with respect to two categorical variables. The resulting frequencies can be displayed in an $r \times c$ contingency table, as shown in Table 8.7. If the row and column marginal totals are fixed (either by design or by conditioning), then

$$\{n_{ij}\} \sim H(N, \{n_{i.}\}, \{n_{.j}\}).$$

Let $\boldsymbol{n} = (n_{11}, \ldots, n_{1c}, \ldots, n_{r1}, \ldots, n_{rc})'$ denote the $rc \times 1$ vector of observed frequencies, and let

$$\boldsymbol{m} = \mathrm{E}(\boldsymbol{n}) = (m_{11}, \ldots, m_{1c}, \ldots, m_{r1}, \ldots, m_{rc})'$$

denote the corresponding vector of expected frequencies. The expected value of n_{ij} is

$$m_{ij} = \frac{n_{i.}n_{.j}}{N} = Np_{i.}p_{.j},$$

where $p_{i.} = n_{i.}/N$ for $i = 1, \ldots, r$ and $p_{.j} = n_{.j}/N$ for $j = 1, \ldots, c$. Also let

$$\boldsymbol{p}_{*.} = (p_{1.}, \ldots, p_{r.})'$$

denote the $r \times 1$ vector of row marginal proportions, and let

$$\boldsymbol{p}_{.*} = (p_{.1}, \ldots, p_{.c})'$$

denote the $c \times 1$ vector of column marginal proportions. Using direct (Kronecker) product notation (Searle, 1982, p. 265),

$$\mathrm{E}(\boldsymbol{n}) = N(\boldsymbol{p}_{*.} \otimes \boldsymbol{p}_{.*}).$$

Let $\boldsymbol{\Sigma}$ denote the $rc \times rc$ variance–covariance matrix of $\boldsymbol{n}$; note that this covariance matrix is singular. The elements of $\boldsymbol{\Sigma}$ are given by

$$\begin{aligned}\operatorname{Cov}(n_{ij}, n_{i'j'}) &= \frac{n_{i.}(\delta_{ii'}N - n_{i'.})n_{.j}(\delta_{jj'}N - n_{.j'})}{N^2(N-1)} \\ &= \frac{N^2}{N-1} p_{i.}(\delta_{ii'} - p_{i'.})p_{.j}(\delta_{jj'} - p_{.j'}),\end{aligned}$$

where $\delta_{ij} = 1$ if $i = j$ and 0 otherwise. In matrix notation,

$$\boldsymbol{\Sigma} = \frac{N^2}{N-1}(\boldsymbol{D}_{\boldsymbol{p}_{*.}} - \boldsymbol{p}_{*.}\boldsymbol{p}'_{*.}) \otimes (\boldsymbol{D}_{\boldsymbol{p}_{.*}} - \boldsymbol{p}_{.*}\boldsymbol{p}'_{.*}),$$

where $\boldsymbol{D}_{\boldsymbol{p}_{*.}}$ and $\boldsymbol{D}_{\boldsymbol{p}_{.*}}$ are diagonal matrices with the elements of $\boldsymbol{p}_{*.}$ and $\boldsymbol{p}_{.*}$ on the main diagonal.

The asymptotic distribution of $N^{-1/2}(\boldsymbol{n}-\boldsymbol{m})$ is $N_{rc}\big(\boldsymbol{0}_{rc}, N^{-1}\boldsymbol{\Sigma}\big)$ (Birch, 1965). If the sample size N is large, $\boldsymbol{n}$ has an approximate $N_{rc}(\boldsymbol{m}, \boldsymbol{\Sigma})$ distribution; note that this is a singular multivariate normal distribution.

Let $\boldsymbol{A} = (\boldsymbol{I}_{r-1}, \boldsymbol{0}_{r-1}) \otimes (\boldsymbol{I}_{c-1}, \boldsymbol{0}_{c-1})$ be an $(r-1)(c-1) \times rc$ matrix, and let $\boldsymbol{G} = \boldsymbol{A}(\boldsymbol{n} - \boldsymbol{m})$ denote the $(r-1)(c-1) \times 1$ vector of differences between the observed and expected frequencies (under the null hypothesis of randomness), where the linear transformation matrix $\boldsymbol{A}$ eliminates the last row and last column.

Under the null hypothesis of randomness,

$$\begin{aligned}\mathrm{E}(\boldsymbol{G}) &= \boldsymbol{0}_{(r-1)(c-1)}, \\ \operatorname{Var}(\boldsymbol{G}) &= \boldsymbol{A}\boldsymbol{\Sigma}\boldsymbol{A}'.\end{aligned}$$

Because $\boldsymbol{G}$ has an approximate $N_{(r-1)(c-1)}(\boldsymbol{0}_{(r-1)(c-1)}, \boldsymbol{A}\boldsymbol{\Sigma}\boldsymbol{A}')$ distribution under H_0,

$$Q = \boldsymbol{G}'(\boldsymbol{A}\boldsymbol{\Sigma}\boldsymbol{A}')^{-1}\boldsymbol{G}$$

is the large-sample quadratic form statistic for testing H_0. If the null hypothesis of randomness is true, then the approximate distribution of Q is $\chi^2_{(r-1)(c-1)}$. It can be shown that

$$Q = \frac{N-1}{N}X^2,$$

where X^2 is the usual Pearson chi-square statistic

$$X^2 = \sum_{i=1}^{r}\sum_{j=1}^{c}\frac{n_{ij} - m_{ij}}{m_{ij}}.$$

8.4.3 Test of Randomness for s r × c Tables

Consider a set of s independent $r \times c$ tables, with the counts in the hth table as shown in Table 8.8. The null hypothesis of interest in this situation is

TABLE 8.8. Cell frequencies for table h

Row	Column Variable					
Variable	1	$\cdots$	j	$\cdots$	c	Total
1	n_{h11}	$\cdots$	n_{h1j}	$\cdots$	n_{h1c}	$n_{h1.}$
$\vdots$	$\vdots$		$\vdots$		$\vdots$	$\vdots$
i	n_{hi1}	$\cdots$	n_{hij}	$\cdots$	n_{hic}	$n_{hi.}$
$\vdots$	$\vdots$		$\vdots$		$\vdots$	$\vdots$
r	n_{hr1}	$\cdots$	n_{hrj}	$\cdots$	n_{hrc}	$n_{hr.}$
Total	$n_{h.1}$	$\cdots$	$n_{h.j}$	$\cdots$	$n_{h.c}$	N_h

H_0: no association between the row and column variables in any of the s tables.

The basic idea is to measure components from each stratum, add the components across strata, and compute a chi-square statistic based on these sums.

If the row and column marginal totals in each table are fixed, the vectors $\boldsymbol{n}_h = (n_{h11}, \ldots, n_{hrc})'$ are independent multiple hypergeometric random variables with

$$\boldsymbol{n}_h \sim H\big(N_h, \{n_{hi.}\}, \{n_{h.j}\}\big).$$

If H_0 is true, $\mathrm{E}(n_{hij}) = n_{hi.}n_{h.j}/N_h$ and

$$\mathrm{Cov}(n_{hij}, n_{hi'j'}) = \frac{n_{hi.}(\delta_{ii'}N_h - n_{hi'.})n_{h.j}(\delta_{jj'}N_h - n_{h.j'})}{N_h^2(N_h-1)},$$

where $\delta_{ij} = 1$ if $i = j$ and 0 otherwise.

Let

$$\boldsymbol{p}_{h*.} = (p_{h1.}, \ldots, p_{hr.})'$$

denote the $r \times 1$ vector of row marginal proportions in the hth table, where $p_{hi.} = n_{hi.}/N_h$, for $i = 1, \ldots, r$, and let

$$\boldsymbol{p}_{h.*} = (p_{h.1}, \ldots, p_{h.c})'$$

denote the corresponding $c \times 1$ vector of column marginal proportions, where $p_{h.j} = n_{h.j}/N_h$ for $j = 1, \ldots, c$. Using matrix notation,

$$\boldsymbol{m}_h = \mathrm{E}(\boldsymbol{n}_h) = N_h(\boldsymbol{p}_{h*.} \otimes \boldsymbol{p}_{h.*}), \tag{8.7}$$

$$\boldsymbol{\Sigma}_h = \frac{N_h^2}{N_h-1}(\boldsymbol{D}_{\boldsymbol{p}_{h*.}} - \boldsymbol{p}_{h*.}\boldsymbol{p}_{h*.}') \otimes (\boldsymbol{D}_{\boldsymbol{p}_{h.*}} - \boldsymbol{p}_{h.*}\boldsymbol{p}_{h.*}'), \tag{8.8}$$

where $\boldsymbol{D}_{\boldsymbol{p}_{h*.}}$ and $\boldsymbol{D}_{\boldsymbol{p}_{h.*}}$ are diagonal matrices with the elements of $\boldsymbol{p}_{h*.}$ and $\boldsymbol{p}_{h.*}$ on the main diagonal, respectively.

Also let

$$\boldsymbol{A} = (\boldsymbol{I}_{r-1}, \boldsymbol{0}_{r-1}) \otimes (\boldsymbol{I}_{c-1}, \boldsymbol{0}_{c-1}),$$

and let $\boldsymbol{G}_h = \boldsymbol{A}(\boldsymbol{n}_h - \boldsymbol{m}_h)$ denote the $(r-1)(c-1) \times 1$ vector of differences between the observed and expected frequencies (under the null hypothesis of randomness) in the hth table. Let $\boldsymbol{G} = \sum_{h=1}^{s} \boldsymbol{G}_h$. Because the s tables are independent,

$$\begin{aligned} \mathrm{E}(\boldsymbol{G}) &= \sum_{h=1}^{s} \mathrm{E}(\boldsymbol{G}_h) = \boldsymbol{0}_{(r-1)(c-1)}, \\ \mathrm{Var}(\boldsymbol{G}) &= \boldsymbol{V_G} = \sum_{h=1}^{s} \mathrm{Var}(\boldsymbol{G}_h) = \sum_{h=1}^{s} \boldsymbol{A}\boldsymbol{\Sigma}_h\boldsymbol{A}', \end{aligned}$$

if H_0 is true.

Because $\boldsymbol{G}$ is approximately $N_{(r-1)(c-1)}(\boldsymbol{0}_{(r-1)(c-1)}, \boldsymbol{V_G})$ under H_0, the large-sample quadratic form statistic for testing H_0 is

$$Q_G = \boldsymbol{G}'\boldsymbol{V}_{\boldsymbol{G}}^{-1}\boldsymbol{G}.$$

This is known as the Cochran–Mantel–Haenszel (CMH) general association statistic. If H_0 is true, Q_G has an approximate $\chi^2_{(r-1)(c-1)}$ distribution. The asymptotic distribution of Q_G is linked to the total sample size $N = \sum_{h=1}^{s} N_h$ rather than to the stratum-specific sample sizes. The statistic Q_G can be used when the row and column variables are nominal. The null hypothesis is tested in terms of $(r-1)(c-1)$ linearly independent functions of the observed counts.

If the CMH statistic Q_G is significant, then there is an association between the row and column variables in at least one of the s strata. However, the power of Q_G is directed toward average partial association alternatives. If certain observed frequencies consistently exceed (or are exceeded by) their corresponding expected frequencies, then these quantities reinforce one another when combined across strata. The statistic Q_G has low power for detecting associations that are not consistent across strata.

If $r = c = 2$, Q_G is the Mantel–Haenszel statistic [Equation (8.6)]. If $s = 1$,

$$Q_G = \frac{N-1}{N} X^2,$$

where X^2 is the usual Pearson chi-square statistic.

8.4.4 Cochran–Mantel–Haenszel Mean Score Statistic

Consider a set of s independent $r \times c$ tables with the counts in the hth table as displayed in Table 8.8. Now, suppose that the column variable is ordinal and that appropriate scores $b_{h1}, \ldots, b_{hc}$ can be assigned to the levels of the column variable. In this case, we may wish to test

H_0: no association between the row and column variables in any of the s tables versus the alternative that the r mean scores differ, on average, across tables.

Under H_0, and conditional on the row and column marginal totals in each table, $\boldsymbol{n}_h = (n_{h11}, \ldots, n_{hrc})'$ are independent multiple hypergeometric random variables with

$$\boldsymbol{n}_h \sim H\big(N_h, \{n_{hi.}\}, \{n_{h.j}\}\big).$$

If H_0 is true, $\boldsymbol{m}_h = \mathrm{E}(\boldsymbol{n}_h)$ and $\boldsymbol{\Sigma}_h = \mathrm{Var}(\boldsymbol{n}_h)$ are given by Equations (8.7) and (8.8), respectively.

Let $\boldsymbol{A}_h = (\boldsymbol{I}_{r-1}, \boldsymbol{0}_{r-1}) \otimes (b_{h1}, \ldots, b_{hc})$, and let $\boldsymbol{M}_h = \boldsymbol{A}_h(\boldsymbol{n}_h - \boldsymbol{m}_h)$ denote the $(r-1) \times 1$ vector of differences between the observed and expected mean scores (under the null hypothesis of randomness) in the hth table. Let $\boldsymbol{M} = \sum_{h=1}^{s} \boldsymbol{M}_h$. Because the s tables are independent,

$$\begin{aligned}
\mathrm{E}(\boldsymbol{M}) &= \sum_{h=1}^{s} \mathrm{E}(\boldsymbol{M}_h) = \boldsymbol{0}_{r-1}, \\
\mathrm{Var}(\boldsymbol{M}) &= \boldsymbol{V}_{\boldsymbol{M}} = \sum_{h=1}^{s} \mathrm{Var}(\boldsymbol{M}_h) = \sum_{h=1}^{s} \boldsymbol{A}_h \boldsymbol{\Sigma}_h \boldsymbol{A}_h',
\end{aligned}$$

if H_0 is true. Because the distribution of $\boldsymbol{M}$ under H_0 is approximately $N_{r-1}(\boldsymbol{0}_{r-1}, \boldsymbol{V}_{\boldsymbol{M}})$, the large-sample quadratic form statistic for testing H_0 is

$$Q_M = \boldsymbol{M}' \boldsymbol{V}_{\boldsymbol{M}}^{-1} \boldsymbol{M}.$$

If H_0 is true, Q_M is approximately χ^2_{r-1}.

The statistic Q_M is known as the CMH mean score statistic. The asymptotic distribution of Q_M is linked to the total sample size $N = \sum_{h=1}^{s} N_h$ rather than to the stratum-specific sample sizes. The null hypothesis is tested in terms of $(r-1)$ linearly independent functions of the observed mean scores. The statistic Q_M is directed at location-shift alternatives, and assesses the extent to which the mean scores in certain rows consistently exceed (or are exceeded by) the mean scores in other rows. Note that this statistic can only be used when the column variable is ordinal or interval and when it is possible to assign reasonable scores to the levels of the column variable. In this case, the mean score in each row is interpretable.

If rank scores (using midranks for tied observations) are used, then Q_M is equivalent to well-known nonparametric tests. If $s = 1$ and $r = 2$, Q_M is the Wilcoxon–Mann–Whitney statistic (Wilcoxon, 1945; Mann and Whitney, 1947). If $s = 1$ and $r > 2$, Q_M is the Kruskal–Wallis (1952) statistic. If $s > 1$ and $n_{hi.} = 1$ for $i = 1, \ldots, r$ and $h = 1, \ldots, s$, then Q_M is Friedman's (1937) chi-square statistic.

If $r = 2$ and the rank scores are standardized by dividing by the stratum-specific sample size N_h, then Q_M is equivalent to van Elteren's (1960) test for combining Wilcoxon rank sum tests across a set of strata. These scores are also known as standardized midrank scores or modified ridit scores.

8.4.5 Cochran–Mantel–Haenszel Correlation Statistic

Again, consider a set of s independent $r \times c$ tables with the counts in the hth table as displayed in Table 8.8. Suppose that the row and column variables are both ordinal or interval and that scores $a_{h1}, \ldots, a_{hr}$ and $b_{h1}, \ldots, b_{hc}$ can be reasonably assigned to the row variable and column variable, respectively. In this case, we may wish to test

H_0: no association between the row and column variables in any of the s tables

versus the alternative that there is a consistent positive (or negative) association between the row scores and the column scores across tables.

Let $\boldsymbol{A}_h = (a_{h1}, \ldots, a_{hr}) \otimes (b_{h1}, \ldots, b_{hc})$ be a row vector with rc components, and let $C_h = \boldsymbol{A}_h(\boldsymbol{n}_h - \boldsymbol{m}_h)$ denote the difference between the observed and expected association scores (under the null hypothesis of randomness) in the hth table. Let $C = \sum_{h=1}^{s} C_h$. Because the s tables are independent,

$$\begin{aligned} \mathrm{E}(C) &= \sum_{h=1}^{s} \mathrm{E}(C_h) = 0, \\ \mathrm{Var}(C) &= V_C = \sum_{h=1}^{s} \mathrm{Var}(C_h) = \sum_{h=1}^{s} \boldsymbol{A}_h \boldsymbol{\Sigma}_h \boldsymbol{A}_h', \end{aligned}$$

if H_0 is true. Because C is approximately $N(0, V_C)$ under H_0, the large-sample quadratic form statistic for testing H_0 is $Q_C = C^2/V_C$. The statistic Q_C is the CMH correlation statistic. If H_0 is true, Q_C has an approximate χ_1^2 distribution.

As with the CMH statistics Q_G and Q_M, the asymptotic distribution of Q_C is linked to the total sample size $N = \sum_{h=1}^{s} N_h$ rather than to the stratum-specific sample sizes. Q_C is directed at correlation alternatives, the extent to which there is a consistent positive (or negative) linear association between the row and column scores. If $s = 1$, then $Q_C = (N-1)r^2$, where r is the Pearson correlation coefficient between the row and column scores.

8.5 Application to Repeated Measurements: Polytomous Response, Multiple Time Points

8.5.1 Introduction

Suppose that a categorical response variable with c possible outcomes is measured at t time points for each of n subjects. Let y_{ij} denote the response from subject i at time j for $i = 1, \ldots, n$ and $j = 1, \ldots, t$. Each y_{ij} takes on one of the possible values $1, \ldots, c$. We wish to test whether the marginal distribution of the response is the same at each of the t time points.

TABLE 8.9. Contingency table layout for data from the ith subject

	Response Category			
Time	1	$\cdots$	c	Total
1	n_{i11}	$\cdots$	n_{i1c}	1
$\vdots$	$\vdots$		$\vdots$	$\vdots$
t	n_{it1}	$\cdots$	n_{itc}	1
Total	$n_{i.1}$	$\cdots$	$n_{i.c}$	t

Define the indicator variables

$$n_{ijk} = \begin{cases} 1, & \text{if subject } i \text{ is classified in response category } k \text{ at time } j, \\ 0, & \text{otherwise,} \end{cases}$$

for $i = 1, \ldots, n$, $j = 1, \ldots, t$, $k = 1, \ldots, c$. The data from subject i can be displayed in a $t \times c$ contingency table, as in Table 8.9. In each row of this $t \times c$ table, one of the n_{ijk} values will be equal to 1 and the remaining n_{ijk} values will be equal to 0. The column marginal total $n_{i.k}$ is the number of times that subject i was classified in response category k; note that $0 \leq n_{i.k} \leq t$.

Under the assumption that the column marginal totals $\{n_{i.k}\}$ are fixed, the null hypothesis of "no partial association" between the row dimension (time) and the column dimension (response) can be tested using Q_G. In this context, there are n strata, one for each subject. The "no partial association" hypothesis is the same as the "interchangeability" hypothesis of Madansky (1963). This null hypothesis implies marginal homogeneity in the distribution of the response across the t time points. Although the data in each table are sparse (all counts will be 0 or 1), the asymptotic distribution is linked to the total sample size $N = \sum_{h=1}^{s} N_h$.

When used in the analysis of repeated measurements, the CMH statistic Q_G is equivalent to McNemar's (1947) test if $c = 2$ and $t = 2$. If $c = 2$ and $t > 2$, Q_G is equivalent to Cochran's (1950) Q test. If $c > 2$ and $t > 2$, then Q_G is equivalent to Birch's (1965) Lagrange multiplier test and Madansky's (1963) interchangeability test. The asymptotic distribution of Q_G is $\chi^2_{(t-1)(c-1)}$; both the row variable (repeated measurements factor) and the column variable (response) are treated as nominal.

If the response variable is ordinal, the mean score statistic Q_M is also applicable; the asymptotic distribution of the test statistic is χ^2_{t-1}. If both the repeated measurements factor and the response variable are ordinal, the correlation statistic Q_C can be used. This statistic has an asymptotic χ^2_1 distribution. In repeated measures applications, Q_M tests equality of means across the levels of the repeated measurements factor, and Q_C tests for linear association between the response variable and the repeated measurements factor.

TABLE 8.10. Drug response data from subject i

Drug	Response F	Response U	Total
A	n_{i11}	n_{i12}	1
B	n_{i21}	n_{i22}	1
C	n_{i31}	n_{i32}	1
Total	$n_{i.1}$	$n_{i.2}$	3

8.5.2 The General Association Statistic Q_G

Grizzle et al. (1969) analyze data in which 46 subjects were treated with each of three drugs (A, B, and C). The response to each drug was recorded as favorable (F) or unfavorable (U). Table 7.2 displays the data. In Chapter 7, the weighted least squares approach was used to test the null hypothesis that the marginal probability of a favorable response is the same for all three drugs.

Let $n_{ijk} = 1$ if subject i's response to drug j is category k and 0 otherwise. The data from the ith subject can be displayed in a 3×2 contingency table, as shown in Table 8.10. The CMH statistic Q_G can be used to test the null hypothesis that, for each subject, the total number of favorable responses ($n_{i.1}$) is distributed at random with respect to the three drugs. The result ($Q_G = 8.5$ with 2 df, $p = 0.01$) supports the conclusion that the response profiles of the three drugs are different. The weighted least squares approach (Section 7.3.2) provided a similar conclusion.

8.5.3 The Mean Score Statistic Q_M and the Correlation Statistic Q_C

Table 8.11 displays data from a study of the efficacy of steam inhalation in the treatment of common cold symptoms (Macknin et al., 1990). Eligible subjects had colds of recent onset (symptoms of nasal drainage, nasal congestion, and sneezing for 3 days or less). Subjects were given two 20-minute steam inhalation treatments, after which severity of nasal drainage was self-assessed for four days. The outcome variable at each day was ordinal with four categories:

0 = no symptoms;
1 = mild symptoms;
2 = moderate symptoms;
3 = severe symptoms.

The goal of the analysis is to assess whether symptom severity improves following treatment.

With respect to the methods that have been discussed in previous chapters, normal-theory methods (Chapters 3–6) are not appropriate because

TABLE 8.11. Nasal drainage severity scores from 30 subjects

ID	Day 1	Day 2	Day 3	Day 4
1	1	1	2	2
2	0	0	0	0
3	1	1	1	1
4	1	1	1	1
5	0	2	2	0
6	2	0	0	0
7	2	2	1	2
8	1	1	1	0
9	3	2	1	1
10	2	2	2	3
11	1	0	1	1
12	2	3	2	2
13	1	3	2	1
14	2	1	1	1
16	2	3	3	3
17	2	1	1	1
18	1	1	1	1
20	2	2	2	2
21	3	1	1	1
22	1	1	2	1
23	2	1	1	2
24	2	2	2	2
25	1	1	1	1
26	2	2	3	1
27	2	0	0	0
28	1	1	1	1
29	0	1	1	0
30	1	1	1	1
31	1	1	1	0
32	3	3	3	3

the response is categorical with only four possible values. Because there are

$$c^t = 4^4 = 256$$

potential response profiles, the sample size is too small for validity of the WLS approach. Although randomization model methods appear to be appropriate, the sample size is probably too small to permit use of Q_G with 9 df. In any event, the general association statistic will have low power.

Because the response is ordinal, mean symptom scores across the four days can be compared using Q_M. This test with 3 df requires the assignment of scores to the values of the ordinal outcome variable. Under the assumption that the values none, mild, moderate, and severe are equally spaced, one choice is to use the values 0, 1, 2, 3 as scores (as displayed in Table 8.11). The resulting value of Q_M is 4.93, with a p-value of 0.18. Rank scores could also be considered; this choice yields $Q_M = 3.35$, $p = 0.34$. The null hypothesis of equality of mean scores across the four days would not be rejected at the 5% level of significance using either set of scores.

The correlation statistic Q_C can also be used to test whether there is a significant linear association between time and response. Because the repeated measurements factor is ordered and the values are equally spaced, integer scores are appropriate. Using integer scores for the response gives $Q_C = 4.36$ with 1 df, $p = 0.04$. If rank scores for the response are used instead, $Q_C = 2.68$ with 1 df, $p = 0.10$.

This example illustrates that the conclusion of an analysis can be affected by the choice of scores. In particular, the use of rank scores leads to a less clear conclusion regarding the statistical significance of Q_C. Some authors recommend the routine use of rank scores in preference to the arbitrary assignment of scores; see, for example, Fleiss (1986, pp. 83–84). As demonstrated by Graubard and Korn (1987), however, rank scores can be a poor choice when the column margin is far from uniformly distributed. This is because rank scores also assign a spacing between the levels of the categories. This spacing is generally not known by the data analyst and may not be as powerful as other spacings for certain patterns of differences among distributions. Graubard and Korn (1987) recommend that scores be specified whenever possible. If the choice of scores is not apparent, they recommend integer (or equally spaced) scores.

When there is no natural set of scores, Agresti (1990, p. 294) recommends that the data be analyzed using several reasonably assigned sets of scores to determine whether substantive conclusions depend on the choice of scores. This type of sensitivity analysis seems especially appropriate in this example, because the results assuming equally spaced scores differ from those obtained using rank scores. For example, the scores 0, 1, 3, 5 assume that the "moderate" category is equally spaced between the "mild" and "severe" categories, whereas "no symptoms' and "mild symptoms" are less far apart. Another possibility would be 0, 1, 2, 4; this choice places severe symptoms further from the three other categories.

8.6 Accommodation of Missing Data

8.6.1 *General Association Statistic Q_G*

Consider again the drug response data analyzed in Section 8.5.2. With reference to Table 7.2, the observed responses of subject 1 were favorable to drugs A and B and unfavorable to drug C. Now, suppose that the drug B response was missing. One approach would be to exclude this subject from the analysis. In this case,

$$\boldsymbol{G} = \sum_{h=2}^{46} \boldsymbol{G}_h = \begin{pmatrix} 3.667 \\ 3.667 \end{pmatrix},$$

$$\text{Var}(\boldsymbol{G}) = \sum_{h=2}^{46} \text{Var}(\boldsymbol{G}_h) = \begin{pmatrix} 7.333 & -3.667 \\ -3.667 & 7.333 \end{pmatrix},$$

and $Q_G = \boldsymbol{G}'\left(\text{Var}(\boldsymbol{G})\right)^{-1}\boldsymbol{G} = 7.333$.

The exclusion of subject 1, however, does not allow us to use the information that the response to drug A (C) was favorable (unfavorable). Alternatively, the data from subject 1 can be displayed as shown in Table 8.12. In this case,

$$\boldsymbol{n}_1 = \begin{pmatrix} 1 \\ 0 \\ 0 \\ 0 \\ 0 \\ 1 \end{pmatrix} \qquad \boldsymbol{m}_1 = \begin{pmatrix} .5 \\ .5 \\ .0 \\ .0 \\ .5 \\ .5 \end{pmatrix}.$$

The variance–covariance matrix of $\boldsymbol{n}_1$ is then

$$\boldsymbol{\Sigma}_1 = \begin{pmatrix} 0.25 & -0.25 & 0.00 & 0.00 & -0.25 & 0.25 \\ -0.25 & 0.25 & 0.00 & 0.00 & 0.25 & -0.25 \\ 0.00 & 0.00 & 0.00 & 0.00 & 0.00 & 0.00 \\ 0.00 & 0.00 & 0.00 & 0.00 & 0.00 & 0.00 \\ -0.25 & 0.25 & 0.00 & 0.00 & 0.25 & -0.25 \\ 0.25 & -0.25 & 0.00 & 0.00 & -0.25 & 0.25 \end{pmatrix}.$$

The components of Q_G from subject 1 are

$$\boldsymbol{G}_1 = \boldsymbol{A}(\boldsymbol{n}_1 - \boldsymbol{m}_1) = \begin{pmatrix} 1 & 0 & 0 & 0 & 0 & 0 \\ 0 & 0 & 1 & 0 & 0 & 0 \end{pmatrix} \begin{pmatrix} 0.5 \\ -0.5 \\ 0.0 \\ 0.0 \\ -0.5 \\ 0.5 \end{pmatrix} = \begin{pmatrix} 0.5 \\ 0 \end{pmatrix},$$

$$\text{Var}(\boldsymbol{G}_1) = \boldsymbol{A}\boldsymbol{\Sigma}_1\boldsymbol{A}' = \begin{pmatrix} 0.25 & 0 \\ 0 & 0 \end{pmatrix}.$$

TABLE 8.12. Drug response data from subject 1 (with drug B response assumed to be missing)

	Response		
Drug	F	U	Total
A	1	0	1
B	0	0	0
C	0	1	1
Total	1	1	2

With the addition of the partial data from subject 1,

$$\begin{aligned}
\boldsymbol{G} &= \boldsymbol{G}_1 + \sum_{h=2}^{46} \boldsymbol{G}_h \\
&= \begin{pmatrix} 0.5 \\ 0 \end{pmatrix} + \begin{pmatrix} 3.667 \\ 3.667 \end{pmatrix} \\
&= \begin{pmatrix} 4.167 \\ 3.667 \end{pmatrix}, \\
\mathrm{Var}(\boldsymbol{G}) &= \mathrm{Var}(\boldsymbol{G}_1) + \sum_{h=2}^{46} \mathrm{Var}(\boldsymbol{G}_h) \\
&= \begin{pmatrix} 0.25 & 0 \\ 0 & 0 \end{pmatrix} + \begin{pmatrix} 7.333 & -3.667 \\ -3.667 & 7.333 \end{pmatrix} \\
&= \begin{pmatrix} 7.583 & -3.667 \\ -3.667 & 7.333 \end{pmatrix}.
\end{aligned}$$

Thus, $Q_G = \boldsymbol{G}'\left(\mathrm{Var}(\boldsymbol{G})\right)^{-1}\boldsymbol{G} = 8.094$. In this case, the use of partial data from one of the subjects increased the strength of the evidence against H_0.

As a second example, consider the Muscatine Coronary Risk Factor Study example of Section 7.4.3. Table 7.11 displays the cross-classification of 522 7–9-year-old males by obesity status at survey years 1977, 1979, and 1981. At each survey, the response was "Yes" if the subject was classified as obese, "No" if the subject was not obese, and "Missing" if the subject did not respond to this survey. In Section 7.4.3, these data were analyzed using the WLS approach.

Table 8.13 displays the proportion of boys classified as obese at each year. Results are displayed for all subjects who provided a response at a given year as well as for the subgroup of 225 boys who responded to all three surveys.

The general association statistic Q_G can be used to test the null hypothesis that the marginal probability of obesity is the same across the three survey years. Using only the 225 subjects with complete data, $Q_G = 2.66$ with 2 df, $p = 0.26$. If all available data are used instead, the value of Q_G

TABLE 8.13. Summary of results of Muscatine Coronary Risk Factor Study

	All Data		Complete Cases	
Year	n	% Obese	n	% Obese
1977	356	18.8	225	19.6
1979	375	20.5	225	19.1
1981	380	23.7	225	23.1

TABLE 8.14. Nasal drainage severity scores from two subjects with incomplete data

ID	Day 1	Day 2	Day 3	Day 4
15		3	3	2
19	3		1	0

increases to 4.18, with $p = 0.12$. Although the use of all available data yields a larger value of the test statistic, neither analysis leads to rejection of the null hypothesis of marginal homogeneity. In Section 7.4.3, the use of a model for predicting the marginal probability of obesity as a linear function of survey year provided nearly significant evidence of a linear trend ($p = 0.05$).

8.6.2 *Mean Score Statistic* Q_M

Section 8.5.3 considered data from a study of the efficacy of steam inhalation in the treatment of common cold symptoms. Each of the 30 subjects included in Table 8.11 had complete data. Table 8.14 displays the data from two subjects (ID 15 and ID 19) that were not included in the analyses of Section 8.5.3. Both subjects' data support the hypothesis that symptoms improve over time and can be included in the computation of Q_M.

Using the symptom scores 0, 1, 2, and 3 for the categories none, mild, moderate, and severe, respectively, the mean score statistic for the complete cases is computed as follows:

$$\begin{aligned} \boldsymbol{A}_h &= \begin{pmatrix} 1 & 0 & 0 & 0 \\ 0 & 1 & 0 & 0 \\ 0 & 0 & 1 & 0 \end{pmatrix} \otimes (0 \quad 1 \quad 2 \quad 3), \\ \boldsymbol{M}_h &= \boldsymbol{A}_h(\boldsymbol{n}_h - \boldsymbol{m}_h), \end{aligned}$$

for $h = 1, \ldots, 30$. For the complete cases,

$$\boldsymbol{M} = \sum_{h=1}^{30} \boldsymbol{M}_h = \begin{pmatrix} 4.5 \\ 0.5 \\ 0.5 \end{pmatrix},$$

TABLE 8.15. Observed cell frequencies for subjects 15 and 19

Subject 15						Subject 19					
	Response						Response				
Day	0	1	2	3	Sum	Day	0	1	2	3	Sum
1	0	0	0	0	0	1	0	0	0	1	1
2	0	0	0	1	1	2	0	0	0	0	0
3	0	0	0	1	1	3	0	1	0	0	1
4	0	0	1	0	1	4	1	0	0	0	1
Sum	0	0	1	2	3	Sum	1	1	0	1	3

TABLE 8.16. Expected cell frequencies for subjects 15 and 19

Subject 15						Subject 19					
	Response						Response				
Day	0	1	2	3	Sum	Day	0	1	2	3	Sum
1	0	0	0	0	0	1	1/3	1/3	0	1/3	1
2	0	0	1/3	2/3	1	2	0	0	0	0	0
3	0	0	1/3	2/3	1	3	1/3	1/3	0	1/3	1
4	0	0	1/3	2/3	1	4	1/3	1/3	0	1/3	1
Sum	0	0	1	2	3	Sum	1	1	0	1	3

$$\begin{aligned} \boldsymbol{V_M} &= \sum_{h=1}^{30} \boldsymbol{A}_h \boldsymbol{\Sigma}_h \boldsymbol{A}_h' = \begin{pmatrix} 7.750 & -2.583 & -2.583 \\ & 7.750 & -2.583 \\ & & 7.750 \end{pmatrix}, \\ Q_M &= \boldsymbol{M}' \boldsymbol{V}_{\boldsymbol{M}}^{-1} \boldsymbol{M} = 4.94, \end{aligned}$$

with 3 df ($p = 0.18$). This result was previously reported in Section 8.5.3.

If we now include the two subjects with missing data, Table 8.15 displays the observed contingency tables for subjects 15 and 19. Table 8.16 similarly displays the corresponding tables of expected frequencies. The contribution of subject 15 to Q_M is

$$\begin{aligned} \boldsymbol{A}_{15}(\boldsymbol{n}_{15} - \boldsymbol{m}_{15}) &= (0 \quad 0.333 \quad 0.333)', \\ \boldsymbol{A}_{15} \boldsymbol{\Sigma}_{15} \boldsymbol{A}_{15}' &= \begin{pmatrix} 0 & 0 & 0 \\ & 0.222 & -0.111 \\ & & 0.222 \end{pmatrix}. \end{aligned}$$

Similarly, the contribution of subject 19 to Q_M is

$$\begin{aligned} \boldsymbol{A}_{19}(\boldsymbol{n}_{19} - \boldsymbol{m}_{19}) &= (1.667 \quad 0 \quad -0.333)', \\ \boldsymbol{A}_{19} \boldsymbol{\Sigma}_{19} \boldsymbol{A}_{19}' &= \begin{pmatrix} 1.556 & 0 & -0.778 \\ & 0 & 0 \\ & & 1.556 \end{pmatrix}. \end{aligned}$$

Using both the complete and the incomplete cases,

$$\boldsymbol{M} = \begin{pmatrix} 4.5 \\ 0.5 \\ 0.5 \end{pmatrix} + \begin{pmatrix} 0 \\ 0.333 \\ 0.333 \end{pmatrix} + \begin{pmatrix} 1.667 \\ 0 \\ -0.333 \end{pmatrix} = \begin{pmatrix} 6.167 \\ 0.833 \\ 0.500 \end{pmatrix},$$

$$\begin{aligned} \boldsymbol{V_M} &= \begin{pmatrix} 7.750 & -2.583 & -2.583 \\ & 7.750 & -2.583 \\ & & 7.750 \end{pmatrix} + \begin{pmatrix} 0 & 0 & 0 \\ & 0.222 & -0.111 \\ & & 0.222 \end{pmatrix} \\ &+ \begin{pmatrix} 1.556 & 0 & -0.778 \\ & 0 & 0 \\ & & 1.556 \end{pmatrix} \\ &= \begin{pmatrix} 9.306 & -2.583 & -3.361 \\ & 7.972 & -2.694 \\ & & 9.528 \end{pmatrix}. \end{aligned}$$

The mean score statistic using complete and incomplete cases is

$$Q_M = \boldsymbol{M}'\boldsymbol{V}_{\boldsymbol{M}}^{-1}\boldsymbol{M} = 7.44$$

with 3 df ($p = 0.06$). The inclusion of the two additional subjects (15 and 19) with incomplete data leads to a larger value of the test statistic.

8.6.3 Correlation Statistic Q_C

The two subjects with incomplete data can also be used in computing Q_C. First, the correlation statistic for the complete cases is computed as follows (using the scores 1–4 for time and 0–3 for symptoms):

$$\begin{aligned} \boldsymbol{A}_h &= (1 \;\; 2 \;\; 3 \;\; 4) \otimes (0 \;\; 1 \;\; 2 \;\; 3), \\ C_h &= \boldsymbol{A}_h(\boldsymbol{n}_h - \boldsymbol{m}_h), \\ C &= \sum_{h=1}^{30} C_h = -15, \\ V_C &= \sum_{h=1}^{30} \boldsymbol{A}_h \boldsymbol{\Sigma}_h \boldsymbol{A}_h' = 51.667, \\ Q_C &= C' V_C^{-1} C = (-15)^2/51.667 = 4.355, \end{aligned}$$

as given in Section 8.5.3.

The contributions of subjects 15 and 19 are:

$$\begin{aligned} \boldsymbol{A}_{15}(\boldsymbol{n}_{15} - \boldsymbol{m}_{15}) &= -1, & \boldsymbol{A}_{15}\boldsymbol{\Sigma}_{15}\boldsymbol{A}_{15}' &= 0.667, \\ \boldsymbol{A}_{19}(\boldsymbol{n}_{19} - \boldsymbol{m}_{19}) &= -4.67, & \boldsymbol{A}_{19}\boldsymbol{\Sigma}_{19}\boldsymbol{A}_{19}' &= 10.889. \end{aligned}$$

Using both complete and incomplete cases:

$$C = -15 - 1 - 4.667 = -20.667,$$
$$V_C = 51.667 + 0.667 + 10.889 = 63.222,$$
$$Q_C = (-20.667)^2/63.222 = 6.76,$$

with 1 df ($p = 0.009$). Again, the inclusion of the two subjects with incomplete data leads to a larger value of the test statistic.

8.7 Use of Mean Score and Correlation Statistics for Continuous Data

Although the randomization model tests were originally developed for stratified two-way contingency tables, the statistics Q_M and Q_C can also be used to analyze a continuous response measured at multiple time points or under multiple conditions. Section 8.5.1 described the use of the CMH tests in analyzing a categorical response variable with c possible outcomes measured at t time points. If the response variable is continuous, so that each of the n subjects has a unique response at each time point, then $c = nt$ will be very large. In this case, the $t \times c$ contingency table for each subject (Table 8.9) will have nt columns. Although the general association statistic Q_G will not be applicable, Q_M can be used to test whether the mean scores across the t time points are equal, and Q_C can be used to test whether there is a linear association between time and response.

As an example, Table 3.1 and Figure 3.2 display the data from a dental study in which the height of the ramus bone (mm) was measured in 20 boys at ages 8, 8.5, 9, and 9.5 years (Elston and Grizzle, 1962). In Section 3.3.2, the unstructured multivariate approach was used to assess whether the mean ramus bone heights differed across the four ages and whether the relationship between ramus bone height and age was linear. Growth curve analysis (Section 4.4.3) and analysis using the linear mixed model (Problem 6.2) were also illustrated using this example. If the assumptions of normal-theory methods are not justified, the randomization model statistics Q_M and Q_C can also be used to analyze these data.

Because the response variable has 57 unique values, each subject has an underlying 4×57 contingency table. Using the actual values of the ramus bone height as scores, $Q_M = 41.293$ with 3 df ($p < 0.001$). Thus, there is a highly significant difference among the four means. Additionally using the scores 8, 8.5, 9, and 9.5 for age, $Q_C = 41.290$ with 1 df ($p < 0.001$). This indicates that there is a strong linear association between ramus bone height and age.

If the value of t is very large, or if the number and spacing of the measurements vary among subjects, Q_M will no longer be applicable. The 1-df

TABLE 8.17. Analysis of serum creatinine reciprocals from 619 subjects using the CMH statistic Q_C

Group	Q_C	p-value
1	—	—
2	2.80	0.094
3	4.68	0.031
4	7.31	0.007

test based on Q_C, however, can still be used. As an example, Section 6.4.3 discusses the analysis of data from 619 subjects with and without a single hereditary kidney disease and with and without hypertension (Jones and Boadi-Boateng, 1991). The response variable of interest is the reciprocal of serum creatinine (SCR); the values of this variable range from 0.028 to 2.5. The explanatory variables are group and patient age (which ranges from 18 to 84 years). Observations were taken at arbitrary times from each subject, and the number of observations per subject ranges from 1 to 22. Table 6.6 gives a partial listing of the data.

It is not possible to use CMH statistics to investigate differences among the four groups of subjects or to develop a model for the effect of age on SCR. If normal-theory methods are not appropriate, however, the CMH correlation statistic Q_C can be used in each group to test the null hypothesis of no association between age and SCR versus the alternative hypothesis of a linear association.

Table 8.17 displays the test statistic and p-value in each of the four groups. Group 1 has both the largest sample size and the most numbers of repeated measurements/subject. Thus, it is not possible to compute Q_C using standard computer programs because these are designed for the analysis of categorical data. In each of groups 3 and 4, there is statistically significant evidence of an association between age and SCR.

8.8 Problems

8.1 Suppose that a dichotomous outcome (coded as "+" or "−") is measured at $t = 2$ time points for each of n subjects. The data from subject i can be displayed in a 2×2 contingency table, as shown in Table 8.4. Apply the Mantel and Fleiss (1980) validity criterion described in Section 8.3 to this situation and show that this requirement simplifies to $b + c \geq 10$, where b (c) is the number of subjects with response "+" ("−") at time 1 and response "−" ("+") at time 2.

8.2 Consider the study described in Problem 7.5, in which a dichotomous response with possible values 0 and 1 is measured at months 0, 2, and 5 for each of n subjects from a single population. Suppose that you wish to test the null hypothesis of no association between the probability of response 1 and month using the randomization model approach.

(a) Under what circumstances would this approach be preferred over the weighted least squares approach?

(b) What are the respective degrees of freedom of the statistics Q_G, Q_M, and Q_C?

(c) Discuss the factors you would consider in deciding which one of the statistics Q_G, Q_M, and Q_C you would use.

(d) If you analyzed the data using the correlation statistic Q_C, what scores would you recommend for the row and column variables?

8.3 In a longitudinal study of health effects of air pollution, 1019 children were examined annually at ages 9, 10, 11, and 12 (Ware et al., 1988; Agresti, 1990). At each examination, the response variable was the presence or absence of wheezing. Table 7.4 displays the data; Section 7.3.3 describes the analysis of these data using the weighted least squares approach.

(a) Which, if any, of the randomization model statistics can be used to test whether there is an association between wheezing and age?

(b) Analyze these data using all appropriate randomization model statistics, and summarize the results.

(c) For these data, what are some of the advantages and disadvantages of the randomization model approach relative to the weighted least squares approach?

8.4 Macknin et al. (1990) studied the efficacy of steam inhalation in the treatment of common cold symptoms. In this study, 32 patients with colds of recent onset (symptoms of nasal drainage, nasal congestion, and sneezing for three days or less) were given two 20-minute steam inhalation treatments, and the severity of various types of symptoms was self-assessed for four days. Table 8.18 displays the nasal congestion ratings, where 0 = no symptoms, 1 = mild symptoms, 2 = moderate symptoms, 3 = severe symptoms, and . denotes missing values. Section 8.5.3 discussed the analysis of another response variable from this study.

(a) Which randomization model statistics can be used to test whether nasal congestion severity improves following treatment?

(b) Using the scores 0, 1, 2, and 3 for nasal congestion severity and the scores 1, 2, 3, and 4 for days following treatment, analyze these data using all appropriate randomization model statistics and summarize the results.

(c) Repeat part (b) using rank scores for nasal congestion severity and the scores 1, 2, 3, and 4 for days following treatment.

8.5 Table 8.18 also displays sneezing severity ratings from the Macknin et al. (1990) study previously considered in Section 8.5.3 and Problem 8.4. The scale 0 = no symptoms, 1 = mild symptoms, 2 = moderate symptoms, and 3 = severe symptoms was again used, and . denotes missing values.

(a) Which randomization model statistics can be used to test whether sneezing severity improves following treatment?

(b) Using the scores 0, 1, 2, and 3 for sneezing severity and the scores 1, 2, 3, and 4 for days following treatment, analyze these data using all appropriate randomization model statistics and summarize the results.

(c) Repeat part (b) using rank scores for sneezing severity and the scores 1, 2, 3, and 4 for days following treatment.

8.6 Deal et al. (1979) measured ventilation volumes (l/min) of eight subjects under six different temperatures of inspired dry air. Table 2.1 displays the resulting data.

(a) Which, if any, of the randomization model statistics can be used to test whether there is an association between ventilation volume and temperature?

(b) Analyze these data using all appropriate randomization model statistics and summarize the results.

(c) Sections 2.2, 3.3.2, and 5.3.3 illustrated the analysis of these data using the summary-statistic, unstructured multivariate, and repeated measures ANOVA approaches. Discuss the similarities and differences (and the reasons for differences) between the results of these methods and your results from part (b).

8.7 Problem 5.3 considered the weights of 13 male mice measured at intervals of three days over the 21 days from birth to weaning (Rao, 1987); Table 5.6 displays the data.

(a) Which, if any, of the randomization model statistics can be used to test whether there is an association between weight and age?

(b) Analyze these data using all appropriate randomization model statistics and summarize the results.

TABLE 8.18. Nasal congestion and sneezing severity scores from 32 subjects

	Congestion				Sneezing			
ID	Day 1	Day 2	Day 3	Day 4	Day 1	Day 2	Day 3	Day 4
1	1	1	2	1	1	1	1	1
2	1	1	0	0	0	0	0	0
3	2	2	2	1	1	1	1	1
4	2	2	2	2	0	0	0	0
5	0	0	2	0	1	0	1	0
6	2	2	1	1	1	1	0	0
7	3	2	2	3	0	0	0	0
8	1	1	2	0	0	1	1	0
9	1	1	1	1	0	0	0	0
10	3	2	2	3	2	1	2	2
11	1	1	1	0	0	0	0	0
12	2	3	2	2	2	2	1	1
13	1	2	2	1	0	2	1	1
14	1	1	0	0	1	1	0	0
15	.	3	2	1	.	0	0	0
16	2	3	3	3	1	2	1	0
17	0	2	1	0	0	0	0	0
18	3	1	3	1	1	0	1	1
19	2	.	3	1	.	2	0	0
20	0	0	0	0	0	0	0	0
21	2	1	1	1	2	1	1	1
22	2	2	2	2	0	0	0	0
23	1	1	0	2	0	0	0	0
24	2	1	1	1	1	0	0	0
25	2	2	1	0	1	1	1	0
26	2	3	2	1	.	1	0	1
27	1	0	0	0	1	0	0	0
28	2	2	2	2	1	1	1	0
29	0	1	1	0	3	1	1	0
30	2	1	1	1	1	1	1	1
31	2	2	1	1	1	1	1	0
32	2	3	3	3	1	1	2	2

TABLE 8.19. Lesion severity data from 14 puppies

	Pulse Duration (ms)				
Animal	2	4	6	8	10
6	0	0	5	0	3
7	0	3	3	4	5
8	0	3	4	3	2
9	2	2	3	0	4
10	0	0	4	4	3
12	0	0	0	4	4
13	0	4	4	4	0
15	0	4	0	0	0
16	0	3	0	1	1
17	.	.	0	1	0
19	0	0	1	1	0
20	.	0	0	2	2
21	0	0	2	3	3
22	.	0	0	3	0

8.8 Problem 2.1 describes a study to test whether pH alters action potential characteristics following administration of a drug; Table 2.9 displays the response variable of interest (V_{max}), which was measured at up to four pH levels for each of 25 subjects.

(a) Which, if any, of the randomization model statistics can be used to test whether there is an association between V_{max} and pH?

(b) Analyze these data using all appropriate randomization model statistics and summarize the results.

8.9 Researchers at the C.S. Mott Children's Hospital, Ann Arbor, Michigan, investigated the effect of pulse duration on the development of acute electrical injury during transesophageal atrial pacing in dogs (Landis et al., 1988). This procedure involves placing a pacemaker in the esophagus. Each of the 14 animals available for experimentation then received atrial pacing at pulse durations of 2, 4, 6, 8, and 10 milliseconds (ms), with each pulse delivered at a separate site in the esophagus for 30 minutes. The response variable, lesion severity, was classified according to depth of injury by histologic examination using an ordinal staging scale from 0 to 5 (0 = no lesion, 5 = acute inflammation of extraesophageal fascia). Table 8.19 displays the resulting data (with missing observations denoted by .). Using appropriate statistical methods, determine whether there is an association between lesion severity and pulse duration.

8.10 An investigator from the University of Iowa Department of Speech Pathology and Audiology studied the effects of induced velopharyngeal

TABLE 8.20. Velopharyngeal fatigue measurements from ten subjects

		Air Pressure (cm H_2O)				
Subject	Sex	0	5	15	25	35
1	F	0.012	0.001	−0.029	−0.136	−0.104
2	M	−0.027	−0.096	−0.123	−0.229	−0.322
3	M	0.033	−0.136	−0.214	−0.180	.
4	F	0.049	−0.019	0.024	−0.191	−0.678
5	M	0.009	−0.036	0.050	0.012	0.041
6	F	−0.082	−0.119	−0.041	−0.099	−0.463
7	M	−0.060	0.203	0.045	−0.053	−0.072
8	F	0.013	0.093	−0.251	−0.210	−0.294
9	M	0.090	−0.150	−0.107	−0.326	−0.634
10	F	0.049	−0.110	−0.027	.	.

fatigue in adults with normal speech mechanisms. The subjects' task was to repeat the syllable /si/ 100 times while an external load was placed on the velopharyngeal mechanism. The external load consisted of various levels of air pressure (0 as a control, 5, 15, 25, and 35 cm H_2O relative to atmospheric pressure) delivered to the nasal passages via a tube and nasal mask assembly. Fatigue was defined by the slope of the regression line fit to the data from each subject under each condition. Table 8.20 shows the fatigue measurements from the ten subjects who participated in the study.

(a) Consider these data to be from a single sample of ten subjects; that is, ignore the fact that there are five males and five females. Test whether there is an association between fatigue and air pressure using appropriate statistical methods. Justify the approach you choose.

(b) Again considering these data to be from a single sample of ten subjects, test whether the relationship between fatigue and air pressure is linear; that is, test whether the nonlinear components of the relationship are equal to zero.

(c) Using appropriate statistical methods, test whether the effect of air pressure on fatigue is the same for males and females. Justify your choice of approach.

8.11 As part of a protocol for the University of Iowa Mental Health Clinical Research Center, 44 schizophrenic patients participated in a four-week antipsychotic medication washout (Arndt et al., 1993). The severity of extrapyramidal side effects was assessed just prior to discontinuation of antipsychotic medication and at weeks 1, 2, 3, and 4 during the washout period. Table 2.4 displays the resulting ratings on the Simpson–Angus scale (a score ranging from 0 to 40); Section 2.2 discusses the analysis of these data using the summary-statistic approach.

Use the randomization model mean score and correlation statistics to test whether there is an association between Simpson–Angus ratings and time since medication withdrawal. Justify your choice of scores for the response variable.

8.12 Table 8.21 displays ratings on the Abnormal Involuntary Movement Scale (AIMS) for the 44 schizophrenic patients considered in Problem 8.11 and in Section 2.2. Use the randomization model mean score and correlation statistics to test whether there is an association between AIMS ratings and time since medication withdrawal. Justify your choice of scores for the response variable.

8.13 Table 8.22 displays ratings on the IMPACT scale for the 44 schizophrenic patients considered in Problems 8.11 and 8.12 and in Section 2.2. This rating scale assesses the total impact of symptoms on a patient's functioning. Use the randomization model mean score and correlation statistics to test whether there is an association between IMPACT ratings and time since medication withdrawal. Justify your choice of scores for the response variable.

TABLE 8.21. Weekly AIMS ratings from 44 schizophrenic patients

Patient	Week 0	Week 1	Week 2	Week 3	Week 4
1	6	6	0	0	4
2	8	11	.	19	6
3	3	4	8	8	9
4	14	10	13	23	8
5	3	10	12	3	7
6	2	3	1	0	0
7	7	.	15	9	9
8	.	.	9	12	6
9	8	12	0	0	0
10	2	3	4	3	1
11	1	0	0	0	0
12	0	0	0	0	.
13	2	0	0	0	0
14	9	4	0	4	1
15	0	0	0	0	0
16	3	0	16	9	8
17	2	13	12	19	4
18	0	0	.	.	.
19	0	3	3	1	0
20	0	7	16	13	13
21	0	4	0	0	.
22	0	2	11	14	18
23	0	0	0	0	0
24	3	0	0	4	5
25	2	0	6	4	3
26	9	20	8	6	11
27	0	0	0	.	.
28	0	0	2	2	.
29	9	4	3	3	1
30	2	0	0	1	0
31	0	0	5	2	0
32	0	0	0	0	0
33	0	0	0	2	0
34	0	0	0	0	0
35	0	5	3	3	4
36	0	0	0	0	0
37	5	9	8	5	2
38	0	4	5	2	1
39	0	0	2	1	0
40	0	0	0	.	.
41	0	0	0	0	0
42	0	0	0	0	.
43	0	0	0	0	0
44	3	1	0	0	3

TABLE 8.22. Weekly IMPACT ratings from 44 schizophrenic patients

Patient	Week 0	Week 1	Week 2	Week 3	Week 4
1	2	9	0	0	3
2	3	4	.	9	3
3	2	4	2	2	2
4	9	4	5	9	4
5	0	0	1	0	0
6	0	3	1	0	0
7	5	.	5	5	3
8	.	.	3	4	2
9	3	4	0	0	0
10	2	2	3	4	1
11	1	0	0	0	0
12	0	0	0	0	.
13	4	0	0	0	0
14	7	3	0	2	1
15	0	0	0	0	0
16	4	0	0	0	4
17	3	8	8	8	2
18	0	0	.	.	.
19	0	1	1	1	0
20	0	5	6	6	7
21	0	1	0	0	.
22	0	0	4	4	5
23	0	0	0	0	0
24	3	0	0	1	2
25	2	0	0	0	0
26	4	5	3	2	5
27	0	0	0	.	.
28	0	0	0	0	.
29	5	2	4	2	1
30	0	4	3	0	0
31	0	0	5	2	0
32	0	0	0	0	0
33	0	0	0	0	0
34	0	0	0	0	0
35	0	0	2	2	2
36	0	0	0	0	0
37	4	4	3	4	2
38	0	1	3	1	1
39	0	0	2	2	0
40	0	0	0	.	.
41	0	0	0	0	0
42	0	0	0	0	.
43	0	0	0	0	0
44	0	1	0	0	1

9

Methods Based on Extensions of Generalized Linear Models

9.1 Introduction

In many applications in which the response variable of interest has a continuous distribution, the normal-theory methods described in Chapters 3–6 may be inappropriate. In addition, in situations where the response variable is categorical, the WLS (Chapter 7) and randomization model (Chapter 8) approaches are not always applicable. For example, although the WLS methodology is often a useful approach to the analysis of repeated binary and ordered categorical outcome variables, it can only accommodate categorical explanatory variables. In addition, the WLS methodology requires a sufficiently large sample size for the marginal response functions at each time point within each subpopulation from the multiway cross-classification of the explanatory variables to have an approximately multivariate normal distribution. The randomization model approach is useful only in one-sample problems. Thus, neither of these methodologies for categorical outcomes can be used in the general repeated measurements setting.

In the case of a univariate response for each experimental unit, classical linear models are useful for analyzing normally distributed outcomes with constant variance. The extension to the class of univariate generalized linear models permits the analysis of both categorical and continuous response variables. For example, generalized linear model methodology can be used to analyze normal, Poisson, binomial, and gamma outcome variables; generalizations for ordered categorical data are also available.

This chapter considers extensions of generalized linear model methodology to the repeated measurements setting. As background, Section 9.2 reviews the basic ideas and concepts of univariate generalized linear models, and Section 9.3 discusses the ideas of quasilikelihood. Readers who are already familiar with this material, or those who are only interested in applications to repeated measurements, can skip these two sections. Section 9.4 provides an overview of methods for the analysis of repeated measurements, and Section 9.5 discusses the GEE methodology of Liang and Zeger (1986). Section 9.6 gives a brief overview of subsequent developments and extensions of GEE, and Section 9.7 briefly reviews extensions of generalized linear model methodology that incorporate random effects. Finally, Section 9.8 discusses the analysis of ordered categorical repeated measurements.

9.2 Univariate Generalized Linear Models

9.2.1 Introduction

The term "generalized linear model" was first introduced in a landmark paper by Nelder and Wedderburn (1972). Generalized linear models extend classical linear models for independent normally distributed random variables with constant variance to other types of outcome variables. Wedderburn (1974) further extended the applicability of generalized linear models by introducing quasilikelihood. Generalized linear model methodology enables a wide range of different problems of statistical modeling and inference to be put in an elegant unifying framework; these problems include analysis of variance, analysis of covariance, and regression models for normal, binary, Poisson, and other types of outcomes.

The unifying theory of generalized linear models has impacted the way such statistical methods are taught. It has also provided greater insight into connections between various statistical procedures and has led to considerable further research. McCullagh and Nelder (1989) provide a comprehensive account of the theory and applications of generalized linear models; Aitkin et al. (1989) and Dobson (1990) provide excellent introductions to the subject.

As a simple example, consider a sample of n experimental units. Let y_i be a response variable and let x_i denote an explanatory variable, for $i = 1, \ldots, n$. In the usual (Gaussian) linear model, we assume that

$$y_i = \beta_0 + \beta_1 x_i + \sigma \epsilon_i,$$

where $\epsilon_1, \ldots, \epsilon_n$ are independent $N(0, 1)$ random variables. An equivalent way of writing the model is as

$$y_i \sim N(\mu_i, \sigma^2),$$

where $y_1, \ldots, y_n$ are independent and $\mu_i = \beta_0 + \beta_1 x_i$. The objectives of this model are to use the explanatory variable to characterize the variation in the mean of the response distribution across experimental units and hence to learn about the relationship between the explanatory variable and the response variable.

Frequently, interest lies in formulating regression models for responses that have other continuous or discrete distributions. Although the objective is to model the mean, it often must be modeled indirectly via the use of a transformation. In the case of a single explanatory variable, the model might be of the form

$$g(\mu_i) = \beta_0 + \beta_1 x_i.$$

The error distribution must also be generalized, usually in a way that complements the choice of the transformation g. This leads to a very broad class of regression models.

Generalized linear models have three components: the random component, the systematic component, and the link between the random and systematic components. The random component identifies the response variable y and assumes a specific probability distribution for y. The systematic component specifies the explanatory variables used as predictors in the model. The link function describes the functional relationship between the systematic component and the expected value of the random component. As a whole, a generalized linear model relates a function of the mean to the explanatory variables through a prediction equation having linear form.

9.2.2 Random Component

Let $y_1, \ldots, y_n$ be independent random variables from the distribution

$$f(y; \theta, \phi) = \exp\left\{ \frac{y\theta - b(\theta)}{a(\phi)} + c(y, \phi) \right\} \tag{9.1}$$

for some specific functions $a(\cdot)$, $b(\cdot)$, and $c(\cdot)$. If ϕ is known, this is an exponential-family model with canonical parameter θ. It may or may not be a two-parameter exponential family if ϕ is unknown. Many common discrete and continuous distributions are members of this general family of probability distributions, such as the normal, gamma, binomial, and Poisson distributions.

Let $l(\theta, \phi; y)$ denote the log-likelihood function considered as a function of θ and ϕ:

$$l(\theta, \phi; y) = \log\bigl(f(y; \theta, \phi)\bigr) = \frac{y\theta - b(\theta)}{a(\phi)} + c(y, \phi).$$

It is convenient to find the mean and variance of y using properties of the score function

$$U = \frac{\partial}{\partial\theta}\bigl[l(\theta, \phi; y)\bigr].$$

To find the moments of U, we use the fact that

$$\frac{\partial}{\partial\theta}\Big[\log\big(f(y;\theta,\phi)\big)\Big] = \frac{1}{f(y;\theta,\phi)}\frac{\partial}{\partial\theta}\Big[f(y;\theta,\phi)\Big]. \tag{9.2}$$

Taking the expectation of both sides of Equation (9.2) yields

$$\int \frac{\partial}{\partial\theta}\Big[\log\big(f(y;\theta,\phi)\big)\Big] f(y;\theta,\phi)dy = \int \frac{\partial}{\partial\theta}\Big[f(y;\theta,\phi)\Big]dy. \tag{9.3}$$

Under certain regularity conditions, the right-hand side of Equation (9.3) is

$$\begin{aligned}\int \frac{\partial}{\partial\theta}\Big[f(y;\theta,\phi)\Big]dy &= \frac{\partial}{\partial\theta}\Big[\int f(y;\theta,\phi)dy\Big] \\ &= \frac{\partial}{\partial\theta}[1] = 0\end{aligned}$$

because $\int f(y;\theta,\phi)dy = 1$. Therefore, $\mathrm{E}(U) = 0$.

Differentiating both sides of Equation (9.3) with respect to θ gives

$$\frac{\partial}{\partial\theta}\Big[\int \frac{\partial}{\partial\theta}\Big[\log\big(f(y;\theta,\phi)\big)\Big] f(y;\theta,\phi)dy\Big] = \frac{\partial}{\partial\theta}\Big[\int \frac{\partial}{\partial\theta}\Big[f(y;\theta,\phi)\Big]dy\Big]. \tag{9.4}$$

Provided that the order of differentiation and integration can be interchanged, the right-hand side of Equation (9.4) is

$$\frac{\partial^2}{\partial\theta^2}\Big[\int f(y;\theta,\phi)dy\Big] = 0$$

and the left-hand side is

$$\begin{aligned}&\int \frac{\partial}{\partial\theta}\Big[\frac{\partial}{\partial\theta}\Big[\log\big(f(y;\theta,\phi)\big)\Big] f(y;\theta,\phi)\Big]dy \\ &\quad = \int\Big\{\frac{\partial^2}{\partial\theta^2}\Big[\log\big(f(y;\theta,\phi)\big)\Big] f(y;\theta,\phi) \\ &\qquad + \frac{\partial}{\partial\theta}\Big[\log\big(f(y;\theta,\phi)\big)\Big]\frac{\partial}{\partial\theta}\Big[f(y;\theta,\phi)\Big]\Big\}dy. \end{aligned} \tag{9.5}$$

From Equation (9.2),

$$\frac{\partial}{\partial\theta}\Big[f(y;\theta,\phi)\Big] = f(y;\theta,\phi)\frac{\partial}{\partial\theta}\Big[\log\big(f(y;\theta,\phi)\big)\Big].$$

The second term of the right-hand side of Equation (9.5) then simplifies to

$$\begin{aligned}&\frac{\partial}{\partial\theta}\Big[\log\big(f(y;\theta,\phi)\big)\Big]\ f(y;\theta,\phi)\ \frac{\partial}{\partial\theta}\Big[\log\big(f(y;\theta,\phi)\big)\Big] \\ &\quad = \Big(\frac{\partial}{\partial\theta}\Big[\log\big(f(y;\theta,\phi)\big)\Big]\Big)^2 f(y;\theta,\phi).\end{aligned}$$

Therefore, Equation (9.4) becomes

$$\int \frac{\partial^2}{\partial\theta^2}\Big[\log\big(f(y;\theta,\phi)\big)\Big] f(y;\theta,\phi)dy + \int \left(\frac{\partial}{\partial\theta}\Big[\log\big(f(y;\theta,\phi)\big)\Big]\right)^2 f(y;\theta,\phi)dy = 0,$$

or

$$\mathrm{E}\left[\frac{\partial^2}{\partial\theta^2}\Big[\log\big(f(y;\theta,\phi)\big)\Big]\right] + \mathrm{E}\left[\left(\frac{\partial}{\partial\theta}\Big[\log\big(f(y;\theta,\phi)\big)\Big]\right)^2\right] = 0.$$

In terms of the score function

$$U = \frac{\partial}{\partial\theta}\Big[l(\theta,\phi;y)\Big],$$

we have $\mathrm{E}(U') + \mathrm{E}(U^2) = 0$, where $'$ denotes differentiation with respect to θ. Thus,

$$\begin{aligned}
\mathrm{E}(U) &= 0, \\
\mathrm{Var}(U) &= \mathrm{E}(U^2) - [\mathrm{E}(U)]^2 = \mathrm{E}(U^2) \\
&= -\mathrm{E}(U').
\end{aligned}$$

The variance of U is called the *information*.

Because

$$l(\theta,\phi;y) = \frac{y\theta - b(\theta)}{a(\phi)} + c(y,\phi),$$

the score function is

$$U = \frac{\partial}{\partial\theta}\Big[l(\theta,\phi;y)\Big] = \frac{y - b'(\theta)}{a(\phi)}.$$

Therefore, $\mathrm{E}(Y) = a(\phi)\mathrm{E}(U) + b'(\theta) = b'(\theta)$, because $\mathrm{E}(U) = 0$. The derivative of U with respect to θ is

$$U' = \frac{\partial}{\partial\theta}\left[\frac{y - b'(\theta)}{a(\phi)}\right] = \frac{-b''(\theta)}{a(\phi)}.$$

Because $\mathrm{E}(U^2) = -\mathrm{E}(U')$,

$$\mathrm{E}\left[\left(\frac{Y - b'(\theta)}{a(\phi)}\right)^2\right] = \frac{b''(\theta)}{a(\phi)}$$

and $\mathrm{Var}(Y) = b''(\theta)a(\phi)$. Note that the variance of y is a product of two functions; $b''(\theta)$ is called the variance function and is denoted $V(\mu)$.

As an example, suppose that y is normally distributed with mean μ and variance σ^2. Because

$$\begin{aligned} f(y) &= \frac{1}{\sqrt{2\pi\sigma^2}} \exp\{-(y-\mu)^2/(2\sigma^2)\} \\ &= \exp\left\{-\frac{1}{2\sigma^2}(y^2 - 2y\mu + \mu^2) - \frac{1}{2}\log(2\pi\sigma^2)\right\} \\ &= \exp\left\{\frac{y\mu - \mu^2/2}{\sigma^2} - \frac{1}{2}\left(\frac{y^2}{\sigma^2} + \log(2\pi\sigma^2)\right)\right\}, \end{aligned}$$

$\theta = \mu$, $\phi = \sigma^2$, $b(\theta) = \theta^2/2$, $a(\phi) = \phi$. Therefore,

$$\begin{aligned} \mathrm{E}(Y) &= b'(\theta) = \theta = \mu, \\ \mathrm{Var}(Y) &= b''(\theta)a(\phi) = 1 \times \phi = \sigma^2. \end{aligned}$$

The variance function is $V(\mu) = 1$, and the dispersion parameter is $\phi = \sigma^2$.

As a second example, suppose that y has the Poisson distribution with mean μ. Because

$$\begin{aligned} f(y) &= \mu^y \exp(-\mu)/y! \\ &= \exp\{y\log(\mu) - \mu - \log(y!)\} \\ &= \exp\{y\log(\mu) - \exp(\log(\mu)) - \log(y!)\}, \end{aligned}$$

$\theta = \log(\mu)$, $a(\phi) \equiv 1$, and $b(\theta) = e^\theta$. Therefore,

$$\begin{aligned} \mathrm{E}(Y) &= b'(\theta) = e^\theta = \mu, \\ \mathrm{Var}(Y) &= b''(\theta)a(\phi) = e^\theta = \mu. \end{aligned}$$

In this case, the variance function is $V(\mu) = \mu$ and the dispersion parameter is $\phi = 1$.

As a final example, suppose that y has the binomial distribution with parameters n and π. In this case,

$$\begin{aligned} f(y) &= \binom{n}{y}\pi^y(1-\pi)^{n-y} \\ &= \exp\left\{\log\binom{n}{y} + y\log(\pi) + (n-y)\log(1-\pi)\right\} \\ &= \exp\left\{y\log\left(\frac{\pi}{1-\pi}\right) + n\log(1-\pi) + \log\binom{n}{y}\right\} \end{aligned}$$

and $\theta = \log(\pi/(1-\pi))$, $a(\phi) = 1$. Because

$$n\log(1-\pi) = -n\log\left(\frac{1}{1-\pi}\right) = -n\log\left(1 + \frac{\pi}{1-\pi}\right),$$

$b(\theta) = n\log(1 + \exp(\theta))$. Therefore,

$$\begin{aligned} \mathrm{E}(Y) &= b'(\theta) = ne^\theta/(1+e^\theta) = n\pi, \\ \mathrm{Var}(Y) &= b''(\theta)a(\phi) = ne^\theta/(1+e^\theta)^2 = n\pi(1-\pi). \end{aligned}$$

9.2.3 Systematic Component

The systematic component of a generalized linear model specifies the explanatory variables. These enter linearly as predictors on the right-hand side of the model equation. For example, suppose that each y_i has an associated $p \times 1$ vector of covariates $\boldsymbol{x}_i = (x_{i1}, \ldots, x_{ip})'$. The linear combination $\eta_i = \beta_0 + \beta_1 x_{i1} + \cdots + \beta_p x_{ip}$ is called the linear predictor.

Some $\{x_j\}$ may be based on others in the model. For example, $x_3 = x_1 x_2$ allows for interaction between x_1 and x_2 in their effects on y. As another example, $x_3 = x_1^2$ allows for a curvilinear effect of x_1.

9.2.4 Link Function

The link between the random and systematic components specifies how

$$\mu = \mathrm{E}(y)$$

relates to the explanatory variables in the linear predictor. One can model the mean μ directly or model a monotonic, differentiable function $g(\mu)$ of the mean. The model formula specifies that

$$g(\mu) = \beta_0 + \beta_1 x_1 + \cdots \beta_p x_p.$$

The function g is called the *link function.*

The link function g relates the linear predictor η_i to the expected value μ_i of y_i. Link functions that map the parameter space for the mean to the real line are preferred in order to avoid numerical difficulties in estimation.

The simplest link function is the identity link: $g(\mu) = \mu$. This choice of link models the mean directly. The identity link specifies a linear model for the mean response:

$$\mu = \beta_0 + \beta_1 x_1 + \cdots \beta_p x_p.$$

This is the form of an ordinary regression model for a continuous response.

Other link functions permit the mean to be nonlinearly related to the predictors. For example, $g(\mu) = \log(\mu)$ models the log of the mean. This might be appropriate when μ cannot be negative. A generalized linear model with this link is called a loglinear model.

The function

$$g(\mu) = \log\left(\frac{\mu}{1-\mu}\right)$$

is called the logit link. This choice is often appropriate when μ is between 0 and 1—for example, when μ is a probability. A generalized linear model using this link is called a logit model.

9.2.5 Canonical Links

Each probability distribution for the random component has one special function of the mean that is called its *natural parameter*. For example, the natural parameter for the normal distribution is the mean itself. Similarly, the log of the mean is the natural parameter for the Poisson distribution, and the logit of the success probability is the natural parameter for the Bernoulli distribution.

The link function that uses the natural parameter as $g(\mu)$ is called the *canonical link.* The canonical link functions for the normal, Poisson, and Bernoulli distributions are:

$$\begin{aligned} \text{Normal}: \quad & g(\mu) = \mu; \\ \text{Poisson}: \quad & g(\mu) = \log(\mu); \\ \text{Bernoulli}: \quad & g(\mu) = \log\big(\mu/(1-\mu)\big). \end{aligned}$$

Although other links are possible, the canonical links are most common in practice. Use of the canonical link function leads to inference for the regression parameters based solely on sufficient statistics.

Let $y_1, \ldots, y_n$ be independent random variables with distributions given by Equation (9.1). The log-likelihood function for $y_1, \ldots, y_n$ is

$$l = \sum_{i=1}^{n} l(\theta_i, \phi; y_i) = \frac{1}{a(\phi)} \sum_{i=1}^{n} y_i \theta_i - \frac{1}{a(\phi)} \sum_{i=1}^{n} b(\theta_i) + \sum_{i=1}^{n} c(y_i, \phi).$$

Let $\boldsymbol{x}_i$ denote the vector of covariate values corresponding to the ith observation y_i, and let $\boldsymbol{\beta}$ denote the vector of regression parameters. If

$$\theta_i = \eta_i = g(\mu_i) = \boldsymbol{x}_i' \boldsymbol{\beta},$$

the first term of l is

$$\frac{1}{a(\phi)} \sum_{i=1}^{n} y_i \boldsymbol{x}_i' \boldsymbol{\beta}.$$

Let $\boldsymbol{X} = (\boldsymbol{x}_1, \ldots, \boldsymbol{x}_n)'$ denote the $n \times p$ matrix of covariate values from all n subjects, and let $\boldsymbol{y} = (y_1, \ldots, y_n)'$. The $p \times 1$ vector $\boldsymbol{X}'\boldsymbol{y}$ with jth component $\sum_{i=1}^{n} x_{ij} y_i$ is a sufficient statistic for $\boldsymbol{\beta}$, and $\eta = \theta$ is called the canonical link function.

The canonical links lead to desirable statistical properties of the model, particularly in small samples. There is usually no a priori reason, however, why the systematic effects in a model should be additive on the scale given by that link. Thus, although it is convenient if effects are additive on the canonical link scale, quality of fit should be the primary model-selection criterion. Fortunately, the canonical links are usually quite sensible on scientific grounds.

For example, in classical linear models for normally distributed response variables, the identity link is plausible because both η and μ can take any value on the real line. In other situations, however, the identity link may not be appropriate.

As an example, because the mean μ of the Poisson distribution is greater than zero, the identity link is less attractive (because $\eta = \boldsymbol{x}_i'\boldsymbol{\beta}$ may be negative). In addition, because models for counts based on independence lead naturally to multiplicative effects, the log link $\eta = \log(\mu)$ is reasonable. Because the inverse function is $\mu = e^\eta$, additive effects contributing to η become multiplicative effects contributing to μ, and μ is necessarily positive.

For binary response variables, $0 < \mu < 1$. A desirable link function should map the interval $(0, 1)$ to the real line. The logit function satisfies this requirement. In addition, use of the logit link for binary responses leads to parameters with odds-ratio interpretations.

9.2.6 Parameter Estimation

Overview

Maximum likelihood (ML) estimates of the parameter vector $\boldsymbol{\beta}$ can be obtained by iterative weighted least squares. The dependent variable is z rather than y, where z is a linearized form of the link function applied to y. The weights are functions of the fitted values $\widehat{\mu}$. The process is iterative because both the adjusted dependent variable z and the weight depend on the fitted values, for which only current estimates are available.

Maximum Likelihood Estimation

The log-likelihood for independent responses $y_1, \ldots, y_n$ is

$$l = \sum_{i=1}^{n} l_i = \sum_{i=1}^{n} \left[\frac{y_i\theta_i - b(\theta_i)}{a(\phi)} + c(y_i, \phi) \right].$$

Under certain regularity conditions, the global maximum of l is the solution of

$$\frac{\partial l}{\partial \beta_j} = 0$$

for $j = 1, \ldots, p$. By the chain rule,

$$\frac{\partial l_i}{\partial \beta_j} = \frac{\partial l_i}{\partial \theta_i} \frac{\partial \theta_i}{\partial \mu_i} \frac{\partial \mu_i}{\partial \eta_i} \frac{\partial \eta_i}{\partial \beta_j}$$

for $j = 1, \ldots, p$.

In evaluating this partial derivative, first observe that

$$\frac{\partial l_i}{\partial \theta_i} = \frac{y_i - b'(\theta_i)}{a(\phi)} = \frac{y_i - \mu_i}{a(\phi)}.$$

Because $\mu_i = b'(\theta_i)$,

$$\frac{\partial \mu_i}{\partial \theta_i} = b''(\theta_i) = \frac{\mathrm{Var}(y_i)}{a(\phi)} = V(\mu_i).$$

Because $\eta_i = \sum_{j=1}^{p} x_{ij}\beta_j$,

$$\frac{\partial \eta_i}{\partial \beta_j} = x_{ij}.$$

Therefore,

$$\begin{aligned}\frac{\partial l_i}{\partial \beta_j} &= \frac{y_i - \mu_i}{a(\phi)} \frac{a(\phi)}{\mathrm{Var}(y_i)} \frac{\partial \mu_i}{\partial \eta_i} x_{ij} \\ &= \frac{(y_i - \mu_i)\, x_{ij}}{\mathrm{Var}(y_i)} \frac{\partial \mu_i}{\partial \eta_i}.\end{aligned}$$

Thus, the ML estimate of $\boldsymbol{\beta} = (\beta_1, \ldots, \beta_p)'$ is the solution of the equations

$$U_j = \sum_{i=1}^{n} \frac{(y_i - \mu_i)\, x_{ij}}{\mathrm{Var}(y_i)} \frac{\partial \mu_i}{\partial \eta_i} = 0$$

for $j = 1, \ldots, p$. Note that this depends on the density f only through the mean and variance. In general, these equations are nonlinear and must be solved numerically using iterative methods.

ML Estimation Using the Newton–Raphson Method

The multidimensional analog of Newton's method requires the $p \times p$ matrix of second derivatives

$$\frac{\partial^2 l}{\partial \beta_j \partial \beta_k}.$$

The mth approximation to $\widehat{\boldsymbol{\beta}}$ is then given by

$$\boldsymbol{b}^{(m)} = \boldsymbol{b}^{(m-1)} - \left[\frac{\partial^2 l}{\partial \beta_j \partial \beta_k}\right]^{-1}_{\boldsymbol{\beta} = \boldsymbol{b}^{(m-1)}} \times \boldsymbol{U}^{(m-1)},$$

where

$$\left[\frac{\partial^2 l}{\partial \beta_j \partial \beta_k}\right]_{\boldsymbol{\beta} = \boldsymbol{b}^{(m-1)}}$$

is the matrix of second derivatives of l evaluated at the estimate of $\boldsymbol{\beta}$ from the $(m-1)$st iteration and $\boldsymbol{U}^{(m-1)}$ is the vector of first derivatives of l evaluated at the estimate of $\boldsymbol{\beta}$ from the $(m-1)$st iteration.

Score Function and Information Matrix

Before describing an alternative method of ML estimation, we first define the score function and information matrix. Let $y_1, \ldots, y_n$ be independent random variables whose probability distributions depend on parameters $\theta_1, \ldots, \theta_p$, where $p \leq n$. Let $l_i(\boldsymbol{\theta}; y_i)$ denote the log-likelihood function of y_i, where $\boldsymbol{\theta} = (\theta_1, \ldots, \theta_p)'$. The log-likelihood function of $y_1, \ldots, y_n$ is

$$l(\boldsymbol{\theta}, y) = \sum_{i=1}^{n} l_i(\boldsymbol{\theta}; y_i),$$

where $\boldsymbol{y} = (y_1, \ldots, y_n)'$.

The total score with respect to θ_j is defined as

$$U_j = \frac{\partial l(\boldsymbol{\theta}; y)}{\partial \theta_j} = \sum_{i=1}^{n} \frac{\partial l_i(\boldsymbol{\theta}; y_i)}{\partial \theta_j}.$$

By the same argument as for the univariate case,

$$\mathrm{E}\left[\frac{\partial l_i(\boldsymbol{\theta}; y_i)}{\partial \theta_j}\right] = 0,$$

so $\mathrm{E}(U_j) = 0$ for $j = 1, \ldots, p$.

The information matrix $\boldsymbol{\mathcal{I}}$ is defined as the variance–covariance matrix of $\boldsymbol{U} = (U_1, \ldots, U_p)'$. The elements of

$$\boldsymbol{\mathcal{I}} = \mathrm{E}\big[(\boldsymbol{U} - \mathrm{E}(\boldsymbol{U}))(\boldsymbol{U} - \mathrm{E}(\boldsymbol{U}))'\big] = \mathrm{E}[\boldsymbol{U}\boldsymbol{U}']$$

are

$$\boldsymbol{\mathcal{I}}_{jk} = \mathrm{E}[U_j U_k] = \mathrm{E}\left[\frac{\partial l_i}{\partial \theta_j} \frac{\partial l_i}{\partial \theta_k}\right].$$

By an argument analogous to that used in the univariate case (single random variable, single parameter),

$$\mathrm{E}\left[\frac{\partial l_i}{\partial \theta_j} \frac{\partial l_i}{\partial \theta_k}\right] = \mathrm{E}\left[-\frac{\partial^2 l_i}{\partial \theta_j \partial \theta_k}\right].$$

Thus, the elements of the information matrix are also given by

$$\boldsymbol{\mathcal{I}}_{jk} = \mathrm{E}\left[-\frac{\partial^2 l}{\partial \theta_j \partial \theta_k}\right].$$

ML Estimation Using the Method of Scoring

An alternative to the Newton–Raphson approach involves replacing the matrix of second derivatives by the matrix of expected values

$$\mathrm{E}\left[\frac{\partial^2 l}{\partial \beta_j \partial \beta_k}\right].$$

This variation was first introduced in the context of probit analysis by Fisher (1935) in the appendix of a paper by Bliss (1935). Because

$$\mathrm{E}\left[\frac{\partial^2 l}{\partial \beta_j \partial \beta_k}\right] = -\mathrm{E}\left[\frac{\partial l}{\partial \beta_j} \frac{\partial l}{\partial \beta_k}\right] = -\boldsymbol{\mathcal{I}},$$

an alternative iterative procedure is given by

$$\boldsymbol{b}^{(m)} = \boldsymbol{b}^{(m-1)} + \big[\boldsymbol{\mathcal{I}}^{(m-1)}\big]^{-1} \boldsymbol{U}^{(m-1)},$$

where $\mathcal{I}^{(m-1)}$ denotes the information matrix evaluated at $\boldsymbol{b}^{(m-1)}$. Multiplication of both sides of the previous equation by $\mathcal{I}^{(m-1)}$ gives

$$\mathcal{I}^{(m-1)}\boldsymbol{b}^{(m)} = \mathcal{I}^{(m-1)}\boldsymbol{b}^{(m-1)} + \boldsymbol{U}^{(m-1)}.$$

For generalized linear models, the (j,k)th element of $\mathcal{I}$ is

$$\begin{aligned}
\mathcal{I}_{jk} &= \mathrm{E}\left[\frac{\partial l_i}{\partial \beta_j}\frac{\partial l_i}{\partial \beta_k}\right] \\
&= \mathrm{E}\left[\frac{(y_i-\mu_i)\,x_{ij}}{\mathrm{Var}(y_i)}\frac{\partial \mu_i}{\partial \eta_i}\,\frac{(y_i-\mu_i)\,x_{ik}}{\mathrm{Var}(y_i)}\frac{\partial \mu_i}{\partial \eta_i}\right] \\
&= \mathrm{E}\left[\frac{(y_i-\mu_i)^2\,x_{ij}\,x_{ik}}{[\mathrm{Var}(y_i)]^2}\left(\frac{\partial \mu_i}{\partial \eta_i}\right)^2\right] \\
&= \frac{x_{ij}\,x_{ik}}{\mathrm{Var}(y_i)}\left(\frac{\partial \mu_i}{\partial \eta_i}\right)^2.
\end{aligned}$$

Thus, $\mathcal{I} = \boldsymbol{X}'\boldsymbol{W}\boldsymbol{X}$, where $\boldsymbol{W}$ is the $n \times n$ diagonal matrix with elements

$$w_{ii} = \frac{1}{\mathrm{Var}(y_i)}\left(\frac{\partial \mu_i}{\partial \eta_i}\right)^2.$$

The iterative procedure can now be written as

$$\boldsymbol{X}'\boldsymbol{W}\boldsymbol{X}\boldsymbol{b}^{(m)} = \boldsymbol{X}'\boldsymbol{W}\boldsymbol{X}\boldsymbol{b}^{(m-1)} + \boldsymbol{U}^{(m-1)}.$$

The jth row of the $p \times n$ matrix $\boldsymbol{X}'\boldsymbol{W}$ is

$$(x_{1j}w_{11},\ldots,x_{nj}w_{nn}) = \left(\frac{x_{1j}}{\mathrm{Var}(y_1)}\left(\frac{\partial \mu_1}{\partial \eta_1}\right)^2,\ldots,\frac{x_{nj}}{\mathrm{Var}(y_n)}\left(\frac{\partial \mu_n}{\partial \eta_n}\right)^2\right),$$

and the jth component of $\boldsymbol{U}$ is

$$U_j = \sum_{i=1}^{n}\frac{(y_i-\mu_i)\,x_{ij}}{\mathrm{Var}(y_i)}\frac{\partial \mu_i}{\partial \eta_i}.$$

Now, let $\boldsymbol{v}$ denote the $n \times 1$ vector with ith component

$$(y_i-\mu_i)\frac{\partial \eta_i}{\partial \mu_i}.$$

$\boldsymbol{U}^{(m-1)}$ can now be written as $\boldsymbol{X}'\boldsymbol{W}\boldsymbol{v}^{(m-1)}$, and the iterative procedure becomes

$$\boldsymbol{X}'\boldsymbol{W}\boldsymbol{X}\boldsymbol{b}^{(m)} = \boldsymbol{X}'\boldsymbol{W}\boldsymbol{X}\boldsymbol{b}^{(m-1)} + \boldsymbol{X}'\boldsymbol{W}\boldsymbol{v}^{(m-1)} = \boldsymbol{X}'\boldsymbol{W}\boldsymbol{z}.$$

The $n \times 1$ vector $\boldsymbol{z}$ has elements

$$z_i = \boldsymbol{x}_i'\boldsymbol{b}^{(m-1)} + (y_i - \mu_i)\frac{\partial \eta_i}{\partial \mu_i},$$

where μ_i and $\frac{\partial \eta_i}{\partial \mu_i}$ are evaluated at $\boldsymbol{b}^{(m-1)}$.

Provided that $\boldsymbol{X}'\boldsymbol{W}\boldsymbol{X}$ has rank p, the vector of parameter estimates is given by

$$\boldsymbol{b}^{(m)} = (\boldsymbol{X}'\boldsymbol{W}\boldsymbol{X})^{-1}\boldsymbol{X}'\boldsymbol{W}\boldsymbol{z}.$$

This solution has the same form as for a linear model fitted using weighted least squares. However, because $\boldsymbol{z}$ and $\boldsymbol{W}$ depend on $\boldsymbol{b}$, the solution must be obtained iteratively. The adjusted dependent variable z_i can be written as

$$z_i = \widehat{\eta}_i + (y_i - \widehat{\mu}_i)\,\frac{\partial \eta_i}{\partial \mu_i},$$

where the derivative of the link is evaluated at $\widehat{\mu}_i$. Because the first-order approximation to $g(y)$ is

$$g(y) \approx g(\mu) + (y - \mu)g'(\mu) = \eta + (y - \mu)\frac{\partial \eta}{\partial \mu},$$

z_i is a linearized form of the link function applied to the data.

ML Estimation for Canonical Links

When the canonical link

$$\eta_i = \theta_i = \sum_{j=1}^{p} x_{ij}\beta_j = \boldsymbol{x}_i'\boldsymbol{\beta}$$

is used, then

$$\frac{\partial \mu_i}{\partial \eta_i} = \frac{\partial \mu_i}{\partial \theta_i} = \frac{\partial b'(\theta_i)}{\partial \theta_i} = b''(\theta_i).$$

In this case,

$$\frac{\partial l_i}{\partial \beta_j} = \frac{(y_i - \mu_i)\,x_{ij}}{\mathrm{Var}(y_i)}\left(\frac{\partial \mu_i}{\partial \eta_i}\right) = \frac{(y_i - \mu_i)\,x_{ij}}{\mathrm{Var}(y_i)}\,b''(\theta_i) = \frac{(y_i - \mu_i)\,x_{ij}}{a(\phi)}$$

because $\mathrm{Var}(y_i) = b''(\theta_i)a(\phi)$. Thus,

$$U_j = \frac{\partial l}{\partial \beta_j} = \sum_{i=1}^{n} \frac{(y_i - \mu_i)\,x_{ij}}{a(\phi)}$$

for $j = 1, \ldots, p$.

The (j, k) component of the matrix of second derivatives is

$$\frac{\partial^2 l}{\partial \beta_j \partial \beta_k} = -\sum_{i=1}^{n} \frac{x_{ij}}{a(\phi)} \left(\frac{\partial \mu_i}{\partial \beta_k} \right)$$

for $j, k = 1, \ldots, p$. Because these components do not depend on the observations $y_i, \ldots, y_n$,

$$\frac{\partial^2 l}{\partial \beta_j \partial \beta_k} = \mathrm{E}\left[\frac{\partial^2 l}{\partial \beta_j \partial \beta_k} \right].$$

Thus, the Newton–Raphson and Fisher scoring algorithms are identical.

9.3 Quasilikelihood

9.3.1 Introduction

Most statisticians agree on the importance of the likelihood function in statistical inference. To construct a likelihood function, however, we must know (or postulate) probability distributions for random variables. In some cases, there may be no theory available on the specific random mechanism by which the data were generated. In other situations, the appropriate theoretical probability distribution may be inadequate to accommodate the complexities of the observed data. For example, the variance of the response may exceed the nominal variance (overdispersion). Another possibility is that the underlying theoretical model may be too complicated to permit parameter estimation and statistical inference.

In such cases, however, we may still have substantial information about the data, such as:

- type of response variable (discrete, continuous, nonnegative, symmetric, skewed, etc.);
- whether the observations are statistically independent;
- how the variability of the response changes with the average response;
- the likely nature of the relationship between the mean response and one or more covariates.

In such situations, quasilikelihood is a method for statistical inference when it is not possible to construct a likelihood function (Wedderburn, 1974; McCullagh, 1983). This estimation technique possesses many of the advantages of maximum likelihood estimation without requiring full distributional assumptions.

Let $\boldsymbol{y} = (y_1, \ldots, y_n)'$ be a vector of independent random variables with mean vector $\boldsymbol{\mu} = (\mu_1, \ldots, \mu_n)'$. Let $\boldsymbol{\beta} = (\beta_1, \ldots, \beta_p)'$ be a vector of unknown parameters with $p \leq n$. We will assume that the parameters of interest, $\boldsymbol{\beta}$, relate to the dependence of $\boldsymbol{\mu}$ on a vector of covariates $\boldsymbol{x}$. This will be denoted by the notation that y_i has mean $\mu_i(\boldsymbol{\beta})$.

We will also assume that $\text{Var}(y_i) = \phi V(\mu_i)$, where $V(\cdot)$ is a known function and ϕ is a possibly unknown scale parameter. Thus,

$$\text{Var}(y) = \phi \boldsymbol{V}(\mu),$$

where $\boldsymbol{V}(\mu)$ is a matrix with diagonal elements $V(\mu_1), \ldots, V(\mu_n)$ and off-diagonal elements of zero.

It is important to note that ϕ is assumed to be constant for all subjects and does not depend on $\boldsymbol{\beta}$ and that $\text{Var}(y_i)$ depends only on μ_i. This latter assumption is mathematically necessary but is also physically sensible. It would be permissible to have $\text{Var}(y_i) = \phi V_i(\mu_i)$; that is, a possibly different functional relationship for each observation.

9.3.2 Construction of a Quasilikelihood Function

Consider the random variable

$$U_i = \frac{y_i - \mu_i}{\phi V(\mu_i)}.$$

U_i has the following properties in common with a log-likelihood derivative:

$$\begin{aligned}
\text{E}(U_i) &= 0, \\
\text{Var}(U_i) &= \text{E}(U_i^2) = \frac{\text{E}[(y_i - \mu_i)^2]}{[\phi V(\mu_i)]^2} = \frac{1}{\phi V(\mu_i)}, \\
\text{E}\left(\frac{\partial U_i}{\partial \mu_i}\right) &= \text{E}\left[\frac{-\phi V(\mu_i) - (y_i - \mu_i)\phi V'(\mu_i)}{[\phi V(\mu_i)]^2}\right] \\
&= -\frac{1}{\phi V(\mu_i)} = -\text{Var}(U_i).
\end{aligned}$$

Most first-order asymptotic theory connected with likelihood functions is founded on the preceding three properties. Thus, it should not be surprising that the integral

$$Q(\mu_i; y_i) = \int_{y_i}^{\mu_i} \frac{y_i - t}{\phi V(t)}\, dt,$$

if it exists, should behave like a log-likelihood function for μ_i. We refer to $Q(\mu_i; y_i)$ as the quasilikelihood for μ_i based on data y_i (or, more correctly, as the log quasilikelihood). Because the components of $\boldsymbol{y}$ are independent, the quasilikelihood for the complete data is

$$Q(\boldsymbol{\mu}; \boldsymbol{y}) = \sum_{i=1}^{n} Q(\mu_i; y_i).$$

As an example, suppose that the random variable y has the $N(\mu, \sigma^2)$ distribution. Then, $V(\mu) = 1$ and $\phi = \sigma^2$. In this case,

$$U = \frac{y - \mu}{\sigma^2}.$$

The quasilikelihood function is

$$\begin{aligned} Q(\mu, y) &= \int_y^\mu \frac{y-t}{\sigma^2}\, dt \\ &= \frac{1}{\sigma^2}\left[yt - \frac{t^2}{2}\right]_y^\mu \\ &= \frac{1}{\sigma^2}\left[y\mu - \frac{\mu^2}{2} - y^2 + \frac{y^2}{2}\right] \\ &= \frac{1}{2\sigma^2}\left[2y\mu - \mu^2 - y^2\right] \\ &= -\frac{(y-\mu)^2}{2\sigma^2}. \end{aligned}$$

This is equivalent to the log-likelihood for the $N(\mu, \sigma^2)$ distribution.

As a second example, suppose that $y \sim P(\mu)$. In this case, $V(\mu) = \mu$, $\phi = 1$, and

$$U = \frac{y - \mu}{\mu}.$$

The quasilikelihood function is

$$\begin{aligned} Q(\mu, y) &= \int_y^\mu \frac{y-t}{t}\, dt \\ &= \int_y^\mu \left(\frac{y}{t} - 1\right) \\ &= \left[y \log(t) - t\right]_y^\mu \\ &= y\log(\mu) - \mu - y\log(y) + y. \end{aligned}$$

In comparison, the log-likelihood for the $P(\mu)$ distribution is

$$y\log(\mu) - \mu - \log(y!).$$

The log-likelihood and the quasilikelihood differ only with respect to terms not involving the parameter μ.

As a third example, suppose that y has the Bernoulli distribution $B(1, \pi)$. Then, $\mu = \pi$, $V(\mu) = \mu(1-\mu)$, and $\phi = 1$. In this case,

$$U = \frac{y - \pi}{\pi(1-\pi)}.$$

The quasilikelihood function is

$$
\begin{aligned}
Q(\pi, y) &= \int_y^\pi \frac{y-t}{t(1-t)}\,dt \\
&= \int_y^\pi \left[\frac{y}{t} + \frac{y-1}{1-t}\right] dt \\
&= \Big[y\log(t) - (y-1)\log(1-t)\Big]_y^\pi \\
&= y\log\Big(\frac{\pi}{1-\pi}\Big) + \log(1-\pi) - y\log\Big(\frac{y}{1-y}\Big) - \log(1-y).
\end{aligned}
$$

In comparison, the log-likelihood for $B(1,\pi)$ is

$$
y\log\Big(\frac{\pi}{1-\pi}\Big) + \log(1-\pi) + \log\binom{1}{y}.
$$

These differ only with respect to terms not involving the parameter π.

9.3.3 Quasilikelihood Estimating Equations

If we treat the quasilikelihood function as if it were a "true" log-likelihood, the estimate of β_j satisfies the equation

$$
\begin{aligned}
0 &= \frac{\partial Q(\mu; y)}{\partial \beta_j} = \sum_{i=1}^n \frac{\partial Q(\mu_i; y_i)}{\partial \beta_j} \\
&= \sum_{i=1}^n \frac{\partial Q(\mu_i; y_i)}{\partial \mu_i}\Big(\frac{\partial \mu_i}{\partial \beta_j}\Big) = \sum_{i=1}^n \frac{y_i - \mu_i}{\phi V(\mu_i)}\Big(\frac{\partial \mu_i}{\partial \beta_j}\Big).
\end{aligned}
$$

In terms of matrices and vectors, let

$$
\begin{aligned}
\boldsymbol{y}_{(n\times 1)} &= (y_1, \ldots, y_n)', \\
\boldsymbol{\mu}_{(n\times 1)} &= (\mu_1, \ldots, \mu_n)', \\
\boldsymbol{V}_{(n\times n)} &= \begin{pmatrix} V(\mu_1) & 0 & \cdots & 0 \\ 0 & V(\mu_2) & & \\ \vdots & & \ddots & \\ 0 & & & V(\mu_n) \end{pmatrix}, \\
\boldsymbol{D}_{(n\times p)} &= \Big(\frac{\partial \boldsymbol{\mu}}{\partial \boldsymbol{\beta}}\Big),
\end{aligned}
$$

where the (i,j) component of $\boldsymbol{D}$ is

$$
\frac{\partial \mu_i}{\partial \beta_j}.
$$

The quasilikelihood estimating equation is

$$\boldsymbol{U}(\widehat{\boldsymbol{\beta}}) = \mathbf{0}_p, \tag{9.6}$$

where

$$\boldsymbol{U}(\boldsymbol{\beta}) = \boldsymbol{D}'\boldsymbol{V}^{-1}(\boldsymbol{y} - \boldsymbol{\mu})/\phi.$$

$\boldsymbol{U}(\boldsymbol{\beta})$ is called the quasiscore function.

The covariance matrix of $\boldsymbol{U}(\boldsymbol{\beta})$, which is also the negative expected value of

$$\frac{\partial \boldsymbol{U}(\boldsymbol{\beta})}{\partial \boldsymbol{\beta}},$$

is $\boldsymbol{\mathcal{I}} = \boldsymbol{D}'\boldsymbol{V}^{-1}\boldsymbol{D}/\phi$. For quasilikelihood functions, the matrix $\boldsymbol{\mathcal{I}}$ plays the same role as the Fisher information for ordinary likelihood functions. In particular, the asymptotic covariance matrix of the vector $\widehat{\boldsymbol{\beta}}$ is

$$\text{Var}(\widehat{\boldsymbol{\beta}}) = \boldsymbol{\mathcal{I}}^{-1} = \phi(\boldsymbol{D}'\boldsymbol{V}^{-1}\boldsymbol{D})^{-1}.$$

McCullagh (1983) discusses consistency, asymptotic normality, and optimality of the quasilikelihood estimator $\widehat{\boldsymbol{\beta}}$.

Starting with an arbitrary estimate $\boldsymbol{b}^{(0)}$ sufficiently close to $\boldsymbol{\beta}$, the sequence of parameter estimates generated by the Newton–Raphson method with Fisher scoring is

$$\begin{aligned}
\boldsymbol{b}^{(m)} &= \boldsymbol{b}^{(m-1)} + \left[\boldsymbol{\mathcal{I}}^{(m-1)}\right]^{-1}\boldsymbol{U}^{(m-1)} \\
&= \boldsymbol{b}^{(m-1)} + \left[\phi(\boldsymbol{D}'\boldsymbol{V}^{-1}\boldsymbol{D})^{-1}\right] \times \left[\boldsymbol{D}'\boldsymbol{V}^{-1}(\boldsymbol{y} - \boldsymbol{\mu})/\phi\right] \\
&= \boldsymbol{b}^{(m-1)} + (\boldsymbol{D}'\boldsymbol{V}^{-1}\boldsymbol{D})^{-1}\boldsymbol{D}'\boldsymbol{V}^{-1}(\boldsymbol{y} - \boldsymbol{\mu}),
\end{aligned}$$

where $\boldsymbol{\mu}$, $\boldsymbol{D}$, and $\boldsymbol{V}$ are evaluated at $\boldsymbol{\mu}^{(m-1)}$. An important property of the estimation procedure is that it does not depend on the value of ϕ. For theoretical purposes, it is helpful to imagine the iterative procedure starting at $\boldsymbol{b}^{(0)} = \boldsymbol{\beta}$. The preceding iterative procedure now shows that the one-step estimator is a linear function of the data; approximate unbiasedness and asymptotic normality follow.

In the preceding respects, the quasilikelihood behaves just like an ordinary log-likelihood. The one exception is in the estimation of ϕ. The conventional estimator of ϕ is a moment estimator based on the residual vector $\boldsymbol{y} - \widehat{\boldsymbol{\mu}}$, namely

$$\widehat{\phi} = \frac{1}{n-p}\sum_{i=1}^{n}\frac{(y_i - \widehat{\mu}_i)^2}{V(\widehat{\mu}_i)} = \frac{X^2}{n-p},$$

where X^2 is the generalized Pearson statistic (McCullagh and Nelder, 1989, p. 34).

9.3.4 Comparison Between Quasilikelihood and Generalized Linear Models

The random component of a generalized linear model assumes a specific distribution for the response y_i. Quasilikelihood assumes only a form for the functional relationship between the mean and the variance of y_i. The quasilikelihood estimating equations for $\boldsymbol{\beta}$ are

$$\sum_{i=1}^{n} \frac{y_i - \mu_i}{\phi V(\mu_i)} \left(\frac{\partial \mu_i}{\partial \beta_j} \right) = 0, \qquad j = 1, \ldots, p.$$

In comparison, the likelihood equations for generalized linear models are

$$\sum_{i=1}^{n} \frac{(y_i - \mu_i)\, x_{ij}}{\mathrm{Var}(y_i)} \left(\frac{\partial \mu_i}{\partial \eta_i} \right) = 0, \qquad j = 1, \ldots, p.$$

Because

$$\frac{\partial \mu_i}{\partial \beta_j} = \frac{\partial \mu_i}{\partial \eta_i} \frac{\partial \eta_i}{\partial \beta_j} = \frac{\partial \mu_i}{\partial \eta_i} x_{ij}$$

and

$$\mathrm{Var}(y_i) = \phi V(\mu_i),$$

the quasilikelihood estimating equations have the same form as the generalized linear model likelihood equations. Quasilikelihood estimation, however, makes only second-moment assumptions about the distribution of y_i rather than full distributional assumptions. Quasilikelihood can also be motivated in terms of least squares; see, for example, Crowder and Hand (1990).

9.4 Overview of Methods for the Analysis of Repeated Measurements

9.4.1 Introduction

Statistical researchers have developed several related types of extensions of generalized linear model and quasilikelihood methods for the analysis of repeated measurements. These methods are useful for both discrete and continuous response variables, including normal, Poisson, binary, and gamma responses. Generalizations for ordered categorical data have also been studied.

These approaches offer some significant advantages over some of the other types of methods discussed in earlier chapters. First, the number of repeated measurements per experimental unit need not be constant, and the measurement times need not be the same across subjects. The linear mixed models approach (Chapter 6) can accommodate this type of data when the response is normally distributed, and randomization model methods (Chapter 8) can be used for nonnormal and categorical data from a *single* sample. However, the general WLS approach for the analysis of categorical data (Chapter 7) cannot be used in this setting.

In addition, the extensions of generalized linear model methodology for the analysis of repeated measurements accommodate discrete or continuous, time-independent or time-dependent covariates. The categorical-data methods of Chapters 7 and 8 are not applicable in this case. Missing data can also be accommodated, with the restriction that the missing-data mechanism must be MCAR (missing completely at random).

Before discussing specific methods, three general types of extensions of generalized linear model methodology to the analysis of repeated measurements will first be introduced:

- marginal models;
- random-effects models;
- transition models.

This categorization of approaches to the analysis of repeated measurements using extensions of generalized linear models was discussed by Zeger and Liang (1992). The Ashby et al. (1992) annotated bibliography of methods for the analysis of correlated categorical data also classifies methods into one of these three types. The distinctions among these types of models are especially important for categorical response variables.

Neuhaus (1992) reviews generalized linear model methods for the analysis of repeated measurements for the case where the response is a binary variable. In addition to marginal, random effects, and transition models, he also discusses a fourth general category: response conditional models. The model proposed by Rosner (1984) exemplifies this approach. Neuhaus and Jewell (1990) show that response conditional models are useful only when estimation of covariate effects is not of prime interest and attention is instead focused on the dependence of responses within clusters.

9.4.2 Marginal Models

Let y_{ij} denote the response at time j from subject i. In marginal models, the marginal expectation $\mu_{ij} = \mathrm{E}(y_{ij})$ is modeled as a function of explanatory variables. The marginal expectation is the average response over the subpopulation that shares a common value of the covariate vector. Note that this is what is modeled in a cross-sectional study. Associations among repeated observations are modeled separately from the marginal mean and variance of the response vector.

The assumptions can be outlined as follows:

1. The marginal expectation μ_{ij} is related to the covariates through a known link function g:

$$g(\mu_{ij}) = \boldsymbol{x}'_{ij}\boldsymbol{\beta},$$

where $\boldsymbol{x}'_{ij} = (x_{ij1}, \ldots, x_{ijp})$ is a vector of covariates specific to subject i at time j and $\boldsymbol{\beta}$ is a $p \times 1$ vector of regression parameters.

2. The marginal variance of y_{ij} is related to the marginal expectation μ_{ij} via

$$\text{Var}(y_{ij}) = \phi V(\mu_{ij}),$$

where V is a known variance function and ϕ is a possibly unknown scale parameter.

3. The covariance between y_{ij} and $y_{ij'}$ is a known function of μ_{ij}, $\mu_{ij'}$, and a vector of unknown parameters $\boldsymbol{\alpha}$.

Note that the marginal regression coefficients have the same interpretation as coefficients from a cross-sectional analysis.

9.4.3 Random-Effects Models

In random-effects models, heterogeneity between individuals arising from unmeasured variables is accounted for by including subject-specific random effects in the model. These random effects are assumed to account for all of the within-subject correlation present in the data. Conditional on the values of the random effects, the responses are assumed to be independent.

The assumptions can be outlined as follows:

1. Given a vector $\boldsymbol{b}_i$ of subject-specific effects for the ith subject, the conditional mean of y_{ij} satisfies the model

$$g\big(\text{E}(y_{ij}|\boldsymbol{b}_i)\big) = \boldsymbol{x}'_{ij}\boldsymbol{\beta} + \boldsymbol{z}'_{ij}\boldsymbol{b}_i,$$

where g is a known link function and $\boldsymbol{z}_{ij}$ is a vector of covariates for subject i at time j.

2. $y_{i1}, \ldots, y_{it_i}$ are independent given $\boldsymbol{b}_i$ for each $i = 1, \ldots, n$.

3. $\boldsymbol{b}_1, \ldots, \boldsymbol{b}_n$ are independent and identically distributed with probability density function f.

9.4.4 Transition Models

In transition models for the analysis of repeated measurements, the observations $y_{i1}, \ldots, y_{it_i}$ from subject i are correlated because y_{ij} is explicitly influenced by the past values $y_{i1}, \ldots, y_{i,j-1}$. The past outcomes are treated as additional predictor variables. The conditional expectation of the current response, given the past responses, is assumed to follow a generalized linear model. The linear predictor component of the model includes the original covariates as well as additional covariates that are known functions of past responses.

Thus, the general form of the model is

$$g(\mathrm{E}(y_{ij}|y_{i1},\ldots,y_{i,j-1})) = \boldsymbol{x}'_{ij}\boldsymbol{\beta} + \sum_{r=1}^{s} f_r(y_{i1},\ldots,y_{i,j-1};\alpha_1,\ldots,\alpha_s),$$

where $f_1,\ldots,f_s$ are functions of previous observations and, possibly, of an unknown parameter vector $\boldsymbol{\alpha} = (\alpha_1,\ldots,\alpha_s)'$. In addition, the conditional variance of y_{ij}, given the past, is proportional to a known function of the conditional mean; that is,

$$\mathrm{Var}(y_{ij}|y_{i1},\ldots,y_{i,j-1}) = \phi V\left(\mathrm{E}(y_{ij}|y_{i1},\ldots,y_{i,j-1})\right),$$

where V is a known variance function and ϕ is an unknown scale parameter.

Korn and Whittemore (1979), Kalbfleisch and Lawless (1985), Muenz and Rubinstein (1985), Wong (1986), Bonney (1987), Kaufmann (1987), Ware et al. (1988), and Zeger and Qaqish (1988), among others, have proposed and studied the use of transition models for various problems.

9.4.5 Comparisons of the Three Approaches

In the case of linear models for continuous, normally distributed responses, the three approaches can be formulated to have regression coefficients with the same interpretation; that is, coefficients from random effects and transition models can have marginal interpretations. Categorical outcome variables, however, require nonlinear link functions. In this case, the three approaches give different interpretations for the regression coefficients.

Transition models express the conditional mean of y_{ij} as a function of covariates and past responses. Transition models are appropriate when it is reasonable to assume that responses follow a stochastic process depending on the individual only through the values of the measured covariates. As discussed in Neuhaus (1992), transition models are most appropriate for assessing the effects of within-cluster (time-dependent) covariates adjusted for the subject's response history. Because covariate effects must be interpreted as being adjusted for the subject's response history, the effects of cluster-level (time-independent) covariates may be poorly estimated using the transition model approach.

The use of random-effects models is often referred to as a "subject-specific" or "cluster-specific" approach (Zeger et al., 1988; Neuhaus et al., 1991). In random-effects models, heterogeneity among individuals is explicitly modeled using individual-specific effects. The regression coefficients have interpretations in terms of the influence of covariates on both an individual's response and on the average response of the population.

In contrast, the use of marginal models is referred to as a "population-averaged" approach. Parameters in marginal models only have interpretations in terms of the influence of covariates on the population-averaged response. Marginal models are appropriate when statistical inferences about the population average are the focus (i.e., when the scientific objectives are to characterize and contrast populations of subjects). This difference should be considered when deciding between marginal and random-effects models for a particular application. When the scientific focus is on an individual's response, random-effects models are preferable. When the focus is on the population-averaged response, a marginal model may be a better choice.

Although marginal models and random-effects models are both useful, in many types of studies marginal models may be the most appropriate. For example, in a clinical trial comparing a treatment group with a control group, estimation of the average difference between control and treatment is generally most important. In addition, Zeger et al. (1988), Neuhaus et al. (1991), and Graubard and Korn (1994) recommend the use of marginal models when all covariates are time-independent. Lindsey and Lambert (1998), however, present an opposing view that although marginal models may sometimes be appropriate for descriptive observational studies, they should only be used with great care in causal experimental settings, such as clinical trials. A practical advantage is that software for fitting marginal models is more widely available.

Another distinction among these three general approaches is that marginal models model the effects of covariates on the marginal expectations. In addition, a model for the association among observations from each subject must also be specified. Random-effects and transition models model the covariate effects and within-subject associations through a single equation.

9.5 The GEE Method

9.5.1 Introduction

The generalized estimating equations (GEE) methodology for the analysis of repeated measurements is a marginal model approach that was proposed by Liang and Zeger (1986); see also Zeger and Liang (1986). The GEE approach is an extension of quasilikelihood to longitudinal data analysis (an extension of the generalized linear model estimating equation to multivariate responses). The method is semiparametric in that the estimating equations are derived without full specification of the joint distribution of a subject's observations. Instead, we specify only the likelihood for the (univariate) marginal distributions and a "working" covariance matrix for the vector of repeated measurements from each subject. The GEE approach is now sometimes referred to as GEE1 to distinguish it from more recent extensions.

The GEE method yields consistent and asymptotically normal solutions, even with misspecification of the time dependence. The estimating equations reduce to the score equations for multivariate normal outcomes. The method avoids the need for multivariate distributions by only assuming a functional form for the marginal distribution at each time point. The covariance structure is treated as a nuisance. Instead, the GEE approach relies on the independence across subjects to estimate consistently the variance of the regression coefficients (even when the assumed correlation is incorrect).

The GEE method is feasible in many situations where maximum likelihood approaches are not because the full multivariate distribution of the response vector is not required. For example, five binary responses per subject give a multinomial distribution with $2^5 - 1 = 31$ independent parameters. With GEE, however, only the five marginal probabilities and at most $5 \times 4/2 = 10$ correlations are estimated. In addition, the efficiency loss relative to maximum likelihood is often minimal. Another advantage is that continuous and categorical covariates can be handled.

Zeger (1988), Zeger et al. (1988), and Liang et al. (1992) provide further background on the GEE methodology. A related method is to estimate a separate parameter vector at each time point and then combine the estimates (Wei and Stram, 1988; Moulton and Zeger, 1989).

9.5.2 Methodology

Overview

The first step of the GEE method is to relate the marginal response

$$\mu_{ij} = \mathrm{E}(y_{ij})$$

to a linear combination of the covariates,

$$g(\mu_{ij}) = \boldsymbol{x}'_{ij}\boldsymbol{\beta},$$

where y_{ij} is the response for subject i at time j, $\boldsymbol{x}_{ij} = (x_{ij1}, \ldots, x_{ijp})'$ is the corresponding $p \times 1$ vector of covariates, and $\boldsymbol{\beta} = (\beta_1, \ldots, \beta_p)'$ is a $p \times 1$ vector of unknown parameters. The vector $\boldsymbol{\beta}$ characterizes how the cross-sectional response distribution depends on the explanatory variables. Finally, $g(\cdot)$ is the link function.

The second step of the GEE approach is to describe the variance of y_{ij} as a function of the mean,

$$\mathrm{Var}(y_{ij}) = V(\mu_{ij})\phi,$$

where $V(\cdot)$ is the variance function and ϕ is a possibly unknown scale parameter. For normally distributed responses, natural choices are

$$g(\mu_{ij}) = \mu_{ij}, \qquad V(\mu_{ij}) = 1, \qquad \text{Var}(y_{ij}) = \phi.$$

If the response variable is binary, the choices

$$g(\mu_{ij}) = \log\left(\frac{\mu_{ij}}{1-\mu_{ij}}\right), \qquad V(\mu_{ij}) = \mu_{ij}(1-\mu_{ij}), \qquad \phi = 1,$$

are often used. If the response variable is a Poisson count,

$$g(\mu_{ij}) = \log(\mu_{ij}), \qquad V(\mu_{ij}) = \mu_{ij}, \qquad \phi = 1,$$

are often used.

The third step is to choose the form of a $t_i \times t_i$ "working" correlation matrix $\boldsymbol{R}_i(\boldsymbol{\alpha})$ for each $\boldsymbol{y}_i = (y_{i1}, \ldots, y_{it_i})'$. The (j, j') element of $\boldsymbol{R}_i(\boldsymbol{\alpha})$ is the known, hypothesized, or estimated correlation between y_{ij} and $y_{ij'}$. This working correlation matrix may depend on a vector of unknown parameters $\boldsymbol{\alpha}$, which is the same for all subjects. Thus, we assume that $\boldsymbol{R}_i(\boldsymbol{\alpha})$ for each subject is known except for a fixed number of parameters $\boldsymbol{\alpha}$ that we must estimate from the data. Although this correlation matrix can differ from subject to subject, we commonly use a working correlation matrix $\boldsymbol{R} = \boldsymbol{R}(\boldsymbol{\alpha})$ that approximates the average dependence among repeated observations over subjects.

Working Correlation Matrix

We should choose the form of $\boldsymbol{R}$ to be consistent with the empirical correlations. $\boldsymbol{R}$ is called a working correlation matrix because with nonnormal responses the actual correlation among a subject's outcomes may depend on the mean values and hence on $\boldsymbol{x}'_{ij}\boldsymbol{\beta}$. The GEE method yields consistent estimates of the regression coefficients and their variances, even with misspecification of the structure of the covariance matrix. In addition, the loss of efficiency from an incorrect choice of $\boldsymbol{R}$ is inconsequential when the number of subjects is large.

Several choices for the working correlation structure have been suggested (Liang and Zeger, 1986). One choice is the independence working correlation model with $\boldsymbol{R} = \boldsymbol{I}$. This choice is motivated by the fact that when the number of subjects is large relative to the number of observations per subject, the correlation influence is often small enough so that ordinary least squares regression coefficients are nearly efficient. The correlation among repeated measurements, however, may have a substantial effect on the estimated variances of the parameters and hence must be taken into account to make correct inferences. These considerations suggest the independence working model with $\boldsymbol{R} = \boldsymbol{I}$. With this choice, solving the GEE is the same as fitting the usual regression models for independent data. Hence, one can use available software to obtain parameter estimates. The correct variance, however, is not supplied in standard software packages. This working model leads to consistent estimates of the parameter vector and its covariance matrix given only that the regression model is specified correctly.

Another choice of working correlation matrix is to choose $\boldsymbol{R}$ equal to a completely specified matrix $\boldsymbol{R}_0$. Choosing $\boldsymbol{R}_0$ close to the true (unknown) correlation gives increased efficiency. Unfortunately, the choice is usually not obvious.

The exchangeable working correlation model has elements $\boldsymbol{R}_{jj'} = \alpha$. Thus, this model assumes that the correlation between measurements at any two observation times is constant. The exchangeable correlation structure is induced in a normal-theory random-effects model with a random intercept for each subject. Although the assumption of constant correlation between any two repeated measurements may not be justified in a longitudinal study, it is often reasonable in situations in which the repeated measurements are not obtained over time. For example, the exchangeable working correlation model might be reasonable if the independent experimental units were households and responses were obtained from each family member living in the household or if the independent experimental units were classrooms and responses were obtained from each student in the classroom.

The first-order autoregressive model (AR–1) has elements $R_{jj'} = \alpha^{|j-j'|}$. In this model, the correlation decreases as the distance between the time points increases. When the responses y_{ij} are normally distributed, this is the correlation structure of the continuous time analog of the first-order autoregressive process. The AR–1 model is a natural one to consider when measurements are taken repeatedly over time. One shortcoming is that the correlations decay very quickly as the spacing between observations increases; this was illustrated in the example of Section 6.4.2.

Another choice for a working correlation matrix is the stationary m-dependent model with elements

$$R_{jj'} = \begin{cases} \alpha^{|t_j - t_{j'}|} & \text{if } |t_j - t_{j'}| \leq m \\ 0 & \text{if } |t_j - t_{j'}| > m \end{cases},$$

where t_j is the jth observation time.

The most general model is the unspecified working correlation matrix with elements $R_{jj'} = \alpha_{jj'}$. In the case of a common set of t time points for each subject, this model has $t(t-1)/2$ parameters to be estimated. Although the unspecified working correlation model is most efficient, it is useful only when there are relatively few observation times. In addition, the occurrence of missing data complicates estimation of $\boldsymbol{R}$ because the estimate obtained using nonmissing data is not guaranteed to be positive-definite.

In choosing a working correlation matrix, the nature of the problem may suggest a structure. For example, for repeated measurements obtained over time, the AR–1 or unstructured models may be useful. When the repeated measurements are not naturally ordered, such as when measurements are obtained from multiple individuals within a family, the exchangeable model may be useful. When the number of experimental units is large and the cluster sizes are small, the choice of $\boldsymbol{R}$ often has little impact on the estimation of $\boldsymbol{\beta}$. In this case, the independence model may suffice.

When there are many repeated measurements per experimental unit, modeling the correlation structure may result in increased efficiency. Consideration of alternative working correlation structures may be useful in this case.

Generalized Estimating Equation

The fourth step of the GEE approach is to estimate the parameter vector $\boldsymbol{\beta}$ and its covariance matrix. For the ith subject, let $\boldsymbol{A}_i$ be the $t_i \times t_i$ diagonal matrix with $V(\mu_{ij})$ as the jth diagonal element. Also let $\boldsymbol{R}_i(\boldsymbol{\alpha})$ be the $t_i \times t_i$ "working" correlation matrix for the ith subject. The working covariance matrix for $\boldsymbol{y}_i = (y_{i1}, \ldots, y_{it_i})'$ is

$$\boldsymbol{V}_i(\boldsymbol{\alpha}) = \phi \boldsymbol{A}_i^{1/2} \boldsymbol{R}_i(\boldsymbol{\alpha}) \boldsymbol{A}_i^{1/2}.$$

The GEE estimate of $\boldsymbol{\beta}$ is the solution of

$$\boldsymbol{U}(\boldsymbol{\beta}) = \sum_{i=1}^{n} \left(\frac{\partial \boldsymbol{\mu}_i}{\partial \boldsymbol{\beta}} \right)' \left[\boldsymbol{V}_i(\widehat{\boldsymbol{\alpha}}) \right]^{-1} (\boldsymbol{y}_i - \boldsymbol{\mu}_i) = \boldsymbol{0}_p, \tag{9.7}$$

where $\widehat{\boldsymbol{\alpha}}$ is a consistent estimate of $\boldsymbol{\alpha}$ and $\boldsymbol{0}_p$ is the $p \times 1$ vector $(0, \ldots, 0)'$.

The estimating equation given by Equation (9.7) is analogous to the quasilikelihood estimating equation of Equation (9.6) in Section 9.3.3. Because Equation (9.7) depends on unknown parameters $\boldsymbol{\beta}$, $\boldsymbol{\alpha}$, and ϕ, Liang and Zeger (1986) propose replacing ϕ and $\boldsymbol{\alpha}$ by consistent estimators $\widehat{\phi}(\boldsymbol{\beta})$ and $\widehat{\boldsymbol{\alpha}}(\boldsymbol{\beta}, \phi)$. These are estimated using functions of the standardized Pearson residuals

$$r_{ij} = \frac{y_{ij} - \widehat{\mu}_{ij}}{\sqrt{[V_i]_{jj}}}. \tag{9.8}$$

The exact form of the estimator of $\boldsymbol{\alpha}$ depends on the choice of the working correlation matrix $\boldsymbol{R}_i(\boldsymbol{\alpha})$. Liang and Zeger (1986) propose residual-based estimators for the unknown parameters of several different working correlation structures.

The form of the GEE was chosen so that inferences about $\boldsymbol{\beta}$ are insensitive to an incorrect choice of $\boldsymbol{V}_i$. Information in the first sample moment is used to estimate $\boldsymbol{\beta}$; information in the second sample moment is used to weight the data efficiently. Choosing the working correlation matrix to be close to the true correlation structure increases efficiency.

Solving the GEE

The solution is found by iterating between quasilikelihood methods for estimating $\boldsymbol{\beta}$ and a robust method for estimating $\boldsymbol{\alpha}$ as a function of $\boldsymbol{\beta}$. The procedure is as follows:

1. Given current estimates of $\boldsymbol{R}_i(\boldsymbol{\alpha})$ and ϕ, calculate an updated estimate of $\boldsymbol{\beta}$ using iteratively reweighted least squares.

2. Given the estimate of $\boldsymbol{\beta}$, calculate the standardized Pearson residuals r_{ij} given by Equation (9.8).

3. Use the residuals r_{ij} to consistently estimate $\boldsymbol{\alpha}$ and ϕ.

4. Repeat steps 1, 2, and 3 until convergence.

Robust Variance Estimate

One approach to estimating the variance–covariance matrix of $\widehat{\boldsymbol{\beta}}$ would be to use the inverse of the Fisher information matrix,

$$\widehat{\mathrm{Var}}(\widehat{\boldsymbol{\beta}}) = \boldsymbol{M}_0^{-1}, \tag{9.9}$$

where

$$\boldsymbol{M}_0 = \sum_{i=1}^{n} \left(\frac{\partial \widehat{\boldsymbol{\mu}}_i}{\partial \boldsymbol{\beta}}\right)' \boldsymbol{V}_i^{-1} \left(\frac{\partial \widehat{\boldsymbol{\mu}}_i}{\partial \boldsymbol{\beta}}\right)$$

and $\boldsymbol{V}_i = \boldsymbol{V}_i(\widehat{\boldsymbol{\alpha}})$. This is called the "model-based" estimator of $\mathrm{Var}(\widehat{\boldsymbol{\beta}})$. As shown by Royall (1986), Equation (9.9) will not provide a consistent estimator of $\mathrm{Var}(\widehat{\boldsymbol{\beta}})$ unless the underlying model is correct. In the analysis of repeated measurements, we are unlikely to be sure that the chosen working correlation model is the true correlation structure.

Liang and Zeger (1986) recommend that the variance–covariance matrix of $\widehat{\boldsymbol{\beta}}$ be estimated by

$$\widehat{\mathrm{Var}}(\widehat{\boldsymbol{\beta}}) = \boldsymbol{M}_0^{-1} \boldsymbol{M}_1 \boldsymbol{M}_0^{-1}, \tag{9.10}$$

where

$$\boldsymbol{M}_1 = \sum_{i=1}^{n} \left(\frac{\partial \widehat{\boldsymbol{\mu}}_i}{\partial \boldsymbol{\beta}}\right)' \boldsymbol{V}_i^{-1} (\boldsymbol{y}_i - \widehat{\boldsymbol{\mu}}_i)(\boldsymbol{y}_i - \widehat{\boldsymbol{\mu}}_i)' \boldsymbol{V}_i^{-1} \left(\frac{\partial \widehat{\boldsymbol{\mu}}_i}{\partial \boldsymbol{\beta}}\right).$$

This estimator of $\mathrm{Var}(\widehat{\boldsymbol{\beta}})$ was defined by Royall (1986) and is known as the "robust" or "information sandwich" estimator. The estimator given by Equation (9.10) is a consistent estimator of $\mathrm{Var}(\widehat{\boldsymbol{\beta}})$ even if $\boldsymbol{R}_i(\boldsymbol{\alpha})$ is not the true correlation matrix of $\boldsymbol{y}_i$.

Thus, a useful feature of the GEE approach is that the large sample properties of $\widehat{\boldsymbol{\beta}}$ and $\widehat{\text{Var}}(\widehat{\boldsymbol{\beta}})$ depend only on the correct specification of the model for the mean

$$g(\mu_{ij}) = \boldsymbol{x}_{ij}'\boldsymbol{\beta}.$$

In particular, the GEE estimators are robust to departures of the working correlation matrix from the true correlation structure. Note that if the true correlation structure is correctly modeled, then $\text{Var}(\boldsymbol{y}_i) = \boldsymbol{V}_i$ and Equation (9.10) simplifies to

$$\widehat{\text{Var}}(\widehat{\boldsymbol{\beta}}) = \boldsymbol{M}_0^{-1}\boldsymbol{M}_1\boldsymbol{M}_0^{-1} = \boldsymbol{M}_0^{-1}\boldsymbol{M}_0\boldsymbol{M}_0^{-1} = \boldsymbol{M}_0^{-1},$$

which is the model-based estimator given by Equation (9.9).

Hypothesis Tests

After estimating the vector of regression coefficients $\widehat{\boldsymbol{\beta}}$, it may be of interest to test hypotheses concerning the elements of $\boldsymbol{\beta}$. Consider hypotheses of the form

$$H_0\colon \boldsymbol{C}\boldsymbol{\beta} = \boldsymbol{d},$$

where $\boldsymbol{C}$ is a $c \times p$ matrix of constants imposing c linearly independent constraints on the elements of $\boldsymbol{\beta}$ and $\boldsymbol{d}$ is a $p \times 1$ vector of constants. Because $\widehat{\boldsymbol{\beta}}$ is asymptotically normal, the Wald statistic

$$Q_C = (\boldsymbol{C}\widehat{\boldsymbol{\beta}} - \boldsymbol{d})'[\boldsymbol{C}\widehat{\text{Var}}(\widehat{\boldsymbol{\beta}})\boldsymbol{C}']^{-1}(\boldsymbol{C}\widehat{\boldsymbol{\beta}} - \boldsymbol{d})$$

has an asymptotic χ_c^2 distribution if H_0 is true.

9.5.3 Example

Spasmodic torticollis is a chronic neurological disorder that affects the muscles of the neck, causing the head to pull, turn, or jerk toward the shoulder. Some patients also experience shaking movements of the head and arms. The cause is unknown, and there is no known cure. One treatment for spasmodic torticollis is injections of botulinum toxin into multiple sites in the contracting muscles of the neck. This has been found to be helpful both in relieving pain and in lessening spasms.

A randomized, double-blind clinical trial of a new source of botulinum toxin type A was conducted in 75 patients with spasmodic torticollis. Patients previously untreated with botulinum toxin were randomized to one of four groups:

1. placebo (20 subjects);
2. 250 units of botulinum toxin A (19 subjects);
3. 500 units of botulinum toxin A (18 subjects);

TABLE 9.1. Clinical global ratings at weeks 2, 4, and 8 from 75 patients with spasmodic torticollis: First ten subjects

				CGR (0 = poor, 1 = good)		
Subject	Group	Age	Sex	Week 2	Week 4	Week 8
1	Placebo	82	F	0	0	0
2	500	41	F	0	0	0
3	250	62	F	0	0	1
4	1000	63	M	0	0	1
5	500	40	M	1	1	1
6	250	43	F	1	1	1
7	1000	56	F	0	0	0
8	Placebo	48	F	0	0	0
9	1000	34	F	0	1	1
10	500	35	M	0	0	0

4. 1000 units of botulinum toxin A (18 subjects).

Following a single injection, patients were evaluated at weeks 2, 4, and 8.

One of the primary outcome variables was a clinical global rating (CGR), which was coded as a dichotomous variable:

- 1 = symptom free or mild symptoms;
- 0 = moderate or severe symptoms.

The covariates of interest were treatment group, age, sex, and week. Age was quantitative and ranged from 26 to 82 years with a mean of 47 years. There were 39 males and 36 females in the study. With six exceptions, the data are complete:

- two patients (both in the 500-unit group) have no follow-up data;
- one patient in the 1000-unit group has a missing value at week 2;
- one patient in the 1000-unit group has a missing value at week 4;
- two patients from the placebo group have missing values at week 8.

The marginal probabilities of a good response are 32% at week 2, 36% at week 4, and 34% at week 8. Table 9.1 displays the data from the first ten subjects.

Because the response variable is dichotomous and there is a continuous covariate, analysis using a generalized linear model methodology seems appropriate. The first issue is the type of model: marginal, random-effects, or transitional. Marginal models are appropriate when inferences about the average response in the subpopulation sharing a common covariate vector value are the focus. In a clinical trial, estimating the average difference between treatments is generally the most important goal. Thus, a marginal model seems appropriate for this example.

Because the response variable is binary, the logit link function and the binomial variance function will be used. The response variable will be defined to be the logit of the probability of a good response. Let y_{ij} denote the response from subject i at time j for $i = 1, \ldots, 75$ and $j = 1, \ldots, 3$, where

$$y_{ij} = \begin{cases} 1 & \text{if the CGR is "good" (symptom-free or mild symptoms)} \\ 0 & \text{if the CGR is "poor" (moderate or severe symptoms)} \end{cases}.$$

Also, let $\boldsymbol{x}_{ij} = (x_{ij1}, \ldots, x_{ijp})'$ denote a $p \times 1$ vector of covariates for subject i at time j. The regression model is

$$\log\left(\frac{\mu_{ij}}{1 - \mu_{ij}}\right) = \boldsymbol{x}'_{ij}\boldsymbol{\beta},$$

where $\mu_{ij} = \mathrm{E}(y_{ij})$ and $\boldsymbol{\beta} = (\beta_1, \ldots, \beta_p)'$ is a $p \times 1$ vector of unknown parameters.

Using the GEE methodology, a working correlation matrix also must be specified. Because there are only three time points, the unstructured model has only three correlation parameters to be estimated and is thus reasonable to consider. In addition, because the data are nearly complete, there will not likely be difficulties in estimating the parameters of this working correlation model. For purposes of comparison, the independence and exchangeable working correlation structures will also be considered.

The covariates to be considered include treatment group, age, sex, and week. One parameterization of treatment group is in terms of three indicator variables:

$$D250 = \begin{cases} 1 & \text{for 250 units} \\ 0 & \text{otherwise} \end{cases}, \quad D500 = \begin{cases} 1 & \text{for 500 units} \\ 0 & \text{otherwise} \end{cases},$$

$$D1000 = \begin{cases} 1 & \text{for 1000 units} \\ 0 & \text{otherwise} \end{cases}.$$

Using this parameterization, it will be possible to assess the effects of each botulinum toxin dosage relative to the placebo and also to test the linear and nonlinear components of dosage (using the spacing 0, 250, 500, 1000). Age is a quantitative covariate, and the binary covariate for sex will be equal to 1 for males and 0 otherwise. The time effect will be parameterized using two indicator variables:

$$W4 = \begin{cases} 1 & \text{if week} = 4 \\ 0 & \text{otherwise} \end{cases}, \quad W8 = \begin{cases} 1 & \text{if week} = 8 \\ 0 & \text{otherwise} \end{cases}.$$

In addition, interactions among these covariates will also be considered.

TABLE 9.2. Spasmodic torticollis clinical trial: Wald tests of interaction effects from model 1

Effect	Chi-square	df	p-value
Age × week	0.30	2	0.84
Sex × week	0.16	2	0.92
Dose × week	4.83	6	0.56
All interactions	5.97	10	0.82

Model 1 includes the covariates age, sex, dosage (three indicator variables), week (two parameters), and the interactions between week and each of age, sex, and dosage. Based on the parameterization of the week effect, the interaction terms estimate the incremental effects of age, sex, and dosage at each of weeks 4 and 8. Thus, there are 18 regression parameters (including the intercept). The focus of this model is on assessing differential effects of age, sex, and dosage over time.

Table 9.2 displays the Wald chi-square statistic, degrees of freedom (df), and p-value for testing each interaction effect. These are computed as

$$\boldsymbol{\beta}_*' \widehat{\boldsymbol{\Sigma}}_*^{-1} \boldsymbol{\beta}_*,$$

where $\boldsymbol{\beta}_*$ is the subset of $\boldsymbol{\beta}$ of interest and $\widehat{\boldsymbol{\Sigma}}_*$ is the estimated covariance matrix of $\boldsymbol{\beta}_*$. None of these tests of interaction appear to be statistically significant. The results obtained from the independence and exchangeable working correlation structures (not shown) are similar.

Because model 1 has a large number of parameters relative to the number of observations, separate models including all of the main effects and only one of the interaction effects displayed in Table 9.2 were also fit. In each of these four models, there was also no evidence of interactions with week.

Model 2 includes the main effects of age, sex, dosage, and week (eight regression parameters, including the intercept). Table 9.3 displays Wald tests of the effects included in this model. Similar results were obtained using the independence and exchangeable working correlation structures. Relative to the conventional 5% level of significance, the effects of age and sex are not individually statistically significant. The joint test of these two effects, however, is significant. Because the week effect is nonsignificant, these two terms will first be omitted.

Model 3 includes the main effects of age, sex, and dosage (six regression parameters, including the intercept). Table 9.4 displays Wald tests of the effects included in this model. The joint effects of age and sex are again statistically significant at the 5% level of significance. The 3-df test of the dosage effect is also significant ($p = 0.02$), as are the 1-df tests comparing the 500-unit and 1000-unit dosages to the placebo.

Table 9.5 displays the estimated regression parameters from Model 3. The odds of a good response versus a poor response decrease as age increases,

TABLE 9.3. Spasmodic torticollis clinical trial: Wald tests from model 2

Effect	Chi-square	df	p-value
Age	3.45	1	0.06
Sex	2.21	1	0.14
Age and sex	6.47	2	0.04
Dose	9.90	3	0.02
250 vs placebo	1.62	1	0.20
500 vs placebo	6.65	1	0.01
1000 vs placebo	6.83	1	0.01
Nonlinear dose	3.11	2	0.21
Week	0.52	2	0.77

TABLE 9.4. Spasmodic torticollis clinical trial: Wald tests from model 3

Effect	Chi-square	df	p-value
Age	3.41	1	0.06
Sex	2.41	1	0.12
Age and sex	6.64	2	0.04
Dose	9.80	3	0.02
250 vs placebo	1.44	1	0.23
500 vs placebo	6.33	1	0.01
1000 vs placebo	6.76	1	0.01
Nonlinear dose	2.81	2	0.25

TABLE 9.5. Spasmodic torticollis clinical trial: Parameter estimates from model 3

Covariate	Estimate	Standard Error	Odds Ratio
Age	−0.03	0.02	0.97
Male sex	−0.66	0.42	0.52
250 units	0.87	0.72	2.39
500 units	1.87	0.74	6.49
1000 units	1.91	0.73	6.73

TABLE 9.6. Spasmodic torticollis clinical trial: Wald tests from model 4

Effect	Chi-square	df	p-value
Age	3.83	1	0.050
Sex	2.60	1	0.107
Age and Sex	7.19	2	0.027
Linear dose	9.28	1	0.002

TABLE 9.7. Spasmodic torticollis clinical trial: Parameter estimates from model 4

Covariate	Estimate	Standard Error	Odds Ratio
Age	−0.03	0.02	0.97
Male sex	−0.70	0.43	0.50
Linear dose	0.44	0.14	1.55

are lower for males than for females, and increase as dosage increases. In particular, the odds of a favorable response are estimated to be 0.97 times as high for each one-year increase in age. In addition, the odds of a favorable response are 0.52 times as high for males as for females. Although the nonlinear effect of dosage was not statistically significant ($p = 0.25$, Table 9.4), the parameter estimates displayed in Table 9.5 indicate that the effects of the 500-unit and 1000-unit dosages are similar and are both roughly twice as large (on the logit scale) as the effect of the 250-unit dosage.

Because the nonlinear effects of dosage are not statistically significantly different from zero, one might also choose to fit a model with a quantitative effect for dosage. This would allow interpretation of the dosage effect using a single parameter. Model 4 is similar to model 3, with the exception that it includes dosage as a linear term (coded as 0 for placebo, 1 for 250 units, 2 for 500 units, and 4 for 1000 units). Tables 9.6 and 9.7 display the Wald tests and estimated regression parameters, respectively.

The joint effects of age and sex are again statistically significant at the 5% level of significance. The 1-df test of the dosage effect is also significant ($p =$ 0.002). The odds of a good response versus a poor response are estimated to increase by 1.55 for each 250-unit increase in dosage.

In model 3, the test of nonlinearity of the dosage effect is not significant (chi-square= 2.81 with 2 df, $p = 0.24$). However, the parameter estimates of the effects for the two highest dosages (500 and 1000 units) are nearly identical and are roughly twice as large as those for the 250-unit dosage (Table 9.5). Thus, the model with indicator effects for dosage may be most appropriate.

Using the same covariates as were used in model 3, Table 9.8 displays the parameter estimates, standard errors, and z statistics (estimate/standard error) for models fit using the unstructured, exchangeable, and indepen-

TABLE 9.8. Spasmodic torticollis clinical trial: Parameter estimates from model 3 using three different working correlation models

		Regression Coefficient		
Covariate	Working Correlation	Estimate	Standard Error	z
Age	Unstructured	−0.0286	0.0155	−1.85
	Exchangeable	−0.0281	0.0152	−1.85
	Independence	−0.0285	0.0153	−1.86
Male sex	Unstructured	−0.6577	0.4240	−1.55
	Exchangeable	−0.6740	0.4244	−1.59
	Independence	−0.7221	0.4262	−1.69
250 units	Unstructured	0.8698	0.7246	1.20
	Exchangeable	0.9073	0.7320	1.24
	Independence	0.9850	0.7325	1.34
500 units	Unstructured	1.8704	0.7433	2.52
	Exchangeable	1.8517	0.7491	2.47
	Independence	1.9294	0.7508	2.57
1000 units	Unstructured	1.9059	0.7329	2.60
	Exchangeable	1.9062	0.7399	2.58
	Independence	1.9614	0.7393	2.65

dence working correlation models. All three working correlation models give similar estimates of the parameters and their standard errors. The estimated working correlation matrices, however, are quite different. Using the unstructured working correlation model,

$$\boldsymbol{R}_{\text{unstructured}} = \begin{pmatrix} 1.00 & 0.67 & 0.43 \\ 0.67 & 1.00 & 0.45 \\ 0.43 & 0.45 & 1.00 \end{pmatrix}.$$

In comparison,

$$\boldsymbol{R}_{\text{exchangeable}} = \begin{pmatrix} 1.00 & 0.49 & 0.49 \\ 0.49 & 1.00 & 0.49 \\ 0.49 & 0.49 & 1.00 \end{pmatrix}$$

and

$$\boldsymbol{R}_{\text{independence}} = \begin{pmatrix} 1.00 & 0.00 & 0.00 \\ 0.00 & 1.00 & 0.00 \\ 0.00 & 0.00 & 1.00 \end{pmatrix}.$$

It is also of interest to compare the results from the GEE method to those from carrying out separate univariate logistic regression analyses at each of the three time points. Table 9.9 displays the parameter estimates, standard

TABLE 9.9. Spasmodic torticollis clinical trial: Parameter estimates from GEE model 3 and univariate logistic regression models

		Regression Coefficient		
Covariate	Model	Estimate	Standard Error	z
Age	GEE	−0.029	0.016	−1.85
	Week 2	−0.034	0.025	−1.37
	Week 4	−0.020	0.024	−0.81
	Week 8	−0.034	0.025	−1.33
Male sex	GEE	−0.658	0.424	−1.55
	Week 2	−0.824	0.551	−1.50
	Week 4	−0.737	0.547	−1.35
	Week 8	−0.650	0.567	−1.15
250 units	GEE	0.870	0.725	1.20
	Week 2	0.893	0.819	1.09
	Week 4	1.359	0.906	1.50
	Week 8	0.708	0.953	0.74
500 units	GEE	1.870	0.743	2.52
	Week 2	1.300	0.824	1.58
	Week 4	2.314	0.910	2.54
	Week 8	2.220	0.918	2.42
1000 units	GEE	1.906	0.733	2.60
	Week 2	1.379	0.842	1.64
	Week 4	2.348	0.918	2.56
	Week 8	2.187	0.921	2.37

errors, and z statistics (estimate/standard error) for GEE model 3 as well as for univariate logistic regression models fit using the data from week 2 only, week 4 only, and week 8 only. Although the parameter estimates from the univariate models differ somewhat across the three time points, the differences are not large relative to the estimated standard errors. In addition, the standard error estimates from the GEE model are smaller than those from the univariate models.

9.5.4 Hypothesis Tests Using Wald Statistics

In the example of Section 9.5.3, hypotheses concerning regression parameters were tested using Wald statistics. One disadvantage of Wald tests of hypotheses about individual parameters or sets of parameters is that such tests are dependent on the measurement scale (not invariant to transformations). Another disadvantage of Wald tests is that they require estimation of the covariance matrix of the vector of parameter estimates. Estimates of variances and covariances may be unstable if the sample size (number of independent experimental units) is small or if the number of repeated measurements per experimental unit is large. In the example of Section 9.5.3, there were only three time points and 73 subjects from whom the outcome variable was observed on one or more of the three occasions. In this case, Wald tests may perform reasonably well.

In the context of sample-survey analysis, Shah et al. (1977) discuss strategies for making adjustments to Wald statistics based on the number of clusters (independent experimental units) to produce test statistics with better properties for moderate sample sizes. In particular, they propose a modification of the Wald statistic based on the same type of transformation used in transforming Hotelling's T^2 statistic to the F distribution. This test is more conservative than the Wald test. LaVange et al. (2001) suggest that the Wald and F-transform p-values be used as lower and upper bounds for judging the robustness of the actual p-value. As the number of independent experimental units increases, these statistics give similar conclusions.

Rotnitzky and Jewell (1990) and Boos (1992) discuss the use of "working" score and likelihood ratio tests for GEE. Hanfelt and Liang (1995) also consider approximate likelihood ratio tests. Although likelihood ratio tests are not implemented in standard software packages, version 8 of SAS (SAS Institute, 1999) provides the Rotnitzky and Jewell (1990) score tests in the GENMOD procedure.

9.5.5 *Assessing Model Adequacy*

Rotnitzky and Jewell (1990) consider the problem of assessing the closeness of the working correlation matrix $\boldsymbol{R}(\boldsymbol{\alpha})$ to the true correlation structure. Inferences regarding the regression coefficients $\boldsymbol{\beta}$ can be made using:

1. the robust variance estimator $\boldsymbol{M}_0^{-1}\boldsymbol{M}_1\boldsymbol{M}_0^{-1}$;
2. the model-based variance estimator $\boldsymbol{M}_0^{-1}$.

The first estimator is consistent even if $\boldsymbol{R}(\boldsymbol{\alpha})$ is misspecified. It may, however, be inefficient. The second estimator assumes that $\boldsymbol{R}(\boldsymbol{\alpha})$ is correctly specified.

Consider testing the hypothesis that the first q components of $\boldsymbol{\beta}$ are equal to specified values. Rotnitzky and Jewell (1990) show that if variance estimation is based on $\boldsymbol{M}_0^{-1}$, the Wald statistic is asymptotically equal to

$$c_1 X_1 + c_2 X_2 + \cdots c_q X_q,$$

where $c_1 \geq c_2 \geq \cdots \geq c_q \geq 0$ are the eigenvalues of a matrix $\boldsymbol{Q}$ and $\boldsymbol{Q}$ is a function of

$$\left(\frac{\partial \mu_i}{\partial \boldsymbol{\beta}}\right),$$

$\boldsymbol{V}_i$, and $\boldsymbol{A}_i$. In addition, $X_1, \ldots, X_q$ are independent χ_1^2 random variables.

Examination of the weights c_j provides information on how close the working correlation matrix $\boldsymbol{R}(\boldsymbol{\alpha})$ is to the true correlation structure and on the effect of a particular choice of $\boldsymbol{V}_i$ on the inference about the components of $\boldsymbol{\beta}$. The asymptotic mean and variance of the Wald statistic are $\sum c_j$ and $2\sum c_j^2$, respectively.

If $\boldsymbol{V}_i$ is close to $\text{Cov}(\boldsymbol{y}_i)$, then

$$\bar{c}_1 = \sum c_j/q, \qquad \bar{c}_2 = \sum c_j^2/q,$$

will both approximately equal 1. Points close to (1, 1) in a plot of $\bar{c}_1$ versus $\bar{c}_2$ for different choices of $\boldsymbol{R}(\boldsymbol{\alpha})$ indicate reasonable choices of the working correlation structure. Note that $\bar{c}_1$ and $\bar{c}_2$ can be computed without computation of the individual eigenvalues:

$$q\bar{c}_1 = \text{trace}(\boldsymbol{Q}), \qquad q\bar{c}_2 = \text{trace}(\boldsymbol{Q}^2).$$

Probability statements about $\bar{c}_1$ and $\bar{c}_2$ would, however, require the null distribution of $\widehat{\boldsymbol{Q}}$. Hadgu et al. (1997) and Hadgu and Koch (1999) demonstrate the use of this approach.

Pan (2001a) describes another approach for assessing the adequacy of the working correlation matrix. He proposes a modified Akaike criterion for GEE called the QIC, where the likelihood is replaced by the quasilikelihood and the penalty term also takes a modified form. This criterion can be used both for choosing the working correlation matrix in the estimating equation and for selecting explanatory variables to be included in the model. Albert and McShane (1995) assess the correlation structure using variograms, and Heagerty and Zeger (1998) propose a new diagnostic (the lorelogram) for assessing the correlation structure for repeated measurements of a categorical outcome variable.

Preisser and Qaqish (1996) propose regression diagnostics to be used with the GEE approach. They consider leverage and residuals to measure the influence of a subset of observations on the estimated regression parameters and on the estimated values of the linear predictor. In addition, they provide computational formulas that correspond to the influence of a single observation and of an entire cluster of correlated observations. Barnhart and Williamson (1998) propose an overall goodness-of-fit test for GEE when the response is binary; this is based on the Hosmer and Lemeshow (2000) approach for logistic regression.

9.5.6 Sample Size Estimation

Liu and Liang (1997) present a general approach for computing sample size and power for studies involving correlated observations. Their approach is a multivariate extension of work by Self and Mauritsen (1988) and

Self et al. (1992), who proposed methods for sample size and power calculations in the context of generalized linear models. Liu and Liang (1997) use GEE methodology to extend this approach to studies with correlated observations. Based on the GEE method, a quasiscore test statistic is used to derive the sample size needed. Liu and Liang (1997) provide general results as well as simplified sample size formulas for some special cases, including linear regression with repeated measurements and the two-sample problem with a repeated binary response. Their simplified expressions for the binary case assume the exchangeable correlation structure. They demonstrate the adequacy of their formula using simulation.

Shih (1997) and Rochon (1998) describe alternative methodologies for sample size and power calculations in GEE. Shih's approach is based on the standardized statistic (parameter estimate divided by estimate of standard error) using the GEE estimator of the variance of the parameter of interest. Pan (2001b) further describes Shih's (1997) approach and derives explicit formulas for several special cases when the response variable is binary. Rochon (1998) bases his approach on the noncentral version of the Wald chi-square statistic and uses the damped exponential family of correlation structures described by Muñoz et al. (1992) for the working correlation matrix. Rochon (1998) presents applications to repeated binary, count, and continuous outcome variables and provides a table for two-group comparisons when the response is binary. Lee and Dubin (1994) and Lipsitz and Fitzmaurice (1994) also discuss sample size estimation; their approaches are restricted to the case of repeated binary responses.

9.5.7 *Studies of the Properties of GEE*

Several researchers have reported the results of empirical studies of the properties of GEE estimators and test statistics (Paik, 1988; Lipsitz et al., 1991; Emrich and Piedmonte, 1992; Sharples and Breslow, 1992; Park, 1993; Hall, 1994; Li, 1994; Lipsitz et al., 1994a; Gunsolley et al., 1995; Hendricks et al., 1996; among others). Most of these studies have focused on the use of the GEE method for analyzing binary response variables. The results will be briefly summarized in terms of the sample size n (number of independent experimental units), the number of time points t, and the number of covariates p.

Lipsitz et al. (1991) simulated binary data with $n = 100, t = 2, p = 1$, and seven correlation structures. They reported that the parameter estimates were biased slightly upward and that the bias increased as the magnitude of the correlation among repeated measurements increased. Confidence interval coverage probabilities were close to the nominal 95% level. Additional simulations with $n = 40$ led to convergence problems (except with the independence working correlation model).

Emrich and Piedmonte (1992) simulated binary data with $n = 20, t = 64$, $p = 4$, and four correlation structures. In all cases considered, parameter estimates were unbiased. Type I error rates, however, were inflated from the nominal 5% level. These ranged to as high as 8% for tests of individual parameters and to as high as 17% for joint tests.

Lipsitz et al. (1994a) simulated binary data with $n = 15$, 30, and 45, $t = 3$, $p = 4$, and three exchangeable correlation structures. Type I error rates were close to the nominal 5% level, and confidence interval coverage probabilities were close to the nominal 95% level.

Li (1994) simulated binary data with $n = 25$, 50, 100, and 200; $t = 3$, $p = 1$, 2, and 3, and four correlation structures. Empirical test sizes and confidence interval coverage proportions were close to nominal levels. He reported convergence problems using the GEE methodology with the unstructured correlation structure when $n = 25$. Li (1994) also studied the properties of WLS estimates and confidence intervals. The WLS approach performed as well as the GEE approach, even when $n = 25$.

Hall (1994) simulated binary data with $n = 80$, $t = 4$, $p = 3$, and seven correlation structures. He studied the bias and mean square error of the estimates of the regression parameters and concluded that the GEE methodology provides satisfactory performance.

Hendricks et al. (1996) evaluated the properties of GEE in the context of a study with geographic clustering and a binary outcome variable. Although GEE accounted for the intracluster correlation when present, estimates of the intracluster correlation were negatively biased when no intracluster correlation was present. In addition, and possibly related to the negatively biased estimates of intracluster correlation, they also found inflated type I error estimates from the GEE method.

Paik (1988) investigated the small-sample properties of the GEE approach for correlated gamma data. With $t = 4$ and $p = 1$, point estimates and confidence intervals perform satisfactorily if $n \geq 30$. With $t = 4$ and $p = 4$, point estimates and confidence intervals perform satisfactorily if $n \geq 50$.

Park (1993) simulated multivariate normal data with $n = 30$ and 50, $t = 4$, $p = 3$, and missing-data probabilities of 0.1, 0.2, and 0.3. For $n = 30$, confidence interval coverage probabilities were less than nominal levels. For $n = 50$, coverage probabilities are close to nominal levels. Park (1993) compared GEE estimators with normal-theory maximum likelihood estimators and reported that GEE estimators are more sensitive to the occurrence of missing data.

9.5.8 Computer Software

Karim and Zeger (1988) wrote the first widely available program for the GEE method. This was a SAS macro written using the SAS IML procedure. Lipsitz and Harrington (1990) published a SAS macro. Davis (1993) published a FORTRAN program for GEE. Although not as user-friendly as the SAS macros, it can be run on any type of computer. Carey (1994) wrote an S-PLUS program that is available from STATLIB. The SUDAAN software package (SUDAAN, 2001), the SAS GENMOD procedure (SAS Institute, 1999), and the STATA statistical package (Hardin and Hilbe, 2001; STATA Corporation, 2001) can also be used.

9.5.9 Cautions Concerning the Use of GEE

First, the GEE method is semiparametric (not nonparametric). Correct specification of the marginal mean and variance are required. In addition, missing data cannot depend on observed or unobserved responses. A moderate to large number of independent experimental units (n) is required. The bias and efficiency for finite samples may depend on:

- number of experimental units (n);
- distribution of cluster sizes;
- magnitudes of the correlations among repeated measurements;
- number and type of covariates.

Another caution concerns the use of GEE with time-dependent covariates. Pepe and Anderson (1994) show that when there are time-dependent covariates in the regression model, $\widehat{\boldsymbol{\beta}}$ may not always be a consistent estimator of $\boldsymbol{\beta}$. In this case, one must either:

1. use a diagonal working covariance matrix;
2. verify that the marginal expectation $\mathrm{E}(y_{ij}|x_{ij})$ is equal to the partly conditional expectation $\mathrm{E}(y_{ij}|x_{i1}, \ldots, x_{it_i})$.

Condition 2 is that the outcome at a particular time point does not depend on covariate values at other time points, after controlling for the covariate values at the particular time point. Note that the second condition is trivially satisfied when the covariates are time-independent. Pepe and Anderson (1994) describe some general classes of correlation structures for which condition 2 does and does not hold.

Crowder (1995) also points out a potential shortcoming of the GEE methodology. He shows that, in some cases, the parameters involved in the specification of the working correlation matrix are subject to an uncertainty of definition that can lead to a breakdown of the asymptotic properties of the estimators. This situation does not occur when the independence working correlation model is used.

9.6 Subsequent Developments

9.6.1 Alternative Procedures for Estimation of GEE Association Parameters

As described in Section 9.5.2, the second step of the GEE iteration procedure uses the standardized Pearson residuals defined by Equation (9.8). Although this choice may be most appropriate for continuous, normally distributed outcomes, it may not be best for categorical response variables. In univariate generalized linear models, other types of residuals have been considered. Modifying the GEE estimation procedure to use a type of residual more appropriate to the response variable might lead to better properties.

Anscombe (1953) proposed defining a residual using a function $A(y)$ instead of y. The function A is chosen to make the distribution of $A(y)$ more normal and is given by

$$\int \frac{d\mu}{V^{1/3}(\mu)}.$$

Application of this approach to generalized linear models is described in McCullagh and Nelder (1989).

In particular, for Poisson outcomes, Anscombe residuals are defined by

$$r_{ij}^A = \frac{\frac{3}{2}(y_{ij}^{2/3} - \widehat{\mu}_{ij}^{2/3})}{\widehat{\mu}_{ij}^{1/6}}.$$

Similarly, the function $A(y)$ for binary outcomes is

$$A(y) = \int_0^y t^{-1/3}(1-t)^{-1/3}dt.$$

This can be computed using algorithms for computing the incomplete beta function $I(\frac{2}{3}, \frac{2}{3})$.

Another type of residual is the deviance residual. In univariate generalized linear models with outcomes $y_1, \ldots, y_n$, the deviance is often used as a measure of discrepancy. The deviance residual is the signed square root of the contribution of each observation to the likelihood ratio statistic for comparing the model under investigation to the full model with n parameters. For Poisson outcomes, the deviance residual is

$$r_{ij}^D = \text{sign}(y_{ij} - \widehat{\mu}_{ij})\sqrt{2(y_{ij}\log(y_{ij}/\widehat{\mu}_{ij}) - y_{ij} + \widehat{\mu}_{ij})}.$$

For binary outcomes,

$$r_{ij}^D = \begin{cases} -\sqrt{2\,|\log(1-\widehat{\pi}_{ij})|} & \text{if } y_{ij} = 0 \\ \sqrt{2\,|\ln(\widehat{\pi}_{ij})|} & \text{if } y_{ij} = 1 \end{cases},$$

where $\widehat{\pi}_{ij}$ is the predicted probability at the current value of $\boldsymbol{\beta}$.

Park et al. (1998) study the use of alternative residuals in the second step of the GEE estimation procedure. They investigate the use of Pearson, Anscombe, and deviance residuals in a model for generating correlated Poisson and binary responses with arbitrary covariance structure. Park et al. (1998) show that there are no clear distinctions among methods. The properties of the GEE estimates, confidence intervals, and test sizes are satisfactory using all three types of residuals. In particular, empirical test sizes for a nominal test at the 5% level of significance are between 4% and 6% for all sample sizes considered. The only notable difference is that estimation using deviance residuals gives lower power than Pearson or Anscombe residuals. Park et al. (1998) conclude that there is no compelling reason to consider use of alternatives to Pearson residuals.

Lipsitz et al. (1991) propose a different approach to modeling the GEE association parameters. For binary outcomes, they study using the odds ratio as the measure of association instead of the Pearson correlation coefficient. This is also considered by Liang et al. (1992). One advantage of this approach is that the odds ratio may be easier to interpret than the correlation coefficient. Other advantages are that pairwise odds ratios are not constrained by the marginal probabilities and are also not constrained to be in the interval $(-1, 1)$. One shortcoming is that this approach applies only to binary outcomes. In a simulation study with $n = 100$, $t = 2$, and $p = 1$, the parameter estimates from the odds-ratio association model appear to be slightly more efficient. The difference between using the odds ratio and using the Pearson correlation coefficient, however, is not large.

Carey et al. (1993) develop an approach for binary repeated measurements similar to that of Lipsitz et al. (1991). The Carey et al. (1993) alternating logistic regressions (ALR) methodology simultaneously regresses the response on explanatory variables as well as modeling the association among responses in terms of pairwise odds ratios. The ALR algorithm iterates between a logistic regression using first-order generalized estimating equations to estimate regression coefficients and a logistic regression of each response on others from the same experimental unit using an appropriate offset to update the odds-ratio parameters. The ALR algorithm is now implemented in the SAS GENMOD procedure (SAS Institute, 1999).

Chaganty (1997) also presents an alternative method for estimating the vector of GEE association parameters $\boldsymbol{\alpha}$. Chaganty's approach is an extension of the method of generalized least squares. Instead of using moment-based estimators of $\boldsymbol{\alpha}$, Chaganty's quasi-least squares (QLS) method estimates $\boldsymbol{\alpha}$ by minimizing a generalized error sum of squares. Shults and Chaganty (1998) extend the QLS approach to unequally spaced and unbalanced data. Chaganty and Shults (1999) discuss the asymptotic bias of the QLS estimator of $\boldsymbol{\alpha}$ and provide modified QLS estimators that are consistent under several working correlation models.

9.6.2 Other Developments and Extensions

Lipsitz et al. (1994a) propose a one-step estimator to circumvent convergence problems associated with the GEE estimation algorithm. In a simulation study with a binary response, $n = 15$, 30, and 45, $t = 3$, and $p = 4$, the performance of the one-step estimator is similar to that of the fully iterated estimator. They recommend the one-step approach when the sample size is small and the association between binary responses is high. In this case, the fully iterated GEE algorithm often has convergence problems.

Robins et al. (1995) propose an extension of GEE that allows for the missing-data mechanism to be missing at random (MAR) rather than missing completely at random (MCAR). Thus, the probability that y_{ij} is missing may depend on past values of the outcome and covariates. The Robins et al. (1995) approach, however, requires the correct specification of a model for the probability of nonresponse.

Paik (1997) also proposes a modification of GEE to handle missing outcomes when the missing-data mechanism is MAR. Xie and Paik (1997a, 1997b) discuss the situation when the covariates are missing at random and the outcome variable is missing completely at random.

Lipsitz et al. (2000) also discuss missing-data issues. They propose a modification of GEE for the case where the response variable is binary that yields less bias than the standard GEE approach when the missing-data mechanism is MAR rather than MCAR.

Rotnitzky and Wypij (1994) propose a general approach for calculating the asymptotic bias of GEE estimators calculated from incomplete data. In an example, they show that use of the exchangeable working correlation structure can result in a larger bias than the independence working correlation model. Fitzmaurice et al. (2001) compare GEE estimators of the association parameters in terms of finite sample and asymptotic bias under a variety of dropout processes.

9.6.3 GEE1 and GEE2

Prentice (1988) considers the special case of binary data and proposes a GEE estimator of the vector $\boldsymbol{\alpha}$ of correlation parameters. In Prentice's approach, there are two estimating equations: one for the mean structure and one for the correlation structure. Prentice (1988) shows that this leads to improved efficiency relative to the original GEE formulation. Zhao and Prentice (1990), Prentice and Zhao (1991), and Liang et al. (1992) further develop this approach. Hall (2001) summarizes the various extensions proposed by these authors.

The original Liang and Zeger (1986) GEE methodology combines an estimating equation for regression (first-moment) parameters with moment-based estimators for the association (second-moment) parameters $\boldsymbol{\alpha}$. Prentice (1988) and Prentice and Zhao (1991) extend Liang and Zeger's work by replacing the moment-based approach to estimating second-moment parameters with an ad hoc estimating equation for these quantities. This is actually a generalization of the Liang and Zeger (1986) approach because the moment-based estimators can be recovered as special cases of the ad hoc estimating equation. This generalization has two important benefits: increased efficiency—particularly with respect to estimation of second-moment parameters—and increased flexibility to model the covariances among within-subject responses.

This generalization is often called GEE1. The term "GEE1" is also used to refer to either the GEE of Liang and Zeger (1986) or the Prentice and Zhao (1991) generalization. The defining characteristic of both of these methods is that they operate as if regression and association parameters are orthogonal to each other, even when they are not (Liang et al., 1992, p. 10). This ensures consistency of the regression parameter estimates even when the covariance model is misspecified.

Zhao and Prentice (1990), Prentice and Zhao (1991), and Liang et al. (1992) also consider an alternative equation for simultaneous estimation of the regression parameters $\boldsymbol{\beta}$ and covariance parameters $\boldsymbol{\alpha}$. This requires modeling the third and fourth moments of y_{ij} instead of just the mean and variance. This extension is called GEE2.

One distinction between GEE1 and GEE2 is that in GEE1 the regression parameters $\boldsymbol{\beta}$ are considered to be orthogonal to the association parameters $\boldsymbol{\alpha}$ (even though, in general, they are not). The GEE1 approach gives consistent estimates of $\boldsymbol{\beta}$ even when the association structure is modeled incorrectly. In contrast, the GEE2 approach gives consistent estimates of $\boldsymbol{\beta}$ and $\boldsymbol{\alpha}$ only when the marginal means and associations are modeled correctly. In this case, GEE2 provides parameter estimates that have high efficiency relative to maximum likelihood. The GEE1 methodology gives slightly less efficient estimates of $\boldsymbol{\beta}$ but may give inefficient estimates of $\boldsymbol{\alpha}$. GEE2, however, sacrifices the appeal of requiring only first- and second-moment assumptions.

Although one method cannot be recommended uniformly over the other, one criterion is to use GEE1 if estimation of the regression parameters is the primary focus. On the other hand, if efficient estimation of the vector of association parameters is of interest *and* if the model for the covariance structure is known to be correctly specified, then the use of GEE2 is recommended. In practice, because the correct model for the association structure is not often known, GEE1 may be more appropriate in general. In addition, software implementing the GEE1 approach is more widely available.

9.6.4 Extended Generalized Estimating Equations (EGEE)

Hall (1994) and Hall and Severini (1998) also attempt to improve on GEE1 by taking a unified approach to the estimation of the regression and association parameters. Whereas Liang and Zeger's (1986) original work has a close connection to quasilikelihood and Prentice and Zhao (1991) motivated their GEE2 work through the ideas of pseudomaximum likelihood estimation (Gouriéroux et al., 1984), Hall and Severini's (1998) extended GEE (EGEE) approach uses ideas from extended quasilikelihood (Nelder and Pregibon, 1987; McCullagh and Nelder, 1989).

The EGEE approach provides estimating equations for regression and association parameters simultaneously that make only first- and second-moment assumptions. Through simulations and asymptotic relative efficiency comparisons, they show that EGEE has efficiency properties comparable to GEE2 and often substantially better than GEE1. If the correlation structure is correctly specified, the EGEE approach estimates the vector of association parameters $\boldsymbol{\alpha}$ efficiently (like GEE2). Although consistency of $\widehat{\boldsymbol{\alpha}}$ requires correct covariance specification, the EGEE approach does not require the correct covariance structure specification for consistency of the regression parameter estimates.

Hall (2001) shows that the EGEE approach is a special case of GEE1. In particular, EGEE amounts to estimation of the correlation structure by maximizing a Gaussian likelihood function, an approach that Crowder (1992) recommended for the analysis of generalized linear models with clustered data. Hall (2001) also develops a true extended quasilikelihood approach for the clustered data case.

9.6.5 Likelihood-Based Approaches

Fitzmaurice and Laird (1993), Molenberghs and Lesaffre (1994), and Heagerty and Zeger (1996) develop likelihood-based approaches that use a marginal mean regression parameter and require full specification of the joint multivariate distribution through higher-moment assumptions. These marginal approaches are computationally intensive even in situations with a small number of repeated measurements for each independent experimental unit. Heagerty (1999) presents an alternative parameterization of the logistic model for binary repeated measurements and studies both likelihood and estimating equation approaches to parameter estimation. A key feature of Heagerty's (1999) marginal model approach is that individual-level predictions or contrasts are also possible.

9.7 Random-Effects Models

Random-effects models for repeated measurements analysis in the generalized linear model framework are more difficult to fit than marginal models. Evaluation of the likelihood (or even the first two moments) requires numerical methods in most cases. In addition, the properties of the resulting estimates and test statistics have not been studied as extensively as for the

GEE method. Although software for random-effects models is becoming more widely available, this topic will not be covered extensively.

Mauritsen (1984) proposes a mixed-effects model known as the logistic binomial. The logistic binomial model eases the computation burden and is available in the Egret software package (Cytel Software, 2000).

Conaway (1990) develops a random-effects model for binary data based on the complementary log-log link and a log-gamma random-effects distribution. This model yields a closed-form expression for the full likelihood, thus simplifying likelihood analysis. The regression parameters, however, do not have log odds-ratio interpretations. Pulkstenis et al. (1998) extends Conaway's model to the analysis of binary repeated measurements subject to informative dropout.

One approach to avoiding numerical integration is to approximate the integrands with simple expansions whose integrals have closed forms (Stiratelli et al., 1984; Breslow and Clayton, 1993). These approximate techniques give effective estimates of the fixed effects but are biased for estimating random effects and the random-effects variance matrix (Zeger and Liang, 1992).

Waclawiw and Liang (1993) propose an alternative strategy based on optimal estimating equations. Zeger and Karim (1991) describe a Bayesian approach using Gibbs sampling. Other authors who have considered generalized linear models with random effects include Gilmour et al. (1985), Schall (1991), Longford (1994), and Ten Have et al. (1998).

The SAS macro GLIMMIX fits generalized linear mixed models using restricted pseudolikelihood (REPL). This approach is discussed in Wolfinger and O'Connell (1993). The Breslow and Clayton (1993) and Wolfinger and O'Connell (1993) procedures are similar in that both use the generalized mixed-model equations. However, the Breslow–Clayton procedure, which they call penalized quasilikelihood, assumes that the scale parameter ϕ is equal to one. The Wolfinger–O'Connell method assumes that ϕ is an unknown parameter to be estimated.

For the mixed-effects logistic model, estimates of fixed effects and variance components are biased under some common conditions, including situations where there are moderate to large variance components—that is, moderate to large within-cluster correlation—and when the cluster sizes (number of repeated measurements per experimental unit) are small to moderate. This was shown by Breslow and Lin (1995) and Kuk (1995). These authors provide methods that reduce the bias, but these are not yet implemented in GLIMMIX.

Version 8 of SAS (SAS Institute, 1999) provides a procedure, PROC NLMIXED, for fitting nonlinear models with fixed and random effects. Estimation techniques are not the same as those used in the earlier NLINMIX and GLIMMIX macros. Parameters are estimated by maximizing an approximation to the likelihood integrated over the random effects. Different integral approximations are available, including adaptive Gaussian quadrature and a first-order Taylor series approximation. A variety of alternative optimization techniques are available to carry out the maximization; the default is a dual quasi-Newton algorithm.

The general topics of nonlinear mixed models and generalized linear mixed models for repeated measurements are discussed in the books by Davidian and Giltinan (1995), Vonesh and Chinchilli (1996), and McCulloch and Searle (2000). Reviews of a variety of methods for analyzing repeated measurements using extensions of generalized linear model methodology are provided by Neuhaus (1992), Zeger and Liang (1992), Fitzmaurice et al. (1993), Liang and Zeger (1993), and Pendergast et al. (1996).

9.8 Methods for the Analysis of Ordered Categorical Repeated Measurements

9.8.1 *Introduction*

There are at least three general approaches to the analysis of repeated measurements when the response variable at each time point or measurement condition is an ordered categorical response.

One approach is to use the CMH mean score and correlation tests described in Chapter 8. These tests, however, are applicable only in the one-sample setting. Landis et al. (1988) review this approach to the analysis of repeated ordered categorical responses.

The weighted least squares approach described in Chapter 7 can also be used. Models for polytomous logit, cumulative logit, and mean score response functions can be considered for one-sample and multisample repeated measurements settings. Unless sample sizes are quite large, however, only mean score models may be feasible.

This section will briefly introduce and discuss the use of methods based on extensions of generalized linear model methodology. Various extensions of the GEE method have been proposed and studied by Stram et al. (1988), Agresti et al. (1992), Kenward and Jones (1992), Liang et al. (1992), Miller et al. (1993), Kenward et al. (1994), Lipsitz et al. (1994b), Gange et al. (1995), Williamson et al. (1995), Heagerty and Zeger (1996), and Lesaffre et al. (1996). Most of these methods are based on the univariate proportional-odds model (Walker and Duncan, 1967; McCullagh, 1980). Heagerty and Zeger (1996) also extend the Carey et al. (1993) alternating logistic regressions (ALR) methodology to repeated ordered categorical outcome variables.

Random-effects models for the analysis of ordered categorical repeated measurements have also been studied. Ten Have (1996) extends the Conaway (1990) random-effects model based on the complementary log-log link and a log-gamma random-effects distribution to accommodate ordered categorical responses. This approach yields a closed-form marginal likelihood. Pulkstenis et al. (2001) further extend this approach to the analysis of ordered categorical repeated measurements subject to informative dropout. Crouchley (1995) also uses complementary log-log link models with conjugate log-gamma random effects to analyze repeated ordered categorical responses.

Harville and Mee (1984) and Jansen (1990) use the EM algorithm in conjunction with approximations or numerical integration to fit mixed-effects ordinal probit models. Ezzet and Whitehead (1991) and Hedeker and Gibbons (1994) employ numerical integration to fit mixed-effects cumulative logistic regression models. Agresti and Lang (1993) develop a maximum likelihood constrained equations approach for fitting cumulative logit models to clustered ordered categorical data that is analogous to binary response conditional likelihood estimation. Zhaorong et al. (1992) and McGilchrist (1994) describe estimation approaches for mixed-effects cumulative probability models using various link functions. Ten Have et al. (1996), Gibbons and Hedeker (1997), and Sheiner et al. (1997) also study random-effects models for the analysis of ordered categorical repeated measurements.

Although computer programs for analyzing repeated measurements of an ordered categorical response are available, the development and ease of use of such software lags behind that of programs for the analysis of other types of repeated measurements. Lipsitz et al. (1994b) and Shaw et al. (1994) describe SAS macros, and Davis and Hall (1996) give a FORTRAN program. The MULTILOG procedure of the SUDAAN software package can also be used. Hedeker and Gibbons (1996a) provide a computer program for the analysis of ordered categorical outcomes using a random-effects model. More recently, version 8 of the SAS GENMOD procedure (SAS Institute, 1999) now provides the Miller et al. (1993) and Lipsitz et al. (1994) extension of GEE to repeated categorical repeated measurements.

In Section 9.8.4, the Stram et al. (1988) methodology for the analysis of repeated ordered categorical outcomes will be described. As background, cumulative logit models for univariate ordered categorical outcomes and the univariate proportional-odds model will first be introduced in Sections 9.8.2 and 9.8.3, respectively. Section 9.8.5 applies the Miller et al. (1993) and Lipsitz et al. (1994) extension of GEE to the example considered in Section 9.8.4.

9.8.2 Univariate Cumulative Logit Models for Ordered Categorical Outcomes

When the response variable is dichotomous, models in which the response function is the logit of the probability of the outcome of interest are commonly used. For categorical responses with more than two outcomes, multiple logit models can be used. When the categorical response is ordered, however, it is often advantageous to construct logits that account for category ordering and are less affected by the number or choice of categories of the response. For example, if a new category is formed by combining adjacent categories of the old scale, the form of the conclusions should be unaffected.

Although multiple logit models for unordered polytomous outcomes restrict consideration to only two response categories at a time, this is unnecessary when the response categories are ordered. Instead, logits can be formed by grouping categories that are contiguous on the ordinal scale. These considerations lead to models based on cumulative response probabilities, from which cumulative logits are defined.

Consider a response variable Y with $c+1$ ordered categories labeled as $0, 1, \ldots, c$. The cumulative response probabilities are

$$\gamma_j = \Pr(Y \leq j), \qquad j = 0, 1, \ldots, c.$$

Thus, $\gamma_0 = \pi_0$, $\gamma_1 = \pi_0 + \pi_1, \ldots, \gamma_c = 1$, where $\pi_j = \Pr(Y = j)$. Cumulative logits are then defined as

$$\lambda_j = \log\left(\frac{\gamma_{j-1}}{1 - \gamma_{j-1}}\right), \qquad j = 1, \ldots, c.$$

Note that each cumulative logit uses all $c+1$ response categories. A model for λ_j is similar to an ordinary logit model for a binary response, where categories 0 to $j-1$ form the first category and categories j to c form the second category.

9.8.3 The Univariate Proportional-Odds Model

Model

The proportional-odds model is

$$\lambda_j(\boldsymbol{x}) = \alpha_j + \boldsymbol{x}'\boldsymbol{\beta}$$

for $j = 1, \ldots, c$, where $\boldsymbol{x}' = (x_1, \ldots, x_p)$ is a vector of explanatory variables and $\boldsymbol{\beta}' = (\beta_1, \ldots, \beta_p)$ is a vector of unknown parameters. Note that the relationship between x_k and a dichotomized response Y does not depend on j, the point of dichotomization. In this model, ordinality is an integral feature, and it is unnecessary to assign scores to the categories.

Some authors consider the equivalent model

$$\lambda_j(\boldsymbol{x}) = \alpha_j - \boldsymbol{x}'\boldsymbol{\beta}.$$

The negative sign ensures that large values of $\boldsymbol{x}'\boldsymbol{\beta}$ lead to an increase in the probability of higher-numbered categories.

Parameter Interpretation

For individuals with covariate vectors $\boldsymbol{x}^*$ and $\boldsymbol{x}$, the odds ratio for response below category j is

$$\begin{aligned}
\Psi_j(\boldsymbol{x}^*, \boldsymbol{x}) &= \frac{\Pr(Y < j \mid \boldsymbol{x}^*)}{\Pr(Y \geq j \mid \boldsymbol{x}^*)} \Big/ \frac{\Pr(Y < j \mid \boldsymbol{x})}{\Pr(Y \geq j \mid \boldsymbol{x})} \\
&= \frac{\exp\{\lambda_j(\boldsymbol{x}^*)\}}{\exp\{\lambda_j(\boldsymbol{x})\}} \\
&= \exp\{\lambda_j(\boldsymbol{x}^*) - \lambda_j(\boldsymbol{x})\} \\
&= \exp\{(\alpha_j + \boldsymbol{x}^{*\prime}\boldsymbol{\beta}) - (\alpha_j + \boldsymbol{x}'\boldsymbol{\beta})\} \\
&= \exp\{\boldsymbol{x}^{*\prime}\boldsymbol{\beta} - \boldsymbol{x}'\boldsymbol{\beta}\} \\
&= \exp\{(\boldsymbol{x}^* - \boldsymbol{x})'\boldsymbol{\beta}\}.
\end{aligned}$$

Note that $\Psi_j(\boldsymbol{x}^*, \boldsymbol{x})$ does not depend on j.

Motivation

Suppose that the underlying continuous (and perhaps unobservable) response variable is Z and that the ordered categorical response Y is produced via cutoff points $\alpha_1, \ldots, \alpha_c$. The categories of Y are envisaged as contiguous intervals on the continuous scale, and the points of division α_j are assumed to be unknown. In this case,

$$Y = \begin{cases} 0 & \text{if } Z \leq \alpha_1 \\ 1 & \text{if } \alpha_1 < Z \leq \alpha_2 \\ \vdots & \vdots \\ c-1 & \text{if } \alpha_{c-1} < Z \leq \alpha_c \\ c & \text{if } Z > \alpha_c \end{cases}.$$

The common effect $\boldsymbol{\beta}$ for different j in the proportional-odds model can be motivated by assuming that a regression model holds when the response is measured more finely (Anderson and Philips, 1981). First, suppose that Z has the standard logistic distribution under some set of standard baseline conditions, so that

$$\Pr(Y \leq j) = \Pr(Z \leq \alpha_{j+1}) = \frac{e^{\alpha_{j+1}}}{1 + e^{\alpha_{j+1}}}$$

for $j = 0, \ldots, c-1$. Also suppose that the effect of explanatory variables is represented by a simple location shift of the distribution of Z. In this case, $Z + \boldsymbol{x}'\boldsymbol{\beta}$ has the standard logistic distribution.

Under these assumptions,

$$\begin{aligned}
\Pr(Y \leq j-1) &= \Pr(Z \leq \alpha_j) \\
&= \Pr(Z + \boldsymbol{x}'\boldsymbol{\beta} \leq \alpha_j + \boldsymbol{x}'\boldsymbol{\beta}) \\
&= \frac{\exp(\alpha_j + \boldsymbol{x}'\boldsymbol{\beta})}{1 + \exp(\alpha_j + \boldsymbol{x}'\boldsymbol{\beta})}
\end{aligned}$$

for $j = 1, \ldots, c$. Therefore,

$$\begin{aligned}\lambda_j(\boldsymbol{x}) &= \log\left(\frac{\Pr(Y \le j-1)}{1-\Pr(Y \le j-1)}\right)\\ &= \log\left(\frac{\dfrac{\exp(\alpha_j + \boldsymbol{x}'\boldsymbol{\beta})}{1+\exp(\alpha_j + \boldsymbol{x}'\boldsymbol{\beta})}}{1-\dfrac{\exp(\alpha_j + \boldsymbol{x}'\boldsymbol{\beta})}{1+\exp(\alpha_j + \boldsymbol{x}'\boldsymbol{\beta})}}\right)\\ &= \alpha_j + \boldsymbol{x}'\boldsymbol{\beta}\end{aligned}$$

for $j = 1, \ldots, c$.

Comments

Because the $c - 1$ response curves are constrained to have the same shape, the proportional-odds model cannot be fit using separate logit models for each cutpoint. In addition, unlike other logit models, the proportional-odds model is not equivalent to a log-linear model.

Walker and Duncan (1967) and McCullagh (1980) give Fisher scoring algorithms for iterative calculation of maximum likelihood estimates of the parameters of the proportional-odds model. The iterative procedure is similar to the Newton–Raphson method, except expected (rather than observed) values are used in the second-derivative matrix.

One caution concerning the use of the proportional-odds model is that it is not difficult to find examples of nonproportional odds (Peterson and Harrell, 1990). Therefore, the model may not be applicable in every situation in which the response is an ordered categorical variable. On the other hand, Hastie et al. (1989) analyze a study with an ordered categorical outcome with 13 categories. Although ordinary linear regression techniques are commonly used for an ordered response with that many categories, they show that such an analysis gives misleading results and demonstrate the appropriateness of the proportional-odds model.

9.8.4 The Stram–Wei–Ware Methodology for the Analysis of Ordered Categorical Repeated Measurements

Introduction

Stram et al. (1988) proposed one of the first approaches to the analysis of repeated measurements when the response is an ordered categorical variable. Their approach is applicable when the response is obtained at a common set of time points for each experimental unit. At each time point, the marginal distribution of the response variable is modeled using the proportional-odds regression model. The parameters of these models are assumed to be specific to each occasion and are estimated by maximizing the occasion-specific likelihoods.

The joint asymptotic distribution of the estimates of these occasion-specific regression coefficients is obtained without imposing any parametric model of dependence on the repeated observations. The vector of estimated regression coefficients is asymptotically multivariate normal with a covariance matrix that can be estimated consistently. The Stram et al. (1988) approach provides procedures to test hypotheses about covariates at a single time point (occasion-specific) and a single covariate across time points (parameter-specific) and to estimate pooled effects of covariates across time points. This approach allows for both time-dependent covariates and missing data. The missing-data mechanism is, however, assumed to be MCAR (missing completely at random). Davis and Hall (1996) describe a FORTRAN program implementing the Stram et al. (1988) approach.

Methodology

Let y_{ij} denote the response at time j from the ith experimental unit (subject) for $i = 1, \ldots, n$ and $j = 1, \ldots, t$. Also, let K denote the number of levels of the ordered categorical response variable; these will be indexed by $k = 1, \ldots, K$. Now, let

$$y^*_{ijk} = \begin{cases} 1 & \text{if } y_{ij} = k, \\ 0 & \text{otherwise,} \end{cases}$$

for $k = 1, \ldots, K$. It is now possible to consider the vectors of indicator variables

$$\boldsymbol{y}^*_{ij} = (y^*_{ij1}, \ldots, y^*_{ijK})'$$

instead of the y_{ij} values.

In addition, at each time j and for each individual i, suppose that a p-dimensional vector of covariates $\boldsymbol{x}_{ij} = (x_{ij1}, \ldots, x_{ijp})'$ is observed. When $\boldsymbol{x}_{ij}$ takes the observed value $\boldsymbol{x}$, let $\zeta_{jk}(\boldsymbol{x}) = \Pr(y^*_{ijk} = 1)$, and let

$$\gamma_{jk}(\boldsymbol{x}) = \sum_{l=1}^{k} \zeta_{jl}(\boldsymbol{x})$$

for each j and k. Thus, $\gamma_{jk}(\boldsymbol{x})$ is the cumulative probability $\Pr(y_{ij} \leq k)$ for all i. According to the proportional-odds model,

$$\lambda_{jk}(\boldsymbol{x}) = \alpha_{jk} - \boldsymbol{x}'\boldsymbol{\beta}_j$$

for $j = 1, \ldots, t$ and $k = 1, \ldots, K$, where

$$\lambda_{jk}(\boldsymbol{x}) = \log\left(\frac{\gamma_{jk}(\boldsymbol{x})}{1 - \gamma_{jk}(\boldsymbol{x})}\right)$$

and $\boldsymbol{\beta}_j$ is a p-dimensional vector of unknown parameters that may depend on j. Notice that in this model a positive regression parameter implies that the odds of observing a large value of y_{ij} increase as the covariate increases. Because $\boldsymbol{\beta}_j$ does not depend on k, the model makes the strong assumption that the additive effect of a covariate on the log odds that $y_{ij} \leq k$ does not depend on k.

To accommodate missing data, let

$$\delta_{ij} = \begin{cases} 1 & \text{when } \boldsymbol{x}_{ij} \text{ and } y_{ij} \text{ are observed,} \\ 0 & \text{otherwise.} \end{cases}$$

It is assumed that, for each i and j, δ_{ij} may depend on $\boldsymbol{x}_{ij}$ but is conditionally independent of y_{ij} given $\boldsymbol{x}_{ij}$. In addition, given $\boldsymbol{x}_{ij}$, the indicator variables δ_{ij} are assumed to be independent of α_{jk} and $\boldsymbol{\beta}_j$. For each time $j = 1, \ldots, t$, $(\boldsymbol{y}^*_{ij}, \boldsymbol{x}_{ij}, \delta_{ij})$ are assumed to be independent and identically distributed across individuals $i = 1, \ldots, n$. Under the MCAR assumption, the missing-data mechanism can be ignored, and occasion-specific estimates of the parameters $\boldsymbol{\beta}_j$ and $\boldsymbol{\alpha}_j = (\alpha_{j1}, \ldots, \alpha_{jK})'$ can be obtained by maximizing the log-likelihood function at time j, as given in Equation (A.1) on page 636 of Stram et al. (1988). The vector $(\widehat{\boldsymbol{\alpha}}'_j, \widehat{\boldsymbol{\beta}}'_j)'$ is asymptotically normal with mean $(\boldsymbol{\alpha}'_j, \boldsymbol{\beta}'_j)'$ and a covariance matrix that can be estimated consistently using expression (A.2) on p. 636 of Stram et al. (1988).

Hypotheses concerning occasion-specific parameters of the form

$$H_0\colon \boldsymbol{C}_j \boldsymbol{\beta}_j = \boldsymbol{0}_c$$

can be tested using the Wald statistic

$$W_j = (\boldsymbol{C}_j \widehat{\boldsymbol{\beta}}_j)'(\boldsymbol{C}_j \widehat{\text{Var}}(\widehat{\boldsymbol{\beta}}_j) \boldsymbol{C}'_j)^{-1} (\boldsymbol{C}_j \widehat{\boldsymbol{\beta}}_j),$$

where $\boldsymbol{C}_j$ is a $c \times p$ matrix of constants. Under H_0, the statistic W_j has an asymptotic χ^2_c distribution. With $\boldsymbol{\beta}_l = (\beta_{1l}, \ldots, \beta_{tl})'$ and $\boldsymbol{C}_l$ a $c \times t$ matrix of constants, parameter-specific hypotheses of the form $H_0\colon \boldsymbol{C}_l \boldsymbol{\beta}_l = \boldsymbol{0}_c$ can be similarly tested.

Parameters specific to the lth covariate, $\boldsymbol{\beta}_l$, can be combined to obtain a pooled estimate

$$\overline{\beta}_l = \sum_{j=1}^{t} w_j \widehat{\beta}_{jl}$$

of the covariate's effect across time. In general, $\boldsymbol{w} = (w_1, \ldots, w_t)'$ is any vector of weights summing to one. However, the estimator $\overline{\beta}^*_l$, which uses

$$\boldsymbol{w}^* = \left(\boldsymbol{1}'_t \widehat{\text{Var}}(\widehat{\boldsymbol{\beta}}_l) \boldsymbol{1}_t\right)^{-1} \widehat{\text{Var}}(\widehat{\boldsymbol{\beta}}_l)^{-1} \boldsymbol{1}_t,$$

has the smallest asymptotic variance among all linear estimators $\overline{\beta}_l$.

Example

In a clinical trial comparing the effects of varying dosages of an anesthetic on postsurgical recovery, 60 young children undergoing outpatient

TABLE 9.10. Recovery room scores from a clinical trial in 60 children undergoing outpatient surgery: First five subjects from each group

Dosage (mg/kg)	ID	Age (months)	Surgery Duration (minutes)	Recovery Room Scores at Minute 0	5	15	30
15	1	36	128	3	5	6	6
	2	35	70	3	4	6	6
	3	54	138	1	1	1	4
	4	47	67	1	3	3	5
	5	42	55	5	6	6	6
20	1	22	75	1	1	1	6
	2	49	42	1	1	1	6
	3	36	58	2	3	3	6
	4	43	60	1	1	2	3
	5	23	64	5	6	6	6
25	1	26	103	1	1	0	3
	2	28	89	3	6	6	6
	3	41	51	2	3	4	4
	4	46	93	1	1	5	6
	5	37	45	2	3	6	6
30	1	46	72	4	6	6	6
	2	38	85	2	4	6	6
	3	59	54	4	5	5	6
	4	16	100	1	1	1	1
	5	65	113	2	3	3	5

surgery were randomized to one of four dosages (15, 20, 25, and 30 mg/kg) of an anesthetic, with 15 children assigned to each dosage group (Davis, 1991). Recovery scores were assigned upon admission to the recovery room (minute 0) and at minutes 5, 15, and 30 following admission. The response at each of the four time points was an ordered categorical variable ranging from 0 (least favorable) to 6 (most favorable). In addition to the dosage, patient age (in months) and duration of surgery (in minutes) were two covariates of potential interest. Table 9.10 displays the data from the first five subjects in each group.

In the first model we will fit to these data (model 1), the covariate vector for subject i at time j includes:

$$x_{ij1} = \begin{cases} 1 & \text{20 mg/kg dose} \\ 0 & \text{otherwise} \end{cases},$$

$$x_{ij2} = \begin{cases} 1 & \text{25 mg/kg dose} \\ 0 & \text{otherwise} \end{cases},$$

$$x_{ij3} = \begin{cases} 1 & \text{30 mg/kg dose} \\ 0 & \text{otherwise} \end{cases},$$

TABLE 9.11. Anesthesia clinical trial: Parameter estimates from model 1

Covariate	Time Point	Regression Coefficient Estimate	Standard Error	Est./S.E.
20 mg/kg	1	−0.105	0.799	−0.13
vs.	2	−0.249	0.758	−0.33
15 mg/kg	3	−0.558	0.724	−0.77
	4	0.194	0.897	0.22
25 mg/kg	1	−0.634	0.770	−0.82
vs.	2	−0.441	0.771	−0.57
15 mg/kg	3	−0.072	0.688	−0.10
	4	−0.371	0.837	−0.44
30 mg/kg	1	−1.010	0.751	−1.34
vs.	2	−0.675	0.735	−0.92
15 mg/kg	3	−0.701	0.708	−0.99
	4	−0.465	0.884	−0.53
Age	1	−0.011	0.018	−0.61
(months)	2	−0.011	0.018	−0.61
	3	−0.028	0.020	−1.45
	4	−0.014	0.020	−0.70
Duration	1	−0.012	0.008	−1.40
of	2	−0.003	0.007	−0.41
surgery	3	−0.008	0.007	−1.14
(minutes)	4	−0.018	0.009	−1.92

$$x_{ij4} = \text{age (months)},$$
$$x_{ij5} = \text{duration of surgery (minutes)}.$$

Note that all covariates are time-independent.

Table 9.11 displays the parameter estimates from Model 1. Because Stram et al. (1988) use the parameterization

$$\lambda_{jk}(\boldsymbol{x}) = \alpha_{jk} - \boldsymbol{x}'\boldsymbol{\beta}_j$$

at each time point j, parameter estimates with positive signs are associated with an increased probability of higher (more favorable) responses.

Nearly all of the estimated regression coefficients are negative. This indicates that the probability of a more favorable outcome decreases as the dosage, age of the patient, or duration of the surgical procedure increases. There is no consistent evidence (across time) of statistically significant effects due to dosage, age, or duration of surgery. The test statistics "Est./S.E." in Table 9.11 are approximately $N(0, 1)$, and none are individually significant based on a two-sided test at the 5% level of significance.

The Stram et al. (1988) procedure permits time-specific hypothesis tests. In particular, the hypothesis that the joint effect of all covariates is not significantly different from zero can be tested at each time point. This hypothesis is

$$H_0: \beta_{j1} = \cdots = \beta_{j5} = 0$$

for $j = 1, \ldots, 4$. The resulting p-values at times 1–4 are 0.44, 0.91, 0.46, and 0.31, respectively.

Hypotheses concerning subsets of the parameters at each time point can also be tested. For example, the hypothesis that the overall dosage effect is not significantly different from zero at each time point is

$$H_0: \beta_{j1} = \beta_{j2} = \beta_{j3} = 0.$$

The p-values from this test at times 1–4 are 0.55, 0.82, 0.68, and 0.86, respectively. One might also wish to test whether the nonlinear components of the dosage effect are significantly different from zero. Because the dosages are equally spaced, this hypothesis is

$$H_0: \beta_{j1} = \beta_{j2} - \beta_{j1}, \beta_{j1} = \beta_{j3} - \beta_{j2}$$

for $j = 1, \ldots, 4$. The resulting p-values at times 1–4 are 0.95, 0.99, 0.63, and 0.88, respectively.

Although the results of model 1 give little evidence of any statistically significant effects of covariates on recovery scores, a simpler model treating dosage as a quantitative variable may also be of interest. This is justified based on the fact that the nonlinear dosage effects are nonsignificant at all four time points. Model 2 thus includes the covariates:

$$\begin{aligned} x_{ij1} &= \text{dosage (mg/kg)}, \\ x_{ij2} &= \text{age (months)}, \\ x_{ij3} &= \text{duration of surgery (minutes)}. \end{aligned}$$

Table 9.12 displays the parameter estimates.

The Stram et al. (1988) procedure also permits parameter-specific hypothesis tests. Table 9.13 displays the null hypotheses and p-values from several parameter-specific tests from model 2. For each of the three covariates, the hypothesis that the parameters at the four time points are jointly equal to zero is not rejected. Because it is also true that the hypothesis of equality of effects across time is not rejected for any of the covariates, pooled estimates of effect may still be of interest.

Table 9.14 displays the pooled estimates of the effects of dosage, age, and surgery duration. The odds of having a recovery score higher than a given cutpoint are estimated to be:

- $e^{-0.0460} = 0.955$ times as high per 1 mg/kg increase in dosage;

TABLE 9.12. Anesthesia clinical trial: Parameter estimates from model 2

		Regression Coefficient		
Covariate	Time Point	Estimate	Standard Error	Est./S.E.
Dosage	1	−0.070	0.049	−1.43
	2	−0.044	0.047	−0.95
	3	−0.033	0.046	−0.72
	4	−0.037	0.056	−0.66
Age	1	−0.013	0.016	−0.81
	2	−0.011	0.017	−0.62
	3	−0.025	0.019	−1.32
	4	−0.017	0.019	−0.93
Duration of surgery	1	−0.012	0.007	−1.57
	2	−0.003	0.007	−0.45
	3	−0.008	0.007	−1.12
	4	−0.017	0.009	−1.94

TABLE 9.13. Anesthesia clinical trial: Parameter-specific hypothesis tests from model 2

Hypothesis	Chi-square	df	p-value
No dosage effect H_0: $\beta_{11} = \beta_{21} = \beta_{31} = \beta_{41} = 0$	2.10	4	0.72
No age effect H_0: $\beta_{12} = \beta_{22} = \beta_{32} = \beta_{42} = 0$	2.84	4	0.58
No surgery duration effect H_0: $\beta_{13} = \beta_{23} = \beta_{33} = \beta_{43} = 0$	7.95	4	0.09
Equality of dosage effects H_0: $\beta_{11} = \beta_{21} = \beta_{31} = \beta_{41}$	0.89	3	0.83
Equality of age effects H_0: $\beta_{12} = \beta_{22} = \beta_{32} = \beta_{42}$	1.82	3	0.61
Equality of surgery duration effects H_0: $\beta_{13} = \beta_{23} = \beta_{33} = \beta_{43}$	5.84	3	0.12

TABLE 9.14. Anesthesia clinical trial: Pooled estimates of effects from model 2

Variable	Estimate	S.E.	Est./S.E.
Dosage	−0.0460	0.0424	−1.09
Age	−0.0143	0.0162	−0.88
Surgery duration	−0.0091	0.0065	−1.40

TABLE 9.15. Anesthesia clinical trial: Parameter estimates from GEE model

Variable	Estimate	S.E.	Est./S.E.
Dosage	0.0380	0.0297	1.28
Age	0.0139	0.0109	1.28
Surgery duration	0.0071	0.0046	1.55

- $e^{-0.0143} = 0.986$ times as high per 1 month increase in age;
- $e^{-0.0091} = 0.991$ times as high per 1 minute increase in surgery duration.

Although there is modest evidence of an effect due to surgery duration, there is essentially no evidence that dosage or age influence postsurgical recovery.

9.8.5 *Extension of GEE to Ordered Categorical Outcomes*

The Stram et al. (1988) methodology models the data at each time point and then combines the resulting parameter estimates. This approach requires a common set of time points for each experimental unit. The SAS GENMOD procedure (SAS Institute, 1999) now provides the capability to analyze repeated ordered categorical outcomes using the GEE approach as extended by Miller et al. (1993) and Lipsitz et al. (1994). Using the GEE approach, the number of repeated measurements per experimental unit need not be constant, and the measurement times need not be the same across experimental units. As with the Stram et al. (1988) methodology, the proportional-odds model is used for the marginal distribution. At this time, the only working correlation model available for the analysis of repeated ordered categorical outcomes using the GENMOD procedure is the independence model.

Table 9.15 displays the results from fitting a model including the covariates dosage (mg/kg), age (months), and surgery duration (minutes). This model includes the same covariates as were included in model 2 fit using the Stram et al. (1988) methodology (Section 9.8.4). The parameter estimates from the GEE approach (Table 9.15) are similar in magnitude (but of opposite sign) to the pooled estimates of effects displayed in Table 9.14. Although the standard errors displayed in Table 9.15 are somewhat smaller than those in Table 9.14, the conclusions from the two approaches are the same. Based on the parameterization used by the SAS GENMOD procedure, the odds of having a recovery score *higher* than a given cutpoint are estimated to be:

- $e^{-0.0380} = 0.963$ times as high per 1 mg/kg increase in dosage;
- $e^{-0.0139} = 0.986$ times as high per 1 month increase in age;

TABLE 9.16. Anesthesia clinical trial: Parameter estimates from GEE model including time in the recovery room as an additional covariate

Variable	Estimate	S.E.	Est./S.E.
Dosage	0.0428	0.0364	1.18
Age	0.0163	0.0132	1.24
Surgery duration	0.0096	0.0054	1.77
Time in recovery room	−0.0946	0.0109	−8.66

- $e^{-0.0071} = 0.993$ times as high per 1 minute increase in surgery duration.

The GEE approach would also allow one to include the main effect of time in the recovery room (minutes) as a factor in the model. This variable takes on the values 0, 5, 15, and 30. Table 9.16 displays the results from this model. The effect of time in the recovery room is highly significant ($p < 0.0001$). The odds of having a recovery score higher than a given cutpoint are estimated to be $e^{0.0946} = 1.1$ times as high per minute spent in the recovery room. Interactions between the other covariates and time in the recovery room could also be investigated using the GEE approach.

9.9 Problems

9.1 Let $y_1, \ldots, y_n$ be a random sample from a distribution with mean μ and variance proportional to μ^2; that is, $\text{Var}(y_i) = \phi\mu^2$.

(a) Find the quasilikelihood function $Q(\mu, y)$ for estimating μ.

(b) For the special case where the variance of y_i is equal to μ^2 (i.e., when $\phi = 1$), derive the quasilikelihood estimator of μ.

(c) Now, suppose that the distribution of y_i is exponential with parameter μ; that is,

$$f(y) = \frac{1}{\mu}e^{-y/\mu}, \quad y > 0.$$

In this case, $\text{E}(y_i) = \mu$ and $\text{Var}(y_i) = \mu^2$. Show that the log-likelihood function for $y_1, \ldots, y_n$ is equivalent to the quasilikelihood function from part (b).

(d) With reference to part (c), express the distribution of y in terms of Equation (9.1). Find the mean, variance, variance function, and dispersion parameter of y using the properties of the score function from Section 9.2.2.

9.2 Let $y_1, \ldots, y_n$ be a random sample from a distribution with mean μ and variance proportional to μ^3; that is, $\text{Var}(y_i) = \phi\mu^3$.

(a) Find the quasilikelihood function $Q(\mu, y)$ for estimating μ.

(b) For the special case where the variance of y_i is equal to μ^3 (i.e., when $\phi = 1$), derive the quasilikelihood estimator of μ.

(c) Now, suppose that the distribution of y_i is inverse Gaussian with parameter μ; that is,

$$f(y) = \left(\frac{1}{2\pi y^3}\right)^{1/2} \exp\left(\frac{-(y-\mu)^2}{2\mu^2 y}\right), \quad y > 0.$$

In this case, $\text{E}(y_i) = \mu$ and $\text{Var}(y_i) = \mu^3$. Show that the log-likelihood function for $y_1, \ldots, y_n$ is equivalent to the quasilikelihood function from part (b).

9.3 Consider the experiment described in Problem 4.4. Let y_{ij} denote the amount of iron absorbed at condition j from pair i for $i = 1, \ldots, 17$ and $j = 1, \ldots, 6$, where $j = 1, 2, 3$ refer to low, medium, and high pH for ethionine and $j = 4, 5, 6$ refer to low, medium, and high pH for control. Suppose that the GEE approach is to be used to assess the effect of group, compound, and pH on iron absorption. Specify a single working correlation matrix that incorporates all of the following constraints:

- Ethionine observations are equally correlated.
- Control observations are equally correlated.
- The correlation between observations for which the pH levels are equal, but the compounds are different, is constant.
- There is no correlation between observations for which the pH levels and compounds are different.

9.4 Suppose that repeated measurements of a time-to-event variable are obtained in a study and that the repeated failure times are always observed (i.e., there are no censored failure times). Assume that the marginal distributions of these repeated failure times are approximately exponentially distributed, and consider the use of the GEE methodology for analysis of these data.

(a) What variance function would you recommend?

(b) What link function would you recommend? Why?

9.5 In a clinical trial comparing two treatments for a respiratory illness, patients from two investigative sites were randomly assigned to active treatment or placebo. Of the 111 subjects included in the study, 54 were assigned to the active treatment group and 57 were assigned to the placebo group. During treatment, respiratory status was determined at four visits using a five-point ordered categorical scale (0 = worst, 4 = best). Covariates of potential interest are site, sex, age, and baseline respiratory status (coded on the same five-point ordered categorical scale). Table 9.17 displays the data from the first ten subjects from each of the two sites. Every subject had complete data for the response and covariates at all four visits.

Davis (1991) and other authors treated respiratory status at baseline and at the four subsequent visits as a dichotomous variable, categorized as "poor" (values of 0, 1, and 2) versus "good" (values of 3 and 4).

(a) Fit a marginal model using the logit of the probability of a good response as the outcome variable and including treatment, site, sex, age, and baseline respiratory status as covariates. Justify your choice of working correlation matrix.

(b) Report estimated odds ratios (good response versus a poor response) for the effects of treatment, site, sex, age, and baseline status.

(c) Summarize the results of your analyses.

9.6 In the Iowa 65+ Rural Health Survey, elderly individuals were followed over a six-year period (at years 0, 3, and 6). One question asked at each survey was "Do you regularly (at least once a month) attend religious meetings or services?" Table 7.6 displays the answers to this question from 1973 individuals who responded at years 0, 3, and 6.

(a) Use the GEE approach and the independence working correlation model to fit a logistic model for predicting church attendance as a function of sex, survey year, and the sex × year interaction.

(b) Based on the results of tests of nonlinearity and parallelism, fit an appropriate reduced model to the data.

(c) Comment on how the results from parts (a) and (b) are affected by the choice of alternative working correlation structures.

(d) How do your results compare with those from the marginal logit model fit using weighted least squares (Section 7.3.5)? Which method seems more appropriate for these data?

9.7 Potthoff and Roy (1964) describe a study conducted at the University of North Carolina Dental School in which the distance (mm) from the center of the pituitary gland to the pterygomaxillary fissure was measured at ages 8, 10, 12, and 14 in 16 boys and 11 girls. Table 3.3 lists the individual measurements as well as the sample means and standard deviations in both groups. Sections 3.4.2, 4.3.2, 4.4.3, and 6.4.1, as well as Problems 5.8 and 6.3, considered other methods for the analysis of these data.

TABLE 9.17. Respiratory status at four visits: First ten subjects from each of the two sites

Site	ID	Trt.	Sex	Age	Baseline	Visit 1	Visit 2	Visit 3	Visit 4
1	1	P	M	46	2	2	2	2	2
	2	P	M	28	2	0	0	0	0
	3	A	M	23	3	3	4	4	3
	4	P	M	44	3	4	3	4	2
	5	P	F	13	4	4	4	4	4
	6	A	M	34	1	1	2	1	1
	7	P	M	43	2	3	2	4	4
	8	A	M	28	1	2	2	1	2
	9	A	M	31	3	3	4	4	4
	10	P	M	37	3	2	3	3	2
2	1	P	F	39	1	2	1	1	2
	2	A	M	25	2	2	4	4	4
	3	A	M	58	4	4	4	4	4
	4	P	F	51	3	4	2	4	4
	5	P	F	32	3	2	2	3	4
	6	P	M	45	3	4	2	1	2
	7	P	F	44	3	4	4	4	4
	8	P	F	48	2	2	1	0	0
	9	A	M	26	2	3	4	4	4
	10	A	M	14	1	4	4	4	4

(a) Use the GEE approach and the independence working correlation structure to model the pituitary–pterygomaxillary fissure distance as a linear function of age. Parameterize the model in terms of an overall intercept and slope with separate intercept and slope increments for females. Test the following null hypotheses:

H_0: equality of intercepts and slopes for males and females;

H_0: equality of intercepts for males and females;

H_0: equality of slopes for males and females.

(b) Compare the estimated coefficients of the resulting linear relationships for males and females with those from growth curve analysis and mixed linear models, as presented in Sections 4.4.3 and 6.4.1.

(c) Repeat part (a) using the exchangeable and unspecified working correlation structures, and compare the results to those from the independence working correlation structure.

(d) Use the GEE approach and the independence working correlation structure to model the pituitary–pterygomaxillary fissure distance as a cubic function of age. Parameterize the model in terms of an overall intercept and linear, quadratic, and cubic age effects, with separate corresponding incremental effects for females. Test the null hypothesis that the nonlinear age effects are jointly equal to zero.

9.8 In a longitudinal study conducted in a group of 188 nuns, dietary balance and bone measurement tests were scheduled to be completed at five-year intervals. All of the study participants were between 35 and 45 years of age at the start of the study (in the mid-1960s). Due to dropouts and missed visits, the number of repeated measurements per participant ranges from 1 to 4. The outcome variable of interest was the adjusted absorption of calcium (CA Abs.); the covariates of potential interest were age, body surface area (BSA), body-mass index (BMI), dietary calcium (Diet. CA), urine calcium (Urine CA), endogenous fecal calcium (EFC), total intestinal calcium (TIC), dietary phosphorus, caffeine intake, and calcium balance (CA Bal.). All of the covariates are time-dependent. Table 9.18 displays the data from the first ten subjects.

(a) Develop a regression model for predicting calcium absorption as a parsimonious function of the covariates.

(b) Summarize the effects of the covariates included in your final model on the outcome.

9.9 Vonesh and Carter (1987) describe a study of the ultrafiltration characteristics of hollow fiber dialyzers. A total of 41 dialyzers were evaluated

TABLE 9.18. Calcium measurements at five-year intervals from a cohort of 188 nuns: First ten subjects

ID	Age	CA Abs.	BSA	BMI	Diet. CA	Urine CA	EFC	TIC	Diet. Phos.	Caff.	CA Bal.
1	45.17	0.442	1.80	27.14	0.222	0.052	0.076	0.124	0.658	371.3	−0.053
1	50.25	0.566	1.83	28.54	0.167	0.056	0.050	0.091	0.637	371.3	−0.012
1	55.25	0.195	1.91	30.56	0.422	0.063	0.076	0.106	0.857	210.7	−0.002
2	41.00	0.308	1.71	22.14	0.776	0.109	0.142	0.170	1.035	482.0	−0.110
2	46.33	0.322	1.72	20.62	0.902	0.160	0.151	.	1.192	185.7	.
2	51.25	0.205	1.75	21.30	0.648	0.108	0.116	0.162	0.935	389.2	−0.005
2	56.42	0.330	1.76	22.73	0.519	0.155	0.114	0.147	0.702	634.0	−0.132
3	44.08	0.302	1.96	25.55	0.518	0.046	0.146	0.178	0.996	175.0	−0.084
3	49.83	0.235	1.95	25.86	0.701	0.064	0.126	0.185	1.224	103.5	0.089
3	54.00	0.145	1.97	27.60	0.627	0.090	0.108	0.130	1.096	229.2	−0.069
3	58.92	0.180	1.98	28.03	0.525	0.023	0.157	0.201	0.928	548.0	−0.045
4	35.67	0.219	1.81	22.30	1.354	0.034	0.158	0.189	1.594	160.7	0.068
4	40.92	0.230	1.80	20.98	1.302	0.184	0.124	0.158	1.581	.	0.063
4	45.92	0.165	1.74	19.47	1.256	0.130	0.140	0.159	1.502	179.6	−0.084
4	50.75	0.135	1.82	21.47	0.773	0.151	0.101	.	1.051	779.0	.
5	37.25	0.527	1.66	19.64	0.261	0.055	0.119	0.169	0.690	321.3	−0.077
5	42.42	0.314	1.62	18.75	0.353	0.071	0.065	0.093	0.888	285.6	−0.019
5	49.08	0.280	1.68	20.42	0.689	0.162	0.088	0.120	1.065	464.1	−0.032
6	37.25	0.503	1.63	19.91	0.234	0.067	0.080	0.123	0.753	260.7	−0.050
6	43.50	0.411	1.65	18.76	0.649	0.154	0.086	.	1.043	150.0	.
7	39.83	0.253	1.68	25.49	1.220	0.161	0.058	0.064	1.526	.	−0.041
7	51.17	0.305	1.54	20.18	0.523	0.136	0.093	0.144	1.175	25.0	−0.007
7	55.17	0.170	1.66	25.16	0.599	0.082	0.101	0.131	1.015	41.0	−0.019
8	38.58	0.201	1.65	23.42	1.041	0.250	0.105	0.136	1.456	.	−0.084
8	43.42	0.300	1.68	24.31	0.552	0.217	0.061	0.097	0.948	.	−0.024
8	48.42	0.250	1.68	24.23	1.216	0.310	0.115	0.169	1.628	.	0.046
8	53.33	0.210	1.69	25.78	1.196	0.263	0.147	0.176	1.464	24.0	−0.144
9	36.83	0.327	1.62	22.29	0.494	0.052	0.134	0.163	1.069	482.0	−0.082
10	38.67	0.259	1.56	20.95	0.720	0.079	0.131	0.149	1.004	210.7	−0.108
10	43.83	0.240	1.58	21.49	0.526	0.071	0.085	0.129	0.900	150.0	0.053
10	48.75	0.310	1.55	20.98	0.517	0.106	0.101	0.148	0.813	210.7	−0.017
10	54.00	0.150	1.52	21.07	0.637	0.092	0.129	0.145	1.080	366.0	−0.140

among three sites, with each site using a different type of dialysate delivery system to monitor transmembrane pressure. For each dialyzer, the ultrafiltration rate (UFR) was measured at several different values of the transmembrane pressure (TMP). Table 9.19 displays the data from the first five units at each of the three sites. Use the GEE methodology to assess the effects of site and TMP on UFR.

9.10 In a longitudinal study of fluoride intake, infants were enrolled at birth and followed over time. During the first nine months of the study, total fluoride intake (mg/kg body weight) was assessed at months 1.5, 3, 6, and 9. The data set contains 4151 observations from 1363 infants. Table 9.20 lists the variables in the file.

(a) Descriptively summarize the data; that is, describe the number and pattern of observations per subject and the distributions of the covariates and outcome variable (total fluoride intake).

(b) Fit a marginal model for predicting fluoride intake as a function of age and the covariates. Test nonlinearity of the age effect and simplify the model accordingly.

(c) Starting from the model incorporating the appropriate effect of age, as well as all other covariates, find a parsimonious reduced model. Interpret the resulting parameter estimates.

(d) Augment your final model by including interactions between age and each of the covariates in your final model. Test for interactions with age and use the results to develop a final model. Interpret the resulting parameter estimates and compare them with part (c).

9.11 Fitzmaurice and Lipsitz (1995) discuss a clinical trial in which 51 patients with arthritis were randomized to one of two treatments: auranofin (A) or placebo (P). Each subject had at most five binary self-assessment measurements of arthritis (0 = poor, 1 = good). The self-assessments were scheduled at baseline (week 0) and at weeks 1, 5, 9, and 13. Randomization to auranofin or placebo occurred following the week 1 assessment. Thus, the treatment remains the same at all time points for patients in the placebo group. In the auranofin group, however, treatment is a time-dependent covariate with the change from placebo to auranofin occurring at week 5. Table 9.21 displays the data from this study.

(a) Using the logit of the probability of a good response as the outcome variable, fit a model including the main effects of time, sex, age, and treatment.

(b) Based on the results of part (a), fit and interpret the results of an appropriate reduced model.

TABLE 9.19. Ultrafiltation rates (ml/hour) at various transmembrane pressures from 41 dialyzers: First five units from each site

Site	Unit	TMP	UFR	Site	Unit	TMP	UFR
1	1	160.0	600	2	3	365.0	1470
	1	265.0	1026		3	454.0	1890
	1	365.0	1470		4	146.0	570
	1	454.0	1890		4	265.0	1026
	2	164.0	516		4	365.0	1470
	2	260.5	930		4	454.0	1890
	2	355.0	1380		5	149.0	360
	2	451.0	1770		5	265.0	1026
	3	156.0	480		5	365.0	1470
	3	260.0	1026		5	454.0	1890
	3	363.0	1470	3	1	183.0	600
	3	466.0	1890		1	265.0	1026
	4	160.0	528		1	365.0	1470
	4	265.0	1026		1	454.0	1890
	4	365.0	1470		2	160.5	480
	4	454.0	1890		2	265.0	1026
	5	157.0	540		2	365.0	1470
	5	265.0	1026		2	454.0	1890
	5	365.0	1470		3	149.5	510
	5	454.0	1890		3	265.0	1026
2	1	166.0	540		3	365.0	1470
	1	265.0	1026		3	454.0	1890
	1	365.0	1470		4	188.5	600
	1	454.0	1890		4	265.0	1026
	1	444.5	1716		4	365.0	1470
	2	156.0	426		4	454.0	1890
	2	265.0	1026		5	208.0	720
	2	365.0	1470		5	265.0	1026
	2	454.0	1890		5	365.0	1470
	3	143.5	390		5	454.0	1890
	3	265.0	1026				

TABLE 9.20. Variables included in the data set from the longitudinal study of fluoride intake

Col.	Variable	Comments
1–4	ID	subject identifier
7–9	age	months; values are 1.5, 3, 6, 9
11	sex	1 = male, 0 = female
13	race	1 = white, 0 = non-white, . = missing
15	mother's age	1 = 30+ years, 0 = less than 30 years
17	mother's education	1 = high school graduate (but not college graduate), 0 = otherwise
19		1 = college graduate, 0 = otherwise
21	first child in the family	1 = yes, 0 = no
23	number of children in the family	1 = two children at home, 0 = otherwise
25		1 = three or more, 0 = otherwise
27	annual household income	1 = \$30,000 or more, 0 = less than \$30,000, . = missing
29–40	total fluoride intake	mg/kg (. = missing)

TABLE 9.21. Self-assessments at five time points from 51 subjects in an arthritis clinical trial

ID	Sex	Age	Group	Week 0	Week 1	Week 5	Week 9	Week 13
1	M	48	A	1	1	1	1	1
2	M	29	A	1	1	1	1	1
3	M	59	P	1	1	1	1	1
4	F	56	P	1	1	1	1	1
5	M	33	P	1	1	1	1	1
6	M	61	P	1	1	0	1	1
7	M	63	A	0	0	1	.	.
8	M	57	P	1	0	1	1	1
9	M	47	P	1	1	1	0	1
10	F	42	A	0	0	1	.	0
11	M	62	A	1	1	1	1	1
12	M	42	P	1	1	1	1	1
13	M	50	A	1	1	1	1	1
14	F	47	A	1	1	.	.	.
15	M	45	P	0	0	0	1	1
16	M	55	A	1	1	1	1	1
17	M	56	A	1	1	1	1	1
18	M	57	P	1	1	1	1	1
19	F	57	P	1	1	1	0	.
20	M	45	A	1	0	1	0	1
21	M	29	A	1	1	0	.	.
22	F	51	A	0	0	1	1	0
23	F	65	P	1	1	0	1	0
24	F	50	A	1	1	1	0	1
25	M	65	A	1	1	1	1	1
26	F	58	P	1	1	0	0	0
27	F	62	A	0	1	1	1	1
28	F	35	A	1	1	1	1	1
29	M	28	A	1	1	1	1	1
30	M	41	A	1	1	1	.	.
31	M	40	P	1	0	1	0	1
32	M	33	P	0	0	0	0	0
33	F	60	P	0	0	0	0	0
34	M	62	A	1	0	1	1	1
35	M	45	P	1	1	0	1	1
36	M	64	P	0	0	0	0	0
37	M	55	P	0	0	0	1	1
38	M	57	A	1	1	1	1	.
39	M	51	P	1	1	0	1	1
40	F	57	A	1	1	1	1	1
41	M	37	P	1	0	1	.	1
42	M	52	A	0	1	1	1	.
43	M	52	P	1	1	.	1	1
44	M	46	A	1	1	1	1	1
45	M	63	A	0	0	1	0	.
46	M	60	P	1	1	0	0	0
47	M	63	A	0	1	.	0	0
48	F	33	P	1	0	0	1	.
49	M	60	A	0	0	1	1	1
50	M	58	A	1	1	1	1	1
51	M	37	P	0	0	0	1	0

TABLE 9.22. Number of hospital visits per quarter during a one-year period for 73 children: First ten subjects

ID	Age (months)	Sex	Maternal Smoking	Quarter 1	2	3	4
1	63	M	Yes	5	0	0	1
2	8	M	Yes	3	4	2	2
3	31	M	Yes	0	0	1	2
4	33	M	Yes	2	0	1	1
5	24	F	Yes	1	0	0	0
6	34	F	Yes	2	0	2	0
7	16	M	Yes	7	0	1	2
8	20	M	Yes	2	4	5	2
9	57	M	Yes	0	0	0	0
10	59	M	Yes	2	0	2	0

9.12 In an example considered by Karim and Zeger (1988), quarterly data were obtained from 73 children over a one-year period. The response of interest was the number of visits to the hospital. Because complete data were obtained from each child, there are a total of $73 \times 4 = 292$ observations. Potential covariates include sex, maternal smoking status, and age of the child at the beginning of the study (in months); each of these covariates is time-independent. In addition, the effect of quarter (1–4) is also of interest. Table 9.22 displays the data from the first ten subjects.

(a) Fit a regression model investigating the relationship between the number of hospital visits and age, sex, maternal smoking status, and quarter.

(b) Based on the results of part (a), fit a reduced model and summarize the results.

9.13 Hadgu and Koch (1999) discuss a dental clinical trial conducted in 109 healthy adult volunteers, aged 18–55 years, with preexisting plaque but without advanced periodontal disease. Prior to enrollment in the study, subjects were screened for a minimum of 20 sound natural teeth. The subjects were then randomized to one of two new mouthrinses (A and B) or to a control mouthrinse (C). The sample sizes in groups A, B, and C were 39, 34, and 36 subjects, respectively. During the study, subjects used their assigned mouthrinse twice daily for six months. Plaque was scored at baseline, at three months, and at six months using the Turesky modification of the Quigley–Hein index. Other variables of interest are sex, age, and smoking status. Table 9.23 displays the data from the first ten subjects.

TABLE 9.23. Dental plaque measurements from 109 subjects in a clinical trial comparing three mouthrinses: First ten subjects

					Month		
Subject	Sex	Age	Smoker	Group	0	3	6
1	F	23	No	B	2.33	0.56	0.90
2	F	24	Yes	C	2.46	1.73	1.58
3	F	42	No	A	2.65	1.42	1.25
4	F	29	Yes	C	2.89	2.61	1.91
5	F	48	Yes	A	2.13	2.48	1.63
6	M	27	No	C	3.00	2.75	1.89
7	F	38	Yes	B	2.53	1.00	0.89
8	M	24	No	B	2.61	2.11	1.61
9	F	27	No	A	2.70	0.00	0.59
10	F	33	No	A	2.48	0.10	0.12

(a) The distributions of the plaque measurements are skewed, especially at months 3 and 6. Suggest appropriate link and variance functions for analyzing these data.

(b) Using your recommended link and variance functions from part (a), carry out analyses to provide answers to the following questions:

- Are the experimental mouthrinses more effective than the control mouthrinse in inhibiting the development of dental plaque?
- What are the effects of sex, age, smoking status, and time?

9.14 Problem 6.8 described a study conducted to determine whether use of an experimental dopamine D_2 agonist can replace the use of levodopa. In this study, 25 patients with Stage II through IV Parkinson's disease were randomized to one of five groups: placebo or 8.4 mg, 16.8 mg, 33.5 mg, or 67 mg of the experimental drug. One of the outcome variables was a clinical global rating (CGI), which was assessed at days 2, 7, and 14. This was an ordered categorical variable and was coded as follows:

1 = very much worse;

2 = much worse;

3 = slightly worse;

4 = no change;

5 = slightly improved;

6 = much improved;

7 = very much improved.

Table 9.24 displays the data. The placebo group is denoted by dose = 0.0.

TABLE 9.24. Clinical global impression ratings from 25 patients with Parkinson's disease

ID	Dose	Day 2	Day 7	Day 14
1	33.5	2	4	4
2	67.0	2	3	4
3	0.0	3	3	4
4	8.4	3	3	2
5	16.8	3	3	3
6	67.0	5	5	5
7	16.8	4	4	4
8	8.4	4	3	2
9	33.5	3	3	3
10	0.0	4	4	3
11	8.4	4	4	4
12	33.5	5	4	3
13	0.0	5	3	4
14	67.0	3	7	6
15	33.5	5	5	5
16	8.4	3	6	4
17	16.8	3	3	3
18	0.0	6	5	6
19	67.0	5	3	3
20	67.0	3	3	4
21	33.5	3	5	5
22	16.8	6	5	5
23	8.4	3	3	3
24	0.0	4	4	5
25	16.8	3	3	3

(a) Fit the proportional-odds model with CGI as the outcome variable and treatment group, day, and the group × day interaction as covariates.

(b) Based on the results of part (a), fit an appropriate reduced model.

9.15 Problem 9.5 considered a clinical trial comparing two treatments for a respiratory illness; Table 9.17 displays the data from the first ten subjects from each of the two sites.

(a) Fit the proportional-odds model with respiratory status as the outcome variable, and treatment, center, sex, age, and baseline respiratory status as covariates. As in Problem 9.5, treat baseline respiratory status as a dichotomous covariate ("poor" versus "good").

(b) Based on the results of part (a), fit an appropriate reduced model. For each covariate included in this model, test the null hypothesis that the effects of the covariate are the same at the four measurement times.

(c) Summarize the results of your analyses.

10

Nonparametric Methods

10.1 Introduction

Most of the methods considered in previous chapters require distributional assumptions on either the joint distribution of a subject's repeated measurements or on the marginal distributions at each time point. For example, Chapters 3, 4, 5, and 6 assume that the vectors of repeated measurements have a multivariate normal joint distribution, either with an arbitrary covariance structure (Chapters 3 and 4) or with some type of structured covariance matrix (Chapters 5 and 6). In Chapter 7, the underlying model for the weighted least squares (WLS) approach is the multinomial distribution. Although the distributional assumptions are much weaker for the methods discussed in Chapter 9, one still must make some basic assumptions concerning the marginal distributions at each time point.

Although the methods of these previous chapters are adequate and appropriate for many types of studies, there are several reasons why the use of nonparametric methods may be indicated. First, when the response variable is continuous, the assumption of multivariate normality is not always reasonable. In other situations involving a continuous outcome variable, the actual distribution may be unknown. Thus, the use of standard parametric procedures is subject to criticism regarding both validity and optimality.

Another situation where nonparametric approaches may be useful is when the response is an ordered categorical variable with a relatively large number of possible outcomes. In such situations, the WLS approach is likely to be inapplicable due to sample size limitations. In addition, the assumptions of specific ordinal data methods such as the proportional-odds model may be inappropriate.

In all of these situations, nonparametric methods for analyzing repeated measurements may be of use. In addition, nonparametric methods may be of interest as a means of confirming the results of a parametric analysis or in assessing the sensitivity of the results to the assumptions of the selected parametric model.

This chapter discusses the use of nonparametric methods for the analysis of repeated measurements. Section 10.2 provides a brief overview of a variety of nonparametric approaches, and the remainder of the chapter considers some specific approaches that are likely to be useful in the analysis of repeated measurements. Section 10.3 reviews multivariate multisample tests for complete data, and Section 10.4 discusses two-sample tests for incomplete data. Although these approaches are not included in standard statistical software packages, special-purpose computer programs are available.

10.2 Overview

A wide variety of nonparametric methods for the analysis of repeated measurements have been developed and studied. Koch et al. (1980) provided an early review and bibliography.

Perhaps the simplest nonparametric approach is to use the summary-statistic method (Chapter 2) in conjunction with nonparametric summary measures of association and nonparametric tests. For example, in the one-sample setting (Table 1.3), interest may focus on assessing the extent of association between the response variable and the repeated measurements factor. If the Spearman rank correlation coefficient between the response variable and the repeated measurements variable is used as the summary statistic for each subject, then the sign test or the Wilcoxon signed rank test can be used to test whether the median of the distribution of the summary statistic is equal to zero. In the multisample setting (Table 1.2), similar methods can be used. For example, the Wilcoxon–Mann–Whitney (if $s = 2$) or Kruskal–Wallis (if $s > 2$) tests can be used to assess whether the distribution of the summary statistic is the same across the s groups.

One general class of nonparametric methods includes procedures that can be classified as multivariate generalizations of univariate distribution-free methods. This approach includes standard asymptotically distribution-free tests for multivariate one-sample and multisample problems that can be used in the repeated measurements setting. There are several such rank-based methods appropriate for the analysis of data from continuous multivariate distributions. When there are no missing values, multivariate one-sample tests for complete data can be used to analyze repeated measurements. These include multivariate generalizations of the sign and Wilcoxon signed rank tests. Puri and Sen (1971, Chapter 4) and Hettmansperger (1984, Chapter 6) discuss these approaches. For complete repeated measurements from multiple samples, multivariate multisample tests are available. These nonparametric analogs of MANOVA include multivariate generalizations of the Kruskal–Wallis and Brown–Mood (Brown and Mood, 1951) median tests and related methods discussed in Puri and Sen (1971, Chapter 5). Section 10.3.2 describes these methods.

Another type of nonparametric approach is the use of asymptotically distribution-free analogs of general parametric procedures for the analysis of multivariate normally distributed outcome variables. Bhapkar (1984) discusses nonparametric counterparts of Hotelling's T^2 statistic and profile analysis. Sen (1984) studies nonparametric analogs of the Potthoff and Roy (1964) growth curve model.

The use of randomization model methods is another nonparametric approach to the analysis of repeated measurements. Chapter 8 describes randomization model analyses for one-sample repeated measurements based on Cochran–Mantel–Haenszel (CMH) statistics. Several common nonparametric test procedures are special cases of CMH tests. These include the tests of Friedman (1937), Durbin (1951), Benard and van Elteren (1953), and Page (1963) as well as the aligned ranks test introduced by Hodges and Lehmann (1962) and further studied by Koch and Sen (1968). Finally, Zerbe and Walker (1977) and Zerbe (1979a, 1979b) discuss methods for randomization analysis of growth curves.

Wei and Lachin (1984) and Wei and Johnson (1985) study distribution-free methods for the two-sample case (Table 1.2 with $s = 2$) when the data are incomplete. These approaches allow the missing-value patterns in the two samples to be different but require the assumption that the missing-value mechanism be independent of the response. Davis (1991, 1994) provides a further discussion of these methods and a computer program. Lachin (1992) proposes additional test statistics and provides estimators of the treatment difference. Palesch and Lachin (1994) extend these methods to more than two groups, and Thall and Lachin (1988), Davis and Wei (1988), and Davis (1996) study related methods for special types of situations with incomplete data. Section 10.4 describes the Wei–Lachin and Wei–Johnson procedures.

Another potential approach to the analysis of repeated measurements when the underlying parametric assumptions are not satisfied is the rank transform method, which consists of replacing observations by their ranks and performing a standard parametric analysis on the ranks (Conover and Iman, 1981). Unfortunately, the rank transform method has been shown to be inappropriate for many common hypotheses (Akritas 1991, 1993). Thompson (1991) and Akritas and Arnold (1994) provide valid asymptotic tests based on the rank transform for selected hypotheses of interest in several repeated measurements models. Kepner and Robinson (1988) consider the one-sample situation of Table 1.3 under the assumption that the repeated measurements y_{ij} from the ith subject are equally correlated. They show the relationships between the rank transform method and the rank tests of Koch (1969) and Agresti and Pendergast (1986) for testing the null hypothesis of no time effect.

Müller (1988), Diggle et al. (1994, Chapter 3), and Kshirsagar and Smith (1995, Chapter 10) discuss nonparametric regression methods for the analysis of repeated measurements, including kernel estimation, weighted local least squares estimation, and smoothing splines. Hart and Wehrly (1986) study the theoretical properties of kernel regression estimation for repeated measurements and show how the case of correlated errors changes the behavior of a kernel estimator. Altman (1990) demonstrates that the standard techniques for bandwidth selection perform poorly when the errors are correlated. Raz (1989) describes an analysis procedure for repeated measurements that combines nonparametric regression methods and the randomization tests of Zerbe (1979b).

10.3 Multivariate One-Sample and Multisample Tests for Complete Data

10.3.1 One Sample

For the one-sample case with no missing data, Hettmansperger (1984, Chapter 6) and Puri and Sen (1971, Chapter 4) study multivariate generalizations of the sign and Wilcoxon signed rank tests. In the one-sample repeated measurements setting of Table 1.3 with no missing data, let θ_j denote the median of the marginal distribution of the response at time j for $j = 1, \ldots, t$. By transforming each of the n vectors $\boldsymbol{y}_i = (y_{i1}, \ldots, y_{it})'$ to a $(t-1)$-component vector of differences $\boldsymbol{y}_i^* = (y_{i1}-y_{i2}, \ldots, y_{i,t-1}-y_{it})'$, these methods can then be used to test the null hypothesis that $\theta_1 = \cdots = \theta_t$. Hettmansperger (1984) provides an example of this approach.

10.3.2 Multiple Samples

Hettmansperger (1984) considers the two-sample situation with complete data; the test statistic is a multivariate version of the Wilcoxon–Mann–Whitney test. Puri and Sen (1971, Chapter 5) discuss multivariate generalizations of the Brown–Mood (1951) and Kruskal–Wallis (1952) tests for the multivariate multisample situation with complete data. Based on these results, Schwertman (1982) provides a computer algorithm for two of these tests, the multivariate multisample rank sum test and the multivariate multisample median test. These methods can be applied to the situation where repeated measurements are obtained from multiple samples

(Table 1.2), as described later. Schwertman (1985) describes this approach in further detail and gives an example of its application to the analysis of repeated measurements.

The general problem considered by Puri and Sen (1971) is that of testing the equality of s multivariate distributions $F_1, \ldots, F_s$, where F_h is a t-variate cumulative distribution function (cdf). When the underlying distributions $F_1, \ldots, F_s$ are multivariate normal, they can differ only in their mean vectors and covariance matrices. For nonnormal F_h, however, differences among distributions may be due to a variety of reasons. In particular, equality of location vectors and covariance matrices does not imply that $F_1 = \cdots = F_s$.

Puri and Sen (1971) assume that the cdfs F_h have a common unspecified form but differ in their location (or scale) vectors. They consider the general null hypothesis $H_0\colon F_1(\boldsymbol{x}) = \cdots = F_s(\boldsymbol{x})$ for all $\boldsymbol{x} = (x_1, \ldots, x_t)'$, where $F_h \in \Omega$ and Ω is the class of continuous cdfs. The general alternative hypothesis is that the distributions F_h are not all equal.

In the context of repeated measurements, suppose that responses are obtained at t time points from subjects in s groups, where n_h is the sample size (number of independent experimental units) in group h for $h = 1, \ldots, s$. Let $F_h(\boldsymbol{x})$ denote the t-variate cdf in group h. Assume that the cdfs $F_h(\boldsymbol{x})$ have a common unspecified form with possible differences in their location (or scale) parameters. For example, suppose that $F_h(\boldsymbol{x}) = F(\boldsymbol{x} + \boldsymbol{\Delta}_h)$, where $\boldsymbol{\Delta}_h = (\Delta_{h1}, \ldots, \Delta_{ht})'$. The null hypothesis of no difference among groups across all time points tests

$$H_0\colon \boldsymbol{\Delta}_1 = \cdots = \boldsymbol{\Delta}_s = (0, \ldots, 0)'.$$

The omnibus alternative hypothesis is that $\boldsymbol{\Delta}_1, \ldots, \boldsymbol{\Delta}_s$ are not all equal.

Let $n = n_1 + \cdots + n_s$ and consider the $n \times t$ data matrix organized as in Table 1.2. Let $\boldsymbol{R}$ denote the $n \times t$ matrix of ranks resulting from ranking each of the t columns of the data matrix (all groups combined) in ascending order. Under H_0, each column of $\boldsymbol{R}$ is a random permutation of the numbers $1, \ldots, n$; thus, $\boldsymbol{R}$ has $(n!)^t$ possible realizations. Two such matrices are said to be *permutationally equivalent* if one can be obtained from the other by a rearrangement of its rows. Let $\boldsymbol{R}^*$ denote the matrix that has the same row vectors as $\boldsymbol{R}$ but is arranged so that its first column is ordered $1, \ldots, n$. The matrix $\boldsymbol{R}^*$ has $(n!)^{t-1}$ possible realizations.

The t components of $\boldsymbol{y}_{hi} = (y_{hi1}, \ldots, y_{hit})'$ are, in general, stochastically dependent. Thus, the joint distribution of the elements of $\boldsymbol{R}$ (or $\boldsymbol{R}^*$) will depend on the unknown distribution F, even when

$$H_0\colon F_1(\boldsymbol{x}) = \cdots = F_s(\boldsymbol{x}) = F(\boldsymbol{x})$$

is true. Let $\mathcal{R}^*$ denote the set of all $(n!)^{t-1}$ possible realizations of $\boldsymbol{R}^*$. The unconditional distribution of $\boldsymbol{R}^*$ over $\mathcal{R}^*$ depends on $F_1, \ldots, F_s$. When

$F_1(\boldsymbol{x}) = \cdots = F_s(\boldsymbol{x})$, the n random vectors

$$\boldsymbol{y}_{11}, \ldots, \boldsymbol{y}_{1n_1}, \boldsymbol{y}_{21}, \ldots, \boldsymbol{y}_{2n_2}, \ldots, \boldsymbol{y}_{s1}, \ldots, \boldsymbol{y}_{sn_s}$$

are independent and identically distributed.

The joint distribution of the $\boldsymbol{y}_{hi}$ is invariant under any permutation among themselves. Thus, the conditional distribution of $\boldsymbol{R}$ over the set of $n!$ possible permutations of the columns of $\boldsymbol{R}^*$ is uniform under

$$H_0 \colon F_1(\boldsymbol{x}) = \cdots = F_s(\boldsymbol{x}) = F(\boldsymbol{x});$$

that is,

$$\Pr(\boldsymbol{R} = \boldsymbol{r} | S(\boldsymbol{R}^*), H_0) = 1/n!$$

for all $\boldsymbol{r} \in S(\boldsymbol{R}^*)$. Puri and Sen (1971) define $\mathcal{P}$ as the conditional (permutational) probability measure generated by the $n!$ equally likely possible permutations of the columns of $\boldsymbol{R}^*$. They show that any statistic that depends explicitly on $\boldsymbol{R}$ has a completely specified conditional distribution under $\mathcal{P}$.

Let R_{ij} denote the (i,j)th element of $\boldsymbol{R}$, let $E_{ij} = J(R_{ij}/(n+1))$ for some function J satisfying Puri and Sen's (1971, p. 95) conditions, and let $\overline{E}_{hj}$ denote the average rank score at the jth time point in the hth sample. Puri and Sen (1971) derive a general test statistic L, which is a weighted sum of s quadratic forms in $\overline{\boldsymbol{E}}_h - \overline{\boldsymbol{E}}_.$, where $\overline{\boldsymbol{E}}_h$ is the $t \times 1$ vector of average rank scores from the hth sample and $\overline{\boldsymbol{E}}_.$ is the vector of average rank scores from all samples combined. The jth component of $\overline{\boldsymbol{E}}_.$ is $\overline{E}_{.j}$. The conditional distribution of L given $\boldsymbol{R}^*$ is the same under H_0 regardless of $F(\boldsymbol{x})$. Under H_0, the $t(s-1)$ contrasts $\overline{E}_{hj} - \overline{E}_{.j}$ are stochastically small in absolute value.

The test criterion L rejects H_0 if any of these contrasts are numerically too large. Unless n and t are both small, exact application of the permutation test based on L is difficult. Puri and Sen (1971) show that the asymptotic null distribution of L is $\chi^2_{t(s-1)}$. They also note that L is asymptotically equivalent to the likelihood ratio test based on Hotelling's T^2 statistic. Two specific tests of this type are the multivariate multisample rank sum test and the multivariate multisample median test.

Multivariate Multisample Rank Sum Test

For each sample at each time point, the multivariate multisample rank sum test (MMRST) compares the difference between the sample average rank and the combined-data average rank. Let $\boldsymbol{r}_h$ denote the $t \times 1$ vector of average ranks from group h, with elements $r_{hj} = \sum_{i=1}^{n_h} r_{hij}/n_h$, where r_{hij} is the rank of the jth response from the ith subject in sample h. Let $\overline{\boldsymbol{r}}_.$ denote the average rank vector $(t \times 1)$ for the combined samples; the jth component of $\overline{\boldsymbol{r}}_.$ is

$$\overline{r}_{.j} = \frac{\sum_{h=1}^{s}\sum_{i=1}^{n_h} r_{hij}}{\sum_{h=1}^{s} n_h}.$$

The test statistic is

$$L_{RS} = \sum_{h=1}^{s} n_h(\boldsymbol{r}_h - \overline{\boldsymbol{r}}_.)'\boldsymbol{V}^{-1}(\boldsymbol{r}_h - \overline{\boldsymbol{r}}_.),$$

where the covariance matrix $\boldsymbol{V}$ has elements

$$V_{jl} = \left(\sum_{h=1}^{s}\sum_{i=1}^{n_h} r_{hij}r_{hil} \Big/ \sum_{h=1}^{s} n_h\right) - \overline{r}_{.j}\overline{r}_{.l}.$$

The statistic L_{RS} tests the hypothesis of no differences in the multivariate response profiles from the s samples; the asymptotic null distribution of this statistic is $\chi^2_{t(s-1)}$. If $t = 1$, L_{RS} reduces to the Kruskal–Wallis test. Schwertman (1982) provides a FORTRAN subroutine for computing the MMRST.

Multivariate Multisample Median Test

Similarly, for each sample at each time point, the multivariate multisample median test (MMMT) compares differences between proportions of responses less than or equal to the median to the corresponding combined-data proportions. Let $\boldsymbol{p}_h$ denote the $t \times 1$ vector of proportions from the hth sample that are less than or equal to the median of the combined samples. The jth component of $\boldsymbol{p}_h$ is $p_{hj} = \sum_{i=1}^{n_h} x_{hij}/n_h$, where

$$x_{hij} = \begin{cases} 1 & \text{if } r_{hij} \leq \sum_{h=1}^{s} n_h/2 \\ 0 & \text{otherwise} \end{cases}.$$

Let $\overline{\boldsymbol{p}}_.$ denote the $t \times 1$ vector of proportions of observations from the combined samples that are less than or equal to the median of the combined samples, with elements

$$\overline{p}_{.j} = \frac{\sum_{h=1}^{s}\sum_{i=1}^{n_h} x_{hij}}{\sum_{h=1}^{s} n_h}.$$

The test statistic is

$$L_M = \sum_{h=1}^{s} n_h(\boldsymbol{p}_h - \overline{\boldsymbol{p}}_.)'\boldsymbol{V}^{-1}(\boldsymbol{p}_h - \overline{\boldsymbol{p}}_.),$$

where the covariance matrix $\boldsymbol{V}$ has elements

$$V_{jl} = \left(\sum_{h=1}^{s} \sum_{i=1}^{n_h} x_{hij} x_{hil} \Big/ \sum_{h=1}^{s} n_h \right) - \overline{p}_{.j} \overline{p}_{.l}.$$

The statistic L_M tests the hypothesis of no differences in the multivariate response profiles from the s samples. The asymptotic null distribution of L_M is $\chi^2_{t(s-1)}$. If $t = 1$, L_M reduces to the Brown–Mood (1951) several-sample median test. Schwertman (1982) gives a FORTRAN subroutine for computing the MMMT.

Examples

Problem 3.10 considered plasma inorganic phosphate measurements obtained from 13 control and 20 obese patients 0, 0.5, 1, 1.5, 2, and 3 hours after an oral glucose challenge (Zerbe, 1979b). Table 3.10 displays the data, and the sample means are plotted in Figure 3.6. Even though the relationship between plasma inorganic phosphate level and time is not monotonic, the multivariate nonparametric tests of Puri and Sen (1971) can be used to make an overall comparison between the two groups. Using the multivariate multisample rank sum test, the chi-square statistic is 21.5 with 6 df ($p < 0.001$). The multivariate multisample median test gives a less significant result (chi-square $= 16.2$, df $= 6$, $p = 0.013$).

As a second example, Section 2.3 considered a clinical trial conducted in 59 epileptic patients (Leppik et al., 1987). In this study, patients suffering from simple or complex partial seizures were randomized to receive either the antiepileptic drug progabide (31 patients) or a placebo (28 patients). At each of four successive postrandomization visits, the number of seizures occurring during the previous two weeks was reported. The medical question of interest is whether progabide reduces the frequency of epileptic seizures. Table 2.7 displays the seizure counts during the successive two-week periods for the first ten patients in the progabide group and the first ten patients in the placebo group. Figure 2.2 displays side-by-side modified box plots (Moore and McCabe, 1993, pp. 42–43) for the two treatments at each assessment time.

In Section 2.3, these data were analyzed using the summary-statistic approach. The two groups can also be compared using the multivariate nonparametric tests of Puri and Sen (1971). During each two-week period, there appears to be a slight tendency for seizure counts to be lower in progabide-treated patients than in placebo-treated patients. For example, the median number of seizures in the progabide group at weeks 2, 4, 6, and 8 is 4, 5, 4, and 4, respectively. The corresponding medians in the placebo group are 5, 4.5, 5, and 5, respectively. Using the multivariate multisample rank sum test, the chi-square statistic is 5.47 with 4 df ($p = 0.24$). The multivariate multisample median test gives an even less significant result (chi-square $= 3.46$, df $= 4$, $p = 0.48$). As in the analyses presented in

Section 2.3, there is little evidence of significant differences between the two groups.

10.4 Two-Sample Tests for Incomplete Data

10.4.1 Introduction

Wei and Lachin (1984) and Wei and Johnson (1985) studied general methods for comparing two samples of incomplete repeated measurements. The methods make no assumptions concerning the distribution of the response variable. The missing-value patterns in the two groups are allowed to be different, and both "embedded" (within the sequence of repeated measurements from a subject) and "tail" (at the end of the sequence of repeated measurements) missing observations can be accommodated. The missing-data mechanism, however, must be independent of the response, and these methods are limited to two-group comparisons.

10.4.2 The Wei–Lachin Method

Wei and Lachin (1984) propose and study a family of asymptotically distribution-free tests for equality of two multivariate distributions. Their approach, which was motivated and developed for the analysis of multivariate censored failure-time data, provides natural generalizations of the log-rank and Gehan–Wilcoxon tests for survival data. The Wei and Lachin (1984) methodology is based on a commonly used random-censorship model (Kalbfleisch and Prentice, 1980), which assumes that the censoring vectors for each subject are mutually independent and also independent of the underlying failure-time vectors. The methodology is also applicable to the analysis of repeated measurements with missing observations.

Let $\boldsymbol{y}_{hi} = (y_{hi1}, \ldots, y_{hit})'$ denote the repeated observations from subject i in group h, for $h = 1, 2$ and $i = 1, \ldots, n_h$. Let $F_h(\boldsymbol{x})$ denote the multivariate cumulative distribution function (cdf) of the repeated observations from group h, for $h = 1, 2$, where $\boldsymbol{x} = (x_1, \ldots, x_t)'$. The Wei–Lachin statistic for testing

$$H_0\colon F_1(\boldsymbol{x}) = F_2(\boldsymbol{x})$$

against the general alternative that $F_1(\boldsymbol{x}) \neq F_2(\boldsymbol{x})$ is

$$X_W^2 = \boldsymbol{W}'\widehat{\boldsymbol{\Sigma}}_W^{-1}\boldsymbol{W},$$

where $\boldsymbol{W}' = (W_1, \ldots, W_t)$ is a vector of test statistics comparing groups 1 and 2 at each of the t time points, and $\widehat{\boldsymbol{\Sigma}}_W$ is a consistent estimator of $\text{Var}(\boldsymbol{W})$ given by Theorem 1 of Wei and Lachin (1984). Apart from a scale factor, the jth component of W is

$$W_j = \sum_{i=1}^{n_1} \sum_{i'=1}^{n_2} \delta_{1ij}\, \delta_{2i'j}\, \phi(y_{1ij}, y_{2i'j}),$$

where

$$\phi(x, y) = \begin{cases} 1 & \text{if } x > y \\ 0 & \text{if } x = y\,, \\ -1 & \text{if } x < y \end{cases} \tag{10.1}$$

and δ_{hij} is 1 if y_{hij} is observed and 0 otherwise. Thus, at each time point j, comparisons between groups 1 and 2 are made for all i, i' for which y_{1ij} and $y_{2i'j}$ are both observed. The asymptotic null distribution of the statistic X_W^2 is χ_t^2.

In many studies, the detection of stochastic ordering of the distributions F_1 and F_2 is of primary interest. For example, the alternative hypothesis H_1 may be that $F_{1j}(x) \leq F_{2j}(x)$ for each pair (F_{1j}, F_{2j}) of marginal cdfs, $j = 1, \ldots, t$. Under this alternative, the observations from group 1 tend to be larger than those from group 2 at each time point. For this situation, Wei and Lachin (1984) proposed the statistic

$$z_W = \frac{\mathbf{e}'\mathbf{W}}{\sqrt{\mathbf{e}'\widehat{\boldsymbol{\Sigma}}_W\mathbf{e}}},$$

where $\mathbf{e}'$ is the t-component vector $(1, \ldots, 1)$. The asymptotic null distribution of z_W is normal with mean zero and variance one $[N(0, 1)]$. If the alternative hypothesis is $F_{1j}(x) \leq F_{2j}(x)$ for $j = 1, \ldots, t$, the null hypothesis is rejected when z_W is a large positive value. Similarly, if the alternative hypothesis is $F_{1j}(x) \geq F_{2j}(x)$, large negative values lead to rejection.

Makuch et al. (1991) provide a FORTRAN subroutine for computing the Wei–Lachin omnibus statistic X_W^2 and linear combination statistic z_W. Although their interest was in the analysis of multivariate censored failure-time data, they give instructions for adapting their algorithm to the general repeated measures setting. Davis (1994) provides a program for the analysis of repeated measurements that calculates X_W^2, z_W, and other test statistics. The two methods give the same results for X_W^2 and z_W (apart from a sign change).

10.4.3 The Wei–Johnson Method

The Wei and Lachin (1984) methodology is based on a random-censorship model, and the focus is on an omnibus test of equality versus a general alternative. In contrast, Wei and Johnson (1985) focus primarily on optimal methods of combining dependent tests and propose a class of two-sample nonparametric tests for incomplete repeated measurements based on two-sample U statistics. Their motivation is that if a researcher wishes to draw an overall conclusion regarding the superiority of one treatment over another (across time), then a univariate one-sided test that combines the results at individual time points is more appropriate than an omnibus two-sided test of $H_0: F_1(\boldsymbol{x}) = F_2(\boldsymbol{x})$.

Before describing the Wei–Johnson (1985) methodology, we first review one-sample and two-sample U statistics.

One-Sample U Statistics

Let $\mathcal{F}$ denote a family of cumulative distribution functions, let $X_1, \ldots, X_n$ be a random sample from a distribution with cdf $F \in \mathcal{F}$, and let γ denote a parameter to be estimated. The parameter γ is said to be *estimable of degree* r for the family $\mathcal{F}$ if r is the smallest sample size for which there exists a function $h(x_1, \ldots, x_r)$ such that

$$\mathrm{E}[h(X_1, \ldots, X_r)] = \gamma$$

for every distribution $F \in \mathcal{F}$. The function $h(x_1, \ldots, x_r)$ is a statistic that does not depend on F and is called the *kernel* of the parameter γ. The function $h(x_1, \ldots, x_r)$ is assumed to be symmetric in its arguments; that is,

$$h(x_1, \ldots, x_r) = h(x_{\alpha_1}, \ldots, x_{\alpha_r})$$

for every permutation $(\alpha_1, \ldots, \alpha_r)$ of the integers $1, \ldots, r$.

A one-sample U statistic for the estimable parameter γ of degree r is created with the symmetric kernel $h(x_1, \ldots, x_r)$ by forming

$$U(X_1, \ldots, X_n) = \binom{n}{r}^{-1} \sum_{\beta \in B} h(X_{\beta_1}, \ldots, X_{\beta_r}),$$

where $B = \{\beta | \beta$ is one of the $\binom{n}{r}$ unordered subsets of r integers chosen without replacement from the set $\{1, \ldots, n\}\}$.

As an example of a one-sample U statistic, let $\mathcal{F}$ denote the class of all univariate distributions with finite first moment γ, and let $X_1, \ldots, X_n$ be a random sample from a distribution with cdf $F \in \mathcal{F}$. Because $\mathrm{E}(X_1) = \gamma$, the mean γ is an estimable parameter of degree 1 for the family $\mathcal{F}$. Using the kernel $h(x) = x$, the U-statistic estimator of the mean is

$$U(X_1, \ldots, X_n) = \binom{n}{1}^{-1} \sum_{i=1}^{n} h(X_i) = \frac{1}{n} \sum_{i=1}^{n} X_i = \overline{X}.$$

An important theorem due to Hoeffding (1948) (see also Randles and Wolfe, 1979, p. 82) establishes the asymptotic normality of standardized one-sample U statistics; this is an example of a central limit theorem for dependent variables. Let $X_1, \ldots, X_n$ be a random sample from a distribution with cdf $F \in \mathcal{F}$, let γ be an estimable parameter of degree r with symmetric kernel $h(x_1, \ldots, x_r)$, and let

$$U(X_1, \ldots, X_n) = \binom{n}{r}^{-1} \sum_{\beta \in B} h(X_{\beta_1}, \ldots, X_{\beta_r}),$$

where B consists of the unordered subsets of r integers chosen without replacement from $\{1, \ldots, n\}$. If $\mathrm{E}[h^2(X_1, \ldots, X_r)] < \infty$, and if

$$\zeta_1 = \mathrm{E}[h(X_1, \ldots, X_r)h(X_1, X_{r+1}, \ldots, X_{2r-1})] - \gamma^2$$

is positive, then the statistic

$$\sqrt{n}[U(X_1, \ldots, X_n) - \gamma]$$

has a limiting $N(0, r^2\zeta_1)$ distribution.

Two-Sample U Statistics

Let $X_1, \ldots, X_m$ and $Y_1, \ldots, Y_n$ be independent random samples from populations with cumulative distribution functions $F(x)$ and $G(y)$, respectively, from a family of cumulative distribution functions $\mathcal{F}$. A parameter γ is estimable of degree (r, s) for distributions (F, G) in the family $\mathcal{F}$ if r and s are the smallest sample sizes for which there exists a function $h(x_1, \ldots, x_r, y_1, \ldots, y_s)$ such that

$$\mathrm{E}[h(X_1, \ldots, X_r, Y_1, \ldots, Y_s)] = \gamma$$

for all distributions $(F, G) \in \mathcal{F}$. The function $h(x_1, \ldots, x_r, y_1, \ldots, y_s)$ is called the two-sample kernel of the parameter γ. The kernel

$$h(x_1, \ldots, x_r, y_1, \ldots, y_s)$$

is assumed to be symmetric separately in its x_i components and in its y_i components.

A two-sample U statistic for the estimable parameter γ of degree (r, s) is created with the kernel $h(x_1, \ldots, x_r, y_1, \ldots, y_s)$ by forming

$$U(X_1, \ldots, X_m, Y_1, \ldots, Y_n) = \frac{\sum_{\alpha \in A} \sum_{\beta \in B} h(X_{\alpha_1}, \ldots, X_{\alpha_r} Y_{\beta_1}, \ldots, Y_{\beta_s})}{\binom{m}{r}\binom{n}{s}},$$

where A (B) is the collection of subsets of r (s) integers chosen without replacement from the integers $\{1, \ldots, m\}$ $(\{1, \ldots, n\})$. Note that sample sizes $m \geq r$ and $n \geq s$ are required.

As an example of a two-sample U statistic, let $\mathcal{F}$ be the class of univariate distributions with finite first moment γ. Let $X_1, \ldots, X_m$ and $Y_1, \ldots, Y_n$

be independent random samples from distributions with cdfs F and G, respectively, where $F, G \in \mathcal{F}$. Because $\mathrm{E}(X_1) = \mu_X$ and $\mathrm{E}(Y_1) = \mu_Y$, the mean difference $\gamma = \mu_Y - \mu_X$ is an estimable parameter of degree $(1,1)$ for the family $\mathcal{F}$. Using the kernel $h(x,y) = y - x$, the U-statistic estimator of the mean difference is

$$\begin{aligned} U(X_1,\ldots,Y_n) &= \left[\binom{m}{1}\binom{n}{1}\right]^{-1} \sum_{i=1}^{m}\sum_{j=1}^{n} h(X_i,Y_j) \\ &= \frac{1}{mn}\sum_{i=1}^{m}\sum_{j=1}^{n}(Y_j - X_i) \\ &= \overline{Y} - \overline{X}. \end{aligned}$$

Lehmann (1951) established the asymptotic normality of standardized two-sample U statistics by extending Hoeffding's (1948) theorem. Considering only the special case of $r = s = 1$, let $X_1,\ldots,X_m$ and $Y_1,\ldots,Y_n$ be independent random samples from distributions with cdfs F and G, respectively, where $F, G \in \mathcal{F}$, let $h(\cdot)$ be a symmetric kernel for an estimable parameter γ of degree $(1,1)$, and let U be the U-statistic estimator of γ. Also, let $N = m + n$ and let

$$0 < \lambda = \lim_{N\to\infty} \frac{m}{N} < 1.$$

Define $\zeta_{1,0}$ and $\zeta_{0,1}$ by

$$\begin{aligned} \zeta_{1,0} &= \mathrm{E}[h(X_1,Y_1)h(X_1,Y_2)] - \gamma^2, \\ \zeta_{0,1} &= \mathrm{E}[h(X_1,Y_1)h(X_2,Y_1)] - \gamma^2. \end{aligned}$$

If $\mathrm{E}[h^2(X_1,Y_1)] < \infty$, and if

$$\sigma^2 = \frac{\zeta_{1,0}}{\lambda} + \frac{\zeta_{0,1}}{1-\lambda} > 0,$$

then the limiting distribution of the statistic $\sqrt{N}(U - \gamma)$ is $N(0,\sigma^2)$.

Joint Limiting Distribution of Correlated Two-Sample U Statistics

Lehmann (1963) proved a general theorem, which will be stated here for the special case of several two-sample U statistics, each of degree $(1,1)$.

Let $\boldsymbol{X}_1,\ldots,\boldsymbol{X}_m$ and $\boldsymbol{Y}_1,\ldots,\boldsymbol{Y}_n$ be independent random samples from distributions with t-variate cdfs F and G, respectively. Thus,

$$\boldsymbol{X}_i = (X_{i1},\ldots,X_{it})'$$

for $i = 1,\ldots,m$, and

$$\boldsymbol{Y}_j = (Y_{j1},\ldots,Y_{jt})'$$

for $j = 1, \ldots, n$. Let $U_1, \ldots, U_t$ be two-sample U statistics with symmetric kernel $h(x, y)$, where U_k estimates γ_k of degree $(1, 1)$ and is given by

$$U_k = (mn)^{-1} \sum_{i=1}^{m} \sum_{j=1}^{n} h(X_{ik}, Y_{jk})$$

for $k = 1, \ldots, t$. Also, let $N = m + n$ and let

$$\lambda = \lim_{N \to \infty} \frac{m}{N}.$$

The joint limiting distribution of

$$\sqrt{N}(U_1 - \gamma_1), \ldots, \sqrt{N}(U_t - \gamma_t)$$

is t-variate normal with zero mean vector and covariance matrix $\mathbf{\Sigma}$ with elements

$$\sigma_{k,k'} = \frac{\zeta_{1(k,k')}}{\lambda} + \frac{\zeta_{2(k,k')}}{1 - \lambda}.$$

The quantities $\zeta_{1(k,k')}$ and $\zeta_{2(k,k')}$ are defined by

$$\begin{aligned}
\zeta_{1(k,k')} &= \operatorname{Cov}\big[(h(X_{1k}, Y_{1k}) - \gamma_k), (h(X_{1k'}, Y_{2k'}) - \gamma_{k'})\big] \\
&= \mathrm{E}[h(X_{1k}, Y_{1k}) h(X_{1k'}, Y_{2k'})] - \gamma_k \gamma_{k'}, \\
\zeta_{2(k,k')} &= \operatorname{Cov}\big[(h(X_{1k}, Y_{1k}) - \gamma_k), (h(X_{2k'}, Y_{1k'}) - \gamma_{k'})\big] \\
&= \mathrm{E}[h(X_{1k}, Y_{1k}) h(X_{2k'}, Y_{1k'})] - \gamma_k \gamma_{k'},
\end{aligned}$$

for $k, k' = 1, \ldots, t$.

Wei–Johnson Methodology

The Wei–Johnson (1985) procedure for the analysis of repeated measurements is based on the preceding theory for correlated two-sample U statistics. The test statistic at the jth time point is

$$U_j = \frac{\sqrt{n_1 + n_2}}{n_1 n_2} \sum_{i=1}^{n_1} \sum_{i'=1}^{n_2} \delta_{1ij}\, \delta_{2i'j}\, \phi(y_{1ij}, y_{2i'j}),$$

where y_{hij} is the observation at time j from subject i in group h for $h = 1, 2$, $i = 1, \ldots, n_h$, and $j = 1, \ldots, t$. In addition,

$$\delta_{hij} = \begin{cases} 1 & \text{if } y_{hij} \text{ is observed} \\ 0 & \text{otherwise} \end{cases},$$

and $\phi(x, y)$ is a kernel function. If $\mathrm{E}[\phi^2(y_{1ij}, y_{2i'j})] < \infty$ for $j = 1, \ldots, t$ and $n_1/(n_1 + n_2) \to c$, with $0 < c < 1$, as $n_1 + n_2 \to \infty$, then the vector

$$\boldsymbol{U} = (U_1, \ldots, U_t)'$$

has an asymptotic null $N(\mathbf{0}_t, \mathbf{\Sigma}_U)$ distribution. If $\text{E}[\phi^4(y_{1ij}, y_{2i'j})] < \infty$ for $j = 1, \ldots, t$, then the elements of the variance–covariance matrix $\mathbf{\Sigma}_U$ of $\boldsymbol{U} = (U_1, \ldots, U_t)'$ can be estimated consistently by

$$\widehat{\sigma}_{jk} = \frac{n_1 + n_2}{n_1} \widehat{\sigma}_{1jk} + \frac{n_1 + n_2}{n_2} \widehat{\sigma}_{2jk},$$

where

$$\widehat{\sigma}_{1jk} = \frac{1}{n_1 n_2 (n_2 - 1)} \sum_{i=1}^{n_1} \sum_{l \neq l'=1}^{n_2} \delta_{1ij}\, \delta_{1ik}\, \delta_{2lj}\, \delta_{2l'k}\, \phi(y_{1ij}, y_{2lj})\, \phi(y_{1ik}, y_{2l'k})$$

and

$$\widehat{\sigma}_{2jk} = \frac{1}{n_2 n_1 (n_1 - 1)} \sum_{l=1}^{n_2} \sum_{i \neq i'=1}^{n_1} \delta_{1ij}\, \delta_{1i'k}\, \delta_{2lj}\, \delta_{2lk}\, \phi(y_{1ij}, y_{2lj})\, \phi(y_{1i'k}, y_{2lk}).$$

Let $\widehat{\mathbf{\Sigma}}_U$ denote the estimated covariance matrix of the vector of test statistics $\boldsymbol{U}$. Because the null distribution of $\boldsymbol{U}$ is approximately multivariate normal with mean vector $\mathbf{0}_t$ and variance–covariance matrix $\widehat{\mathbf{\Sigma}}_U$, the hypothesis $H_0 \colon F_1(x_1, \ldots, x_t) = F_2(x_1, \ldots, x_t)$ can be tested against a general alternative using the statistic $X_U^2 = \boldsymbol{U}' \widehat{\mathbf{\Sigma}}_U^{-1} \boldsymbol{U}$. If H_0 is true, this statistic has an asymptotic χ_t^2 distribution. A univariate one-sided test that combines the results at individual time points can be based on the linear combination

$$\boldsymbol{c}'\boldsymbol{U} = \sum_{j=1}^{t} c_j U_j,$$

where $\boldsymbol{c}' = (c_1, \ldots, c_t)$ is a vector of weights. Under H_0, the statistic

$$z_U = \frac{\boldsymbol{c}'\boldsymbol{U}}{\sqrt{\boldsymbol{c}' \widehat{\mathbf{\Sigma}}_U \boldsymbol{c}}}$$

is asymptotically $N(0, 1)$.

The simplest choice for the vector $\boldsymbol{c}$ is to weight each component equally; that is, to choose $\boldsymbol{c}' = (1, \ldots, 1)$. Another possibility is to weight by the reciprocals of the variances using

$$\boldsymbol{c}' = \left(\frac{1}{\widehat{\sigma}_{11}}, \ldots, \frac{1}{\widehat{\sigma}_{tt}} \right). \tag{10.2}$$

Under the assumption that the test statistics at the individual time points are estimates of a common effect, the optimal weights are given by

$$\boldsymbol{c}' = (1, \ldots, 1) \widehat{\mathbf{\Sigma}}_U^{-1} \tag{10.3}$$

(O'Brien, 1984; Ashby, Pocock, and Shaper, 1986). In practice, however, this assumption may not hold. In addition, Bloch and Moses (1988) show that, in general, the use of simple weights often results in little loss of efficiency. Note that if the values of the test statistics differ considerably across time points, the weights given by Equation (10.3) may give a result that is quite different from that using equal weights or weighting by precision.

Wei and Johnson (1985) suggest several choices for the kernel function $\phi(x, y)$. If Equation (10.1) is used, the Wei–Johnson vector of test statistics $\boldsymbol{U}$ and the Wei–Lachin vector of test statistics $\boldsymbol{W}$ are equivalent, apart from a scale factor. The consistent estimators of the variances and covariances of the components of the vector of test statistics, however, are different. The two methods will usually give similar results.

10.4.4 Examples

Complete Data

Although the Wei–Lachin (1984) and Wei–Johnson (1985) procedures were developed for the two-sample case with incomplete data, these procedures can also be applied when there are no missing data. Using the data from the Leppik et al. (1987) clinical trial conducted in 59 epileptic patients (partially displayed in Table 2.7 and previously considered in Sections 2.3 and 10.3.2), the Wei–Lachin vector of test statistics at the four time points is $\boldsymbol{W}' = (-0.4700, -0.0375, -0.2008, -0.3685)$ with estimated covariance matrix

$$\widehat{\boldsymbol{\Sigma}}_W = \begin{pmatrix} 0.0788 & 0.0529 & 0.0460 & 0.0509 \\ 0.0529 & 0.0804 & 0.0538 & 0.0556 \\ 0.0460 & 0.0538 & 0.0789 & 0.0501 \\ 0.0509 & 0.0556 & 0.0501 & 0.0775 \end{pmatrix}.$$

The Wei–Lachin omnibus chi-square statistic for testing equality of distributions is $X_W^2 = \boldsymbol{W}'\widehat{\boldsymbol{\Sigma}}_W^{-1}\boldsymbol{W} = 5.66$ with 4 df ($p = 0.23$).

The Wei–Johnson procedure using the kernel function of Equation (10.1) gives a vector $\boldsymbol{U}$ of test statistics equivalent (apart from a scale factor) to the Wei–Lachin $\boldsymbol{W}$ but uses a different estimator of the covariance matrix. Weighting each time point equally, the Wei–Johnson univariate statistic

$$\frac{\boldsymbol{c}'\boldsymbol{U}}{\sqrt{\boldsymbol{c}'\widehat{\boldsymbol{\Sigma}}_U\boldsymbol{c}}},$$

with $\boldsymbol{c}' = (1, \ldots, 1)$, is equal to -1.09. With reference to the $N(0, 1)$ distribution, the two-sided p-value is 0.14.

Incomplete Data

Problem 2.10 describes a clinical trial comparing two treatments for maternal pain relief during labor (Davis, 1991). In this study, 83 women in labor were randomized to receive an experimental pain medication (43 subjects) or placebo (40 subjects). Treatment was initiated when the cervical dilation was 8 cm. At 30-minute intervals, the amount of pain was self-reported by placing a mark on a 100-mm line (0 = no pain, 100 = very much pain). Table 2.18 displays the data from the first 20 subjects in each group.

Because the repeated pain scores are both nonnormal and incomplete, it seems appropriate to compare the two groups using the Wei–Lachin or the Wei–Johnson procedures. Based on the data from minutes 30, 60, 90, 120, 150, and 180, the Wei–Lachin vector of test statistics is

$$\boldsymbol{W}' = (-0.3941, -0.6017, -0.7551, -0.7287, -0.4972, -0.2976),$$

with estimated covariance matrix

$$\widehat{\boldsymbol{\Sigma}}_W = \begin{pmatrix} 0.0794 & 0.0479 & 0.0284 & 0.0178 & 0.0114 & 0.0057 \\ 0.0479 & 0.0585 & 0.0316 & 0.0208 & 0.0155 & 0.0064 \\ 0.0284 & 0.0316 & 0.0368 & 0.0197 & 0.0111 & 0.0036 \\ 0.0178 & 0.0208 & 0.0197 & 0.0265 & 0.0148 & 0.0054 \\ 0.0114 & 0.0155 & 0.0111 & 0.0148 & 0.0132 & 0.0057 \\ 0.0057 & 0.0064 & 0.0036 & 0.0054 & 0.0057 & 0.0052 \end{pmatrix}.$$

The Wei–Johnson procedure using the kernel function of Equation (10.1) gives the vector of test statistics

$$\boldsymbol{U}' = (-1.5784, -2.4100, -3.0245, -2.9185, -1.9916, -1.1918),$$

with estimated covariance matrix

$$\widehat{\boldsymbol{\Sigma}}_U = \begin{pmatrix} 1.3298 & 0.9268 & 0.6557 & 0.4182 & 0.2429 & 0.1433 \\ 0.9268 & 1.1120 & 0.7783 & 0.5576 & 0.3625 & 0.2114 \\ 0.6557 & 0.7783 & 0.9337 & 0.7511 & 0.4985 & 0.2555 \\ 0.4182 & 0.5576 & 0.7511 & 0.7790 & 0.5016 & 0.2528 \\ 0.2429 & 0.3625 & 0.4985 & 0.5016 & 0.4189 & 0.2234 \\ 0.1433 & 0.2114 & 0.2555 & 0.2528 & 0.2234 & 0.1819 \end{pmatrix}.$$

Table 10.1 displays the standardized test statistics (statistic/standard error) for the Wei–Lachin and Wei–Johnson methods at each of the six time points. The signs of the test statistics indicate that, at each time point, the pain scores are lower (better) in the experimental group than in the placebo group. Although the two methods yield similar conclusions, the Wei–Lachin standardized statistic is larger in absolute value (more significant) than the Wei–Johnson statistic at every time point. The Wei–Lachin omnibus chi-square statistic for testing equality of distributions is highly significant ($X_W^2 = \boldsymbol{W}'\widehat{\boldsymbol{\Sigma}}_W^{-1}\boldsymbol{W} = 30.1$ with 6 df, $p < 0.001$), whereas the omnibus Wei–Johnson statistic is marginally significant ($X_U^2 = \boldsymbol{U}'\widehat{\boldsymbol{\Sigma}}_U^{-1}\boldsymbol{U} = 11.9$ with 6 df, $p = 0.065$).

TABLE 10.1. Wei–Lachin and Wei–Johnson analyses of labor pain clinical trial

	Standardized Test Statistic	
	Wei–Lachin	Wei–Johnson
Time point (minute):		
30	−1.40	−1.37
60	−2.49	−2.28
90	−3.94	−3.13
120	−4.47	−3.31
150	−4.33	−3.08
180	−4.11	−2.79
Linear combinations:		
Equal weights	−3.88	−3.06
Reciprocals of variances [Equation (10.2)]	−4.85	−3.28
Optimal [Equation (10.3)]	−4.42	−2.11

Table 10.1 also displays standardized values of three linear combinations of the statistics calculated at the separate time points. For both methods, all three linear combination statistics indicate a significant difference between the two groups with respect to the $N(0,1)$ reference distribution.

10.5 Problems

10.1 Box (1950) describes an experiment in which 30 rats were randomly assigned to three treatment groups. Group 1 was a control group, group 2 had thyroxin added to their drinking water, and group 3 had thiouracil added to their drinking water. Although there were ten rats in each of groups 1 and 3, group 2 consisted of only seven rats (due to an unspecified accident at the beginning of the experiment). The resulting body weights of each of the 27 rats at the beginning of the experiment and at weekly intervals for four weeks were previously considered in Problems 2.4, 4.3, and 5.9 and are displayed in Table 2.12.

(a) Use nonparametric methods to test whether the body-weight distributions differ among the three groups.

(b) Compare your results with those from Problems 2.4, 4.3, and 5.9.

10.2 In an investigation of the effects of various dosages of radiation therapy on psychomotor skills (Danford et al., 1960), 45 cancer patients were trained to operate a psychomotor testing device. Six patients were not given radiation and served as controls, and the remainder were treated with dosages of 25–50 R, 75–100 R, or 125–250 R. The resulting psychomotor test scores on the three days following radiation treatment were previously considered in Problems 2.6, 4.6, and 5.11 and are displayed in Table 2.14.

(a) Use nonparametric methods to test whether the distributions of the psychomotor test scores differ among the four groups.

(b) Compare your results with those from Problems 2.6, 4.6, and 5.11.

10.3 Potthoff and Roy (1964) describe a study conducted at the University of North Carolina Dental School in which the distance (mm) from the center of the pituitary gland to the pterygomaxillary fissure was measured at ages 8, 10, 12, and 14 in 16 boys and 11 girls. Table 3.3 lists the individual measurements as well as the sample means and standard deviations in both groups.

(a) Let F_b and F_g denote the multivariate cumulative distribution functions for boys and girls, respectively. Use nonparametric methods to test $H_0: F_b = F_g$.

(b) Sections 3.4.2, 4.3.2, 4.4.3, and 6.4.1, as well as Problems 5.8, 6.3, and 9.7, considered several other methods for the analysis of these data. Compare the results from part (a) to the tests of equality of groups presented in Sections 3.4.2, 4.3.2, 4.4.3, and 6.4.1.

10.4 Koziol et al. (1981) describe an experiment in which 30 mice were injected with mouse colon carcinoma cells. Five days later, the mice were randomly divided into three groups of ten mice each. The groups were then given different immunotherapy regimens. Group A received injections of tissue culture medium around the growing tumor, group B received injections of tissue culture medium and normal spleen cells, and group C received injections of normal spleen cells, immune RNA, and tumor antigen. Table 10.2 displays tumor volumes (mm^3) at days 7, 11, 12, 13, 14, 15, and 17. Compare the three immunotherapy regimens using an appropriate nonparametric procedure.

10.5 Amini and Patel (1984) report the results of a study to detect differences in the percentage of erythrocyte survival among three genetically different groups of 7–8-week-old female mice. Groups 1, 2, and 3 consisted of 11, 8, and 11 mice, respectively. For each mouse, the percentage of erythrocytes surviving was measured at ionic concentrations of 0.3, 0.35, 0.4, 0.45, 0.5, and 0.55. Table 10.3 displays the data. Use a nonparametric method to test whether the multivariate distributions in the three groups are the same.

10.6 Eighty subjects with multiple sclerosis participated in a randomized, placebo-controlled trial studying the efficacy of fampridine, a compound to enhance nerve conduction. Prior to the initiation of treatment, the time required to walk a specified distance was measured for each subject. The

TABLE 10.2. Tumor volumes (mm^3) in three groups of ten mice

		Day						
Group	ID	7	11	12	13	14	15	17
A	1	35.3	157.1	122.5	217.6	340.3	379.0	556.6
	2	19.6	152.2	129.6	176.6	213.9	317.9	356.4
	3	27.0	122.4	196.1	196.1	332.2	388.9	469.3
	4	55.0	95.0	205.9	205.9	270.0	307.3	405.1
	5	24.6	168.8	135.3	196.0	340.2	340.4	507.3
	6	12.6	85.0	70.1	225.1	225.1	289.0	317.9
	7	35.2	129.8	180.0	274.7	420.1	340.3	507.2
	8	29.8	157.0	126.8	202.5	225.0	307.2	320.1
	9	70.0	129.7	196.0	205.8	375.7	419.1	421.2
	10	29.5	156.9	176.7	225.0	289.0	372.6	379.2
B	1	48.6	115.3	90.8	176.5	317.9	421.2	529.2
	2	66.7	289.0	215.6	268.8	388.8	487.4	551.3
	3	24.5	143.7	115.0	90.7	194.3	559.6	629.3
	4	14.4	84.7	135.2	191.2	176.4	356.4	397.1
	5	10.8	70.0	80.0	118.3	156.8	215.6	268.8
	6	11.3	15.0	205.8	289.0	346.8	529.2	629.2
	7	18.0	56.7	115.3	96.8	177.5	268.8	320.0
	8	60.0	166.6	166.7	324.0	420.0	440.0	634.8
	9	29.4	152.1	122.4	186.3	186.3	274.7	485.1
	10	41.1	186.2	176.6	274.6	361.0	379.1	440.0
C	1	12.5	108.0	96.8	186.2	202.5	213.9	379.1
	2	23.4	129.6	176.5	196.6	320.0	397.1	500.0
	3	22.2	65.0	176.4	191.3	213.8	274.6	405.0
	4	11.2	52.9	70.0	129.6	152.1	303.5	415.0
	5	66.6	147.0	260.1	420.0	460.0	653.4	806.4
	6	11.4	115.2	65.1	32.0	10.8	3.2	1.4
	7	22.1	55.0	115.2	55.0	93.6	118.8	118.3
	8	40.5	156.8	65.0	84.7	191.2	291.5	400.0
	9	32.0	44.6	108.9	258.8	247.5	405.0	372.6
	10	10.0	118.3	166.6	176.4	186.2	340.2	361.0

TABLE 10.3. Percentage of erythrocytes surviving at six ionic concentrations from 30 female mice

		Ionic Concentration					
Group	ID	0.3	0.35	0.4	0.45	0.5	0.55
1	1	94.1	97.2	94.6	87.3	33.1	5.6
	2	100.0	100.0	100.0	93.7	35.6	3.7
	3	100.0	100.0	98.3	90.3	29.1	0.0
	4	100.0	99.9	96.0	87.7	35.9	2.8
	5	100.0	100.0	97.7	82.4	31.8	0.0
	6	88.9	90.3	90.9	81.7	28.7	0.0
	7	100.0	98.4	98.9	79.8	23.1	0.0
	8	100.0	93.9	100.0	92.3	32.1	2.1
	9	96.3	95.2	92.1	82.2	26.6	0.0
	10	99.5	99.8	94.5	84.2	22.5	0.0
	11	97.6	97.3	94.6	90.4	45.9	0.0
2	1	100.0	100.0	94.2	76.9	14.2	0.0
	2	97.5	98.1	92.3	71.3	10.2	0.0
	3	93.2	96.6	89.8	69.2	10.0	0.0
	4	95.7	98.7	89.8	76.4	0.3	0.0
	5	82.9	89.2	82.4	68.8	12.0	0.0
	6	100.0	100.0	92.2	81.2	14.5	0.0
	7	100.0	100.0	98.9	67.1	12.5	0.0
	8	97.9	99.5	94.8	76.4	19.5	0.0
3	1	100.0	96.4	94.4	82.1	19.4	1.3
	2	98.6	97.7	88.1	80.4	11.8	0.0
	3	100.0	100.0	100.0	100.0	17.1	0.0
	4	100.0	95.8	89.2	78.5	17.0	0.0
	5	100.0	100.0	97.3	17.8	17.7	0.0
	6	89.3	92.1	88.4	71.9	14.4	0.0
	7	100.0	100.0	100.0	82.7	21.6	0.0
	8	99.8	95.3	97.7	76.5	10.8	0.0
	9	91.4	95.0	94.4	85.8	30.2	0.0
	10	100.0	99.4	97.9	81.5	7.3	0.0
	11	97.8	100.0	96.2	77.6	10.7	0.0

TABLE 10.4. Ambulation time improvements at weeks 2, 4, and 6 from 80 subjects with multiple sclerosis: Subjects 1–10

		Ambulation Time Improvement (seconds)		
Subject	Treatment	Week 2	Week 4	Week 6
1	Fampridine	7.72	1.42	6.74
2	Fampridine	−8.18	.	.
3	Placebo	−0.45	−1.11	−0.34
4	Placebo	0.65	−1.38	−5.88
5	Fampridine	4.15	4.20	11.04
6	Placebo	1.31	1.15	1.23
7	Placebo	0.59	0.29	0.86
8	Placebo	1.02	2.86	2.61
9	Placebo	−44.09	−20.42	17.99
10	Fampridine	3.30	4.11	1.34

process was repeated at weeks 2, 4, and 6 during treatment, and the outcome variable was the change from baseline in ambulation time. Because this was computed as the baseline value minus the follow-up value, positive numbers indicate improvement. Table 10.4 displays the data from the first ten subjects. Use nonparametric methods to compare the fampridine and placebo groups with respect to the ambulation time changes at weeks 2, 4, and 6.

10.7 In the Iowa Cochlear Implant Project, the effectiveness of two types of cochlear implants was studied in profoundly and bilaterally deaf patients. In one group of 23 subjects, the "type A" implant was used. A second group of 21 subjects received the "type B" implant. In both groups, the electrode array was surgically implanted five to six weeks prior to electrical connection to the external speech processor. A sentence test was then administered at 1, 9, 18, and 30 months after connection. The outcome variable of interest at each time point was the percentage of correct scores. The resulting data were previously considered in Problem 2.9 and are displayed in Table 2.17.

(a) Test whether there is a difference between the two types of implants using nonparametric methods.

(b) Compare your results with those from Problem 2.9.

10.8 Problem 2.11 discussed data from the National Cooperative Gallstone Study, which investigated the safety of the drug chenodiol for the treatment of cholesterol gallstones. Tables 2.19 and 2.20 display serum cholesterol measurements prior to treatment and at 6, 12, 20, and 24 months of follow-up for patients in the placebo and high-dose chenodiol groups, respectively (Wei and Lachin, 1984). Use a nonparametric test to compare the chenodiol and placebo groups with respect to the changes in cholesterol levels (from baseline) at months 6, 12, 20, and 24.

10.9 Crépeau et al. (1985) describe an investigation of the effects of three treatment regimens on induced tumors in mice. In this experiment, 45 mice were injected subcutaneously with mouse colon carcinoma cells. Five days later, when the induced tumors were palpable, the mice were randomly divided into three groups of 15 mice each. Group 1 was a control group, group 2 received normal spleen cells only, and group 3 received normal spleen cells, immune RNA, and tumor antigen. Table 10.5 displays subsequent tumor volumes (mm^3) at days 10, 11, 12, 13, 14, 15, 17, 18, 19, and 20. Compare the three immunotherapy regimens using an appropriate nonparametric procedure.

10.10 Volberding et al. (1990) describe a randomized, placebo-controlled study of AZT in adults with asymptomatic HIV infection. In this study, CD4+ cell counts were measured at weeks 8, 16, 32, and 48 from 497 subjects treated with 1500 mg/day of zidovudine (AZT) and 459 subjects treated with a placebo. There are numerous missing values, especially at the later time points. Table 10.6 displays the data from the first 50 subjects. Use appropriate nonparametric methods to test whether the CD4+ distributions arc the same in the two groups.

TABLE 10.5. Tumor volumes (mm^3) in 45 mice

		Day									
Group	ID	10	11	12	13	14	15	17	18	19	20
1	1	40.5	56.7	72.6	90.8	135.2	151.2	177.5	177.5	172.5	191.3
	2	25.6	32.0	35.2	40.5	72.6	90.8	126.8	126.8	126.8	143.7
	3	32.0	40.5	66.6	96.8	151.2	180.0	270.0	281.6	332.8	356.3
	4	19.6	48.6	70.0	96.8	151.2	180.0	247.5	332.8	487.4	505.4
	5	10.8	25.6	56.7	75.0	129.6	176.4	303.5	420.0	560.0	600.4
	6	50.0	50.0	58.4	65.0	85.0	115.2	202.5	202.5	225.4	258.8
	7	25.6	35.2	52.7	90.8	115.2	129.6	156.8	156.8	176.4	191.3
	8	22.1	48.6	75.0	84.7	90.8	100.8	176.4	277.5	356.4	356.4
	9	10.8	25.6	48.6	50.0	84.7	100.8	180.0	277.5	420.0	487.4
	10	10.8	25.6	60.0	65.0	78.7	90.0	156.8	202.5	361.0	388.8
	11	17.2	25.6	48.6	52.7	143.7	186.2	243.2	243.2	281.6	332.8
	12	25.6	56.7	90.8	90.8	90.8	126.8	191.3	191.3	191.3	217.6
	13	4.8	19.6	65.0	75.0	126.8	180.0	307.8	332.8	356.4	487.4
	14	25.6	40.5	84.7	90.8	147.0	152.1	225.0	247.5	388.8	419.1
	15	5.3	35.2	90.8	90.8	96.8	115.2	152.1	152.1	176.4	247.5
2	1	17.2	25.6	60.0	75.0	156.8	186.2	236.3	281.6	343.0	388.8
	2	48.6	66.6	100.8	115.2	160.6	243.2	317.9	419.1	505.4	556.6
	3	5.3	5.3	6.3	19.6	52.7	129.6	281.6	307.8	388.8	487.4
	4	19.6	25.6	48.6	35.2	78.7	78.7	85.0	156.8	317.9	487.4
	5	25.6	50.0	84.7	84.7	84.7	115.2	205.8	307.8	523.5	556.8
	6	55.0	75.0	100.8	115.2	186.2	247.5	332.8	356.4	419.1	460.0
	7	25.6	40.5	56.7	65.0	84.7	156.8	225.4	225.4	225.4	247.5
	8	17.2	32.0	56.7	65.0	96.8	115.2	169.0	191.3	258.8	343.0
	9	10.8	22.1	48.6	65.0	143.7	176.4	202.8	225.4	292.5	388.8
	10	12.6	25.6	52.7	90.8	202.5	247.5	388.8	419.1	453.6	620.0
	11	25.6	48.6	96.8	96.8	96.8	160.6	247.5	247.5	247.5	303.5
	12	22.1	48.6	78.7	90.8	115.2	126.8	176.4	191.3	281.6	303.5
	13	32.0	56.7	100.8	100.8	115.2	186.2	235.2	281.6	345.6	388.8
	14	65.0	84.7	143.7	143.7	156.8	180.0	225.0	276.0	303.5	303.5
	15	28.8	32.0	52.7	65.0	100.8	180.0	276.0	307.8	346.8	388.8
3	1	4.8	7.5	19.6	28.8	60.0	78.7	100.8	135.2	191.3	191.3
	2	1.4	3.2	6.3	10.8	28.8	32.0	60.0	78.7	115.2	168.8
	3	1.4	2.3	4.8	2.3	1.4	19.6	25.6	28.8	41.6	41.6
	4	4.8	4.8	4.8	10.8	28.8	25.6	22.1	10.8	6.3	2.3
	5	1.8	4.8	12.6	17.2	48.6	70.0	152.1	152.1	156.8	176.4
	6	4.0	7.5	32.0	32.0	55.0	60.0	70.0	84.7	108.9	115.2
	7	0.4	2.3	4.0	6.3	7.5	7.5	7.5	6.3	1.4	1.4
	8	1.4	1.4	3.2	6.3	17.2	32.0	78.7	78.7	86.4	135.2
	9	1.4	4.0	7.5	10.8	14.4	22.1	50.0	70.0	84.7	100.8
	10	1.4	1.4	1.4	6.3	19.6	22.1	28.8	28.8	36.5	40.5
	11	1.4	3.2	7.5	10.8	32.0	48.6	66.6	78.7	118.3	156.8
	12	0.6	0.4	0.0	3.2	10.8	10.8	12.6	19.6	44.8	32.0
	13	1.4	1.4	0.4	0.4	1.4	6.3	12.6	19.6	28.8	28.8
	14	1.4	1.4	1.4	3.2	19.6	28.8	40.5	40.5	44.6	56.7
	15	1.4	1.4	3.2	10.8	32.0	32.0	32.0	22.1	19.6	19.6

TABLE 10.6. CD4+ cell counts at four time points from a clinical trial in adults with asymptomatic HIV infection: First 50 subjects

		Week						Week			
ID	Trt.	8	16	32	48	ID	Trt.	8	16	32	48
1	P	476	432	510	425	26	P	.	423	517	632
2	P	216	337	264	321	27	P	578	575	574	740
3	A	672	614	326	494	28	P	257	244	202	.
4	A	287	329	426	368	29	P	480	528	390	464
5	P	166	250	.	.	30	A	330	412	456	233
6	A	375	312	94	183	31	A	489	787	515	520
7	A	486	475	546	246	32	A	122	70	63	.
8	A	545	226	475	428	33	P	756	414	967	920
9	A	362	332	368	370	34	P	504	483	406	384
10	P	288	215	266	225	35	P	264	480	344	.
11	A	513	344	210	.	36	P	630	714	525	554
12	A	286	354	179	191	37	A	706	728	.	.
13	A	421	371	.	492	38	A	70	.	.	.
14	A	143	192	135	121	39	A	300	299	.	.
15	P	484	350	271	.	40	A	588	464	.	.
16	P	287	405	.	.	41	A	548	446	650	721
17	A	365	278	377	334	42	P	235	220	570	320
18	A	480	390	510	.	43	P	253	.	.	.
19	P	668	320	630	426	44	A	317	270	206	189
20	P	337	306	401	351	45	A	522	378	400	320
21	A	477	556	505	529	46	A	162	308	444	406
22	A	528	477	525	811	47	A	529	399	477	474
23	A	521	458	543	425	48	A	314	276	231	358
24	A	432	483	391	465	49	P	134	203	165	88
25	A	440	392	.	.	50	A	309	.	.	.

Bibliography

Agresti, A. (1988). Logit models for repeated ordered categorical response data. In *Proceedings of the 13th Annual SAS Users Group International Conference*, pages 997–1005, Cary, NC. SAS Institute Inc.

Agresti, A. (1989). A survey of models for repeated ordered categorical response data. *Statistics in Medicine*, 8:1209–1224.

Agresti, A. (1990). *Categorical Data Analysis.* John Wiley and Sons, New York.

Agresti, A. and Lang, J. B. (1993). A proportional odds model with subject-specific effects for repeated ordered categorical responses. *Biometrika*, 80:527–534.

Agresti, A., Lipsitz, S. R., and Lang, J. B. (1992). Comparing marginal distributions of large, sparse contingency tables. *Computational Statistics and Data Analysis*, 14:55–73.

Agresti, A. and Pendergast, J. (1986). Comparing mean ranks for repeated measures data. *Communications in Statistics—Theory and Methods*, 15:1417–1434.

Ahn, C., Overall, J. E., and Tonidandel, S. (2001). Sample size and power calculations in repeated measurement analysis. *Computer Methods and Programs in Biomedicine*, 64:121–124.

Ahn, C., Tonidandel, S., and Overall, J. E. (2000). Issues in use of SAS PROC.MIXED to test the significance of treatment effects in controlled clinical trials. *Journal of Biopharmaceutical Statistics*, 10:265–286.

Aitkin, M., Anderson, D., Francis, B., and Hinde, J. (1989). *Statistical Modelling in GLIM.* Oxford University Press, Oxford.

Akaike, H. (1973). Information theory and an extension of the maximum likelihood principle. In Petrov, B. N. and Csaki, F., editors, *Second International Symposium on Information Theory*, pages 267–281. Akademiai Kiado, Budapest.

Akritas, M. G. (1991). Limitations of the rank transform procedure: A study of repeated measures designs, part I. *Journal of the American Statistical Association*, 86:457–460.

Akritas, M. G. (1993). Limitations of the rank transform procedure: A study of repeated measures designs, part II. *Statistics and Probability Letters*, 17:149–156.

Akritas, M. G. and Arnold, S. F. (1994). Fully nonparametric hypotheses for factorial designs, I: Multivariate repeated measures designs. *Journal of the American Statistical Association*, 89:336–343.

Albert, P. S. (1999). Longitudinal data analysis (repeated measures) in clinical trials. *Statistics in Medicine*, 18:1707–1732.

Albert, P. S. (2000). A transitional model for longitudinal binary data subject to nonignorable missing data. *Biometrics*, 56:602–608.

Albert, P. S. and Follmann, D. A. (2000). Modeling repeated count data subject to informative dropout. *Biometrics*, 56:667–677.

Albert, P. S. and McShane, L. M. (1995). A generalized estimating equations approach for spatially correlated binary data: Applications to the analysis of neuroimaging data. *Biometrics*, 51:627–638.

Altman, N. S. (1990). Kernel smoothing of data with correlated errors. *Journal of the American Statistical Association*, 85:749–759.

Amini, S. B. and Patel, K. M. (1984). A SAS program for nonparametric tests for homogeneity of dose response growth curves. In *Proceedings of the 9th Annual SAS Users Group International Conference*, pages 810–815, Cary, NC. SAS Institute Inc.

Anderson, J. A. and Philips, P. R. (1981). Regression, discrimination and measurement models for ordered categorical variables. *Applied Statistics*, 30:22–31.

Anderson, R. L. and Bancroft, T. A. (1952). *Statistical Theory in Research.* McGraw-Hill, New York.

Anderson, T. W. (1984). *An Introduction to Multivariate Statistical Analysis.* John Wiley and Sons, New York.

Anscombe, F. J. (1953). Contribution to the discussion of H. Hotelling's paper. *Journal of the Royal Statistical Society, Series B*, 15:229–230.

Arndt, S., Davis, C. S., Miller, D. D., and Andreasen, N. C. (1993). Effect of antipsychotic withdrawal on extrapyramidal symptoms: Statistical methods for analyzing single sample repeated measures data. *Neuropsychopharmacology*, 8:67–75.

Ashby, D., Pocock, S. J., and Shaper, A. G. (1986). Ordered polytomous regression: An example relating serum biochemistry and haematology to alcohol consumption. *Applied Statistics*, 35:289–301.

Ashby, M., Neuhaus, J. M., Hauck, W. W., Bacchetti, P., Heilbron, D. C., Jewell, N. P., Segal, M. R., and Fusaro, R. E. (1992). An annotated bibliography of methods for analysing correlated categorical data. *Statistics in Medicine*, 11:67–99.

Barnhart, H. X. and Williamson, J. M. (1998). Goodness-of-fit tests for GEE modeling with binary responses. *Biometrics*, 54:720–729.

Bartlett, M. S. (1937). Properties of sufficiency and statistical tests. *Proceedings of the Royal Society of London A*, 160:268–282.

Bartlett, M. S. (1939). A note on tests of significance in multivariate analysis. *Proceedings of the Cambridge Philosophical Society*, 35:180–185.

Bartlett, M. S. (1966). *Stochastic Processes.* Cambridge University Press, Cambridge.

Benard, A. and van Elteren, P. (1953). A generalization of the method of m rankings. *Proceedings of the Koninklijke Nederlandse Akademie van Wetenschappen A*, 56:358–369.

Bhapkar, V. P. (1984). Univariate and multivariate multisample location and scale tests. In Krishnaiah, P. R. and Sen, P. K., editors, *Handbook of Statistics, Volume 4: Nonparametric Methods*, pages 31–62. Elsevier Science Publishers, Amsterdam.

Birch, M. W. (1965). The detection of partial association, II: The general case. *Journal of the Royal Statistical Society, Series B*, 27:111–124.

Bishop, Y. M. M., Feinberg, S. E., and Holland, P. W. (1975). *Discrete Multivariate Analysis: Theory and Practice.* The MIT Press, Cambridge, MA.

Bliss, C. I. (1935). The calculation of the dosage-mortality curve. *Annals of Applied Biology*, 22:134–167.

Bloch, D. A. (1986). Sample size requirements and the cost of a randomized clinical trial with repeated measurements. *Statistics in Medicine*, 5:663–667.

Bloch, D. A. and Moses, L. E. (1988). Nonoptimally weighted least squares. *The American Statistician*, 42:50–53.

Bock, R. D. (1963). Programming univariate and multivariate analysis of variance. *Technometrics*, 5:95–117.

Bock, R. D. (1975). *Multivariate Statistical Methods in Behavioral Research*. McGraw-Hill, New York.

Bonney, G. E. (1987). Logistic regression for dependent binary observations. *Biometrics*, 43:951–973.

Boos, D. D. (1992). On generalized score tests. *The American Statistician*, 46:327–333.

Box, G. E. P. (1950). Problems in the analysis of growth and wear curves. *Biometrics*, 6:362–389.

Box, G. E. P. (1954). Some theorems on quadratic forms applied in the study of analysis of variance problems. II, Effects of inequality of variance and of correlation between errors in the two-way classification. *Annals of Mathematical Statistics*, 25:484–498.

Breslow, N. E. and Clayton, D. G. (1993). Approximate inference in generalized linear mixed models. *Journal of the American Statistical Association*, 88:9–25.

Breslow, N. E. and Lin, X. (1995). Bias correction in generalised linear mixed models with a single component of dispersion. *Biometrika*, 82:81–91.

Brown, C. H. (1990). Protecting against nonrandomly missing data in longitudinal studies. *Biometrics*, 46:143–155.

Brown, G. W. and Mood, A. M. (1951). On median tests for linear hypotheses. In *Proceedings of the Second Berkeley Symposium on Mathematical Statistics and Probability*, Berkeley, CA. University of California Press.

Byrne, P. J. and Arnold, S. F. (1983). Inference about multivariate means for a nonstationary autoregressive model. *Journal of the American Statistical Association*, 78:850–855.

Carey, V. C. (1994). A shar file for the Liang/Zeger generalized estimating equation approach to GLMs for dependent data. Available from STATLIB at http://lib.stat.cmu.edu.

Carey, V. C., Zeger, S. L., and Diggle, P. (1993). Modelling multivariate binary data with alternating logistic regressions. *Biometrika*, 80:517–526.

Carr, G. J., Hafner, K. B., and Koch, G. G. (1989). Analysis of rank measures of association for ordinal data from longitudinal studies. *Journal of the American Statistical Association*, 84:797–804.

Chaganty, N. R. (1997). An alternative approach to the analysis of longitudinal data via generalized estimating equations. *Journal of Statistical Planning and Inference*, 63:39–54.

Chaganty, N. R. and Shults, J. (1999). On eliminating the asymptotic bias in the quasi-least squares estimate of the correlation parameter. *Journal of Statistical Planning and Inference*, 76:145–161.

Cnaan, A., Laird, N. M., and Slasor, P. (1997). Using the general linear mixed model to analyse unbalanced repeated measures and longitudinal data. *Statistics in Medicine*, 16:2349–2380.

Cochran, W. G. (1950). The comparison of percentages in matched samples. *Biometrika*, 37:256–266.

Cole, J. W. L. and Grizzle, J. E. (1966). Applications of multivariate analysis of variance to repeated measurements experiments. *Biometrics*, 22:810–828.

Conaway, M. R. (1990). A random effects model for binary data. *Biometrics*, 46:317–328.

Conaway, M. R. (1992). The analysis of repeated categorical measurements subject to nonignorable nonresponse. *Journal of the American Statistical Association*, 87:817–824.

Conaway, M. R. (1993). Non-ignorable non-response models for time-ordered categorical variables. *Applied Statistics*, 42:105–115.

Conaway, M. R. (1994). Causal nonresponse models for repeated categorical measurements. *Biometrics*, 50:1102–1116.

Conover, W. J. and Iman, R. L. (1981). Rank transformations as a bridge between parametric and nonparametric statistics. *The American Statistician*, 35:124–133.

Cook, R. D. (1986). Assessment of local influence. *Journal of the Royal Statistical Society, Series B*, 48:133–169.

Cook, R. J. and Lawless, J. F. (1997). Marginal analysis of recurrent events and a terminating event. *Statistics in Medicine*, 16:911–924.

Cornoni-Huntley, J., Brock, D. B., Ostfeld, A., Taylor, J. O., and Wallace, R. B. (1986). *Established Populations for Epidemiologic Studies of the Elderly, Resource Data Book.* National Institutes of Health (NIH Publ. No. 86-2443), Bethesda, MD.

Crépeau, H., Koziol, J., Reid, N., and Yuh, Y. S. (1985). Analysis of incomplete multivariate data from repeated measurement experiments. *Biometrics*, 41:505–514.

Crouchley, R. (1995). A random-effects model for ordered categorical data. *Journal of the American Statistical Association*, 90:489–498.

Crowder, M. J. (1992). Comments on "Multivariate regression analyses for categorical data". *Journal of the Royal Statistical Society, Series B*, 54:26–27.

Crowder, M. J. (1995). On the use of a working correlation matrix in using generalised linear models for repeated measures. *Biometrika*, 82:407–410.

Crowder, M. J. (1996). Keep timing the tablets: Statistical analysis of pill dissolution rates. *Applied Statistics*, 45:323–334.

Crowder, M. J. and Hand, D. J. (1990). *Analysis of Repeated Measures.* Chapman and Hall, London.

Cushny, A. R. and Peebles, A. R. (1905). The action of optical isomers II: Hyoscines. *Journal of Physiology*, 32:501–510.

Cytel Software (2000). *Egret for Windows.* Cytel Software Corporation, Cambridge, MA.

Danford, M. B., Hughes, H. M., and McNee, R. C. (1960). On the analysis of repeated-measurements experiments. *Biometrics*, 16:547–565.

Davidian, M. and Giltinan, D. M. (1995). *Nonlinear Models for Repeated Measurement Data.* Chapman and Hall, London.

Davis, C. S. (1991). Semi-parametric and non-parametric methods for the analysis of repeated measurements with applications to clinical trials. *Statistics in Medicine*, 10:1959–1980.

Davis, C. S. (1992). Analysis of incomplete categorical repeated measures. In *Proceedings of the 17th Annual SAS Users Group International Conference*, pages 1374–1379, Cary, NC. SAS Institute Inc.

Davis, C. S. (1993). A computer program for regression analysis of repeated measures using generalized estimating equations. *Computer Methods and Programs in Biomedicine*, 40:15–31.

Davis, C. S. (1994). A computer program for nonparametric analysis of incomplete repeated measures from two samples. *Computer Methods and Programs in Biomedicine*, 42:39–52.

Davis, C. S. (1996). Non-parametric methods for comparing multiple treatment groups to a control group, based on incomplete non-decreasing repeated measurements. *Statistics in Medicine*, 15:2509–2521.

Davis, C. S. and Hall, D. B. (1996). A computer program for regression analysis of ordered categorical repeated measurements. *Computer Methods and Programs in Biomedicine*, 51:153–169.

Davis, C. S. and Wei, L. J. (1988). Nonparametric methods for analyzing incomplete nondecreasing repeated measurements. *Biometrics*, 44:1005–1018.

Dawson, J. D. (1994). Comparing treatment groups on the basis of slopes, areas-under-the-curve, and other summary measures. *Drug Information Journal*, 28:723–732.

Dawson, J. D. and Lagakos, S. W. (1991). Analyzing laboratory marker changes in AIDS clinical trials. *Journal of Acquired Immune Deficiency Syndromes*, 4:667–676.

Dawson, J. D. and Lagakos, S. W. (1993). Size and power of two-sample tests of repeated measures data. *Biometrics*, 49:1022–1032.

Dawson, K. S., Gennings, C., and Carter, W. H. (1997). Two graphical techniques useful in detecting correlation structure in repeated measures data. *The American Statistician*, 51:275–283.

Deal, E. C., McFadden, E. R., Ingram, R. H., Strauss, R. H., and Jaeger, J. J. (1979). Role of respiratory heat exchange in production of exercise-induced asthma. *Journal of Applied Physiology*, 46:467–475.

Dempster, A. P., Rubin, D. B., and Tsutakawa, R. K. (1981). Estimation in covariance components models. *Journal of the American Statistical Association*, 76:341–353.

Diggle, P. J. (1988). An approach to the analysis of repeated measurements. *Biometrics*, 44:959–971.

Diggle, P. J. (1990). *Time Series: A Biostatistical Introduction.* Oxford University Press, New York.

Diggle, P. J. and Donnelly, J. B. (1989). A selected bibliography on the analysis of repeated measurements and related areas. *Australian Journal of Statistics*, 31:183–193.

Diggle, P. J., Heagerty, P. J., Liang, K. Y., and Zeger, S. L. (2002). *Analysis of Longitudinal Data.* Oxford University Press, Oxford.

Diggle, P. J. and Kenward, M. G. (1994). Informative drop-out in longitudinal data analysis (with discussion). *Applied Statistics*, 43:49–93.

Diggle, P. J., Liang, K. Y., and Zeger, S. L. (1994). *Analysis of Longitudinal Data.* Oxford University Press, Oxford.

Dobson, A. J. (1990). *An Introduction to Generalized Linear Models.* Chapman and Hall, London.

Draper, D. (1987). Comments on "Prediction of future observations in growth curve models". *Statistical Science*, 2:454–461.

Duncan, O. D. (1985). Some models of response uncertainty for panel analysis. *Social Science Research*, 14:126–141.

Duong, Q. P. (1984). On the choice of the order of autoregressive models: A ranking and selection approach. *Journal of Time Series Analysis*, 5:145–157.

Durbin, J. (1951). Incomplete blocks in ranking experiments. *British Journal of Mathematical and Statistical Psychology*, 4:85–90.

Dwyer, J. H., Feinleib, M., Lippert, P., and Hoffmeister, H. (1992). *Statistical Models for Longitudinal Studies of Health.* Oxford University Press, New York.

Elston, R. C. and Grizzle, J. E. (1962). Estimation of time-response curves and their confidence bands. *Biometrics*, 18:148–159.

Emrich, L. J. and Piedmonte, M. R. (1992). On some small sample properties of generalized estimating equation estimates for multivariate dichotomous outcomes. *Journal of Statistical Computation and Simulation*, 41:19–29.

Everitt, B. S. (1994a). Exploring multivariate data graphically: A brief review with examples. *Journal of Applied Statistics*, 21:63–94.

Everitt, B. S. (1994b). *A Handbook of Statistical Analyses Using S-Plus.* Chapman and Hall, London.

Everitt, B. S. (1995). The analysis of repeated measures: A practical review with examples. *Statistician*, 44:113–135.

Ezzet, F. and Whitehead, J. (1991). A random effects model for ordinal responses from a crossover trial. *Statistics in Medicine*, 10:901–906.

Fahrmeir, L. and Tutz, G. (2001). *Multivariate Statistical Modelling Based on Generalized Linear Models*. Springer-Verlag, New York.

Fisher, R. A. (1935). The case of zero survivors. *Annals of Applied Biology*, 22:164–165.

Fitzmaurice, G. M. and Laird, N. M. (1993). A likelihood-based method for analysing longitudinal binary responses. *Biometrika*, 80:141–151.

Fitzmaurice, G. M., Laird, N. M., and Rotnitzky, A. G. (1993). Regression models for discrete longitudinal data. *Statistical Science*, 8:284–309.

Fitzmaurice, G. M. and Lipsitz, S. R. (1995). A model for binary time series data with serial odds ratio patterns. *Applied Statistics*, 44:51–61.

Fitzmaurice, G. M., Lipsitz, S. R., Molenberghs, G., and Ibrahim, J. G. (2001). Bias in estimating association parameters for longitudinal binary responses with drop-outs. *Biometrics*, 57:15–21.

Fleiss, J. L. (1986). *The Design and Analysis of Clinical Experiments*. John Wiley and Sons, New York.

Follmann, D. and Wu, M. (1995). An approximate generalized linear model with random effects for informative missing data. *Biometrics*, 51:151–168.

Follmann, D., Wu, M., and Geller, N. L. (1994). Testing treatment efficacy in clinical trials with repeated binary measurements and missing observations. *Communications in Statistics—Theory and Methods*, 23:557–574.

Friedman, M. (1937). The use of ranks to avoid the assumption of normality implicit in the analysis of variance. *Journal of the American Statistical Association*, 32:675–701.

Frison, L. and Pocock, S. J. (1992). Repeated measures in clinical trials: Analysis using mean summary statistics and its implications for design. *Statistics in Medicine*, 11:1685–1704.

Gange, S. J., Linton, K. L. P., Scott, A. J., DeMets, D. L., and Klein, R. (1995). A comparison of methods for correlated ordinal measures with ophthalmic applications. *Statistics in Medicine*, 14:1961–1974.

Ghosh, M., Grizzle, J. E., and Sen, P. K. (1973). Nonparametric methods in longitudinal studies. *Journal of the American Statistical Association*, 68:29–36.

Gibbons, R. D. and Hedeker, D. (1997). Random effects probit and logistic regression models for three-level data. *Biometrics*, 53:1527–1537.

Gilmour, A. R., Anderson, R. D., and Rae, A. L. (1985). The analysis of binomial data by a generalized linear mixed model. *Biometrika*, 72:593–599.

Girden, E. R. (1992). *ANOVA: Repeated Measures.* Sage Publications, Newbury Park, CA.

Goldstein, H. (1979). *The Design and Analysis of Longitudinal Studies: Their Role in the Measurement of Change.* Academic Press, New York.

Gornbein, J. A., Lazaro, C. G., and Little, R. J. A. (1992). Incomplete data in repeated measures analysis. *Statistical Methods in Medical Research*, 1:275–295.

Gouriéroux, C., Monfort, A., and Trognon, A. (1984). Pseudomaximum likelihood methods: Theory. *Econometrica*, 52:681–700.

Graubard, B. I. and Korn, E. L. (1987). Choice of column scores for testing independence in ordered $2 \times k$ contingency tables. *Biometrics*, 43:471–476.

Graubard, B. I. and Korn, E. L. (1994). Regression analysis with clustered data. *Statistics in Medicine*, 13:509–522.

Greenhouse, S. W. and Geisser, S. (1959). On methods in the analysis of profile data. *Psychometrika*, 24:95–112.

Grizzle, J. E. and Allen, D. M. (1969). Analysis of growth and dose response curves. *Biometrics*, 25:357–381.

Grizzle, J. E., Starmer, C. F., and Koch, G. G. (1969). Analysis of categorical data by linear models. *Biometrics*, 25:489–504.

Groves, L., Shellenberger, M. K., and Davis, C. S. (1998). Tizanidine treatment of spasticity: A meta-analysis of controlled, double-blind, comparative studies with baclofen and diazepam. *Advances in Therapy*, 15:241–251.

Gunsolley, J. C., Getchell, C., and Chinchilli, V. M. (1995). Small sample characteristics of generalized estimating equations. *Communications in Statistics—Simulation and Computation*, 24:869–878.

Hadgu, A. and Koch, G. G. (1999). Application of generalized estimating equations to a dental randomized clinical trial. *Journal of Biopharmaceutical Statistics*, 9:161–178.

Hadgu, A., Koch, G. G., and Westrom, L. (1997). Analysis of ectopic pregnancy data using marginal and conditional models. *Statistics in Medicine*, 16:2403–2417.

Hagenaars, J. A. (1990). *Categorical Longitudinal Data: Log-linear Panel, Trend, and Cohort Analysis.* Sage Publications, Newbury Park, CA.

Hall, D. B. (1994). *Extended Generalized Estimating Equations for Longitudinal Data.* PhD thesis, Northwestern University, Evanston, IL.

Hall, D. B. (2001). On the application of extended quasi-likelihood to the clustered data case. *Canadian Journal of Statistics*, 29:77–97.

Hall, D. B. and Severini, T. A. (1998). Extended generalized estimating equations for clustered data. *Journal of the American Statistical Association*, 93:1365–1375.

Hand, D. J. and Crowder, M. J. (1996). *Practical Longitudinal Data Analysis.* Chapman and Hall, London.

Hand, D. J. and Taylor, C. C. (1987). *Multivariate Analysis of Variance and Repeated Measures.* Chapman and Hall, London.

Hanfelt, J. J. and Liang, K. Y. (1995). Approximate likelihood ratios for general estimating functions. *Biometrika*, 82:461–477.

Hardin, J. and Hilbe, J. (2001). *Generalized Linear Models and Extensions.* Stata Press, College Station, TX.

Hart, J. D. and Wehrly, T. E. (1986). Kernel regression estimation using repeated measurements data. *Journal of the American Statistical Association*, 81:1080–1088.

Harville, D. A. (1977). Maximum likelihood approaches to variance component estimation and to related problems. *Journal of the American Statistical Association*, 72:320–338.

Harville, D. A. and Mee, R. W. (1984). A mixed-model procedure for analyzing ordered categorical data. *Biometrics*, 40:393–408.

Hastie, T. J., Botha, J. L., and Schnitzler, C. M. (1989). Regression with an ordered categorical response. *Statistics in Medicine*, 8:785–794.

Heagerty, P. J. (1999). Marginally specified logistic-normal models for longitudinal binary data. *Biometrics*, 55:688–698.

Heagerty, P. J. and Zeger, S. L. (1996). Marginal regression models for clustered ordinal measurements. *Journal of the American Statistical Association*, 91:1024–1036.

Heagerty, P. J. and Zeger, S. L. (1998). Lorelogram: A regression approach to exploring dependence in longitudinal categorical responses. *Journal of the American Statistical Association*, 93:150–162.

Hedeker, D. and Gibbons, R. D. (1994). A random-effects ordinal regression model for multilevel analysis. *Biometrics*, 50:933–944.

Hedeker, D. and Gibbons, R. D. (1996a). MIXOR: A computer program for mixed-effects ordinal regression analysis. *Computer Methods and Programs in Biomedicine*, 49:157–176.

Hedeker, D. and Gibbons, R. D. (1996b). MIXREG: A computer program for mixed-effects regression analysis with autocorrelated errors. *Computer Methods and Programs in Biomedicine*, 49:229–252.

Henderson, C. R. (1953). Estimation of variance and covariance components. *Biometrics*, 9:226–252.

Hendricks, S. A., Wassell, J. T., Collins, J. W., and Sedlak, S. L. (1996). Power determination for geographically clustered data using generalized estimating equations. *Statistics in Medicine*, 15:1951–1960.

Hettmansperger, T. R. (1984). *Statistical Inference Based on Ranks*. John Wiley and Sons, New York.

Heyting, A., Tolboom, J. T. B. M., and Essers, J. G. A. (1992). Statistical handling of drop-outs in longitudinal clinical trials. *Statistics in Medicine*, 11:2043–2061.

Hills, M. (1968). A note on the analysis of growth curves. *Biometrics*, 24:192–196.

Hirotsu, C. (1991). An approach to comparing treatments based on repeated measures. *Biometrika*, 78:583–594.

Hodges, J. L. and Lehmann, E. L. (1962). Rank methods for combination of independent experiments in analysis of variance. *Annals of Mathematical Statistics*, 33:482–497.

Hoeffding, W. (1948). A class of statistics with asymptotically normal distribution. *Annals of Mathematical Statistics*, 19:293–325.

Hogg, R. V. and Craig, A. T. (1995). *Introduction to Mathematical Statistics*. Prentice-Hall, Englewood Cliffs, NJ.

Hosmer, Jr., D. W. and Lemeshow, S. (2000). *Applied Logistic Regression*. John Wiley and Sons, New York.

Hotelling, H. (1931). The generalization of Student's ratio. *Annals of Mathematical Statistics*, 2:360–378.

Hotelling, H. (1947). Multivariate quality control, illustrated by the air testing of sample bombsights. In Eisenhart, C., Hastay, M., and Wallis, W. A., editors, *Techniques of Statistical Analysis*, pages 111–184. McGraw-Hill, New York.

Hotelling, H. (1951). A generalized T test and measure of multivariate dispersion. In Neyman, J., editor, *Proceedings of the Second Berkeley Symposium on Mathematical Statistics and Probability*, pages 23–41, Los Angeles and Berkeley, CA. University of California.

Huynh, H. (1978). Some approximate tests for repeat measurement designs. *Psychometrika*, 43:161–175.

Huynh, H. and Feldt, L. S. (1970). Conditions under which mean square ratios in repeated measurement designs have exact F-distributions. *Journal of the American Statistical Association*, 65:1582–1589.

Huynh, H. and Feldt, L. S. (1976). Estimation of the Box correction for degrees of freedom from sample data in randomized block and split-plot designs. *Journal of Educational Statistics*, 1:69–82.

Ito, K. (1962). A comparison of the powers of two multivariate analysis of variance tests. *Biometrika*, 49:455–462.

Jansen, J. (1990). On the statistical analysis of ordinal data when extravariation is present. *Applied Statistics*, 39:75–84.

Jennrich, R. I. and Schluchter, M. D. (1986). Unbalanced repeated-measures models with structured covariance matrices. *Biometrics*, 42:805–820.

Johnson, N. L., Kotz, S., and Balakrishnan, N. (1997). *Discrete Multivariate Distributions.* John Wiley and Sons, New York.

Jones, R. H. (1981). Fitting continuous-time autoregressions to discrete data. In Findley, D. F., editor, *Applied Time Series Analysis II*, pages 651–682. Academic Press, New York.

Jones, R. H. (1993). *Longitudinal Data with Serial Correlation: A State-Space Approach.* Chapman and Hall, London.

Jones, R. H. and Boadi-Boateng, F. (1991). Unequally spaced longitudinal data with AR(1) serial correlation. *Biometrics*, 47:161–175.

Kalbfleisch, J. D. and Lawless, J. F. (1985). The analysis of panel data under a Markov assumption. *Journal of the American Statistical Association*, 80:863–871.

Kalbfleisch, J. D. and Prentice, R. L. (1980). *The Statistical Analysis of Failure Time Data.* John Wiley and Sons, New York.

Karim, M. R. and Zeger, S. L. (1988). GEE: A SAS macro for longitudinal data analysis. Technical Report 674, Department of Biostatistics, The Johns Hopkins University, Baltimore.

Kaufmann, H. (1987). Regression models for nonstationary categorical time series: Asymptotic estimation theory. *Annals of Statistics*, 15:79–98.

Kenward, M. G. (1987). A method for comparing profiles of repeated measurements. *Applied Statistics*, 36:296–308.

Kenward, M. G. (1998). Selection models for repeated measurements with non-random dropout: An illustration of sensitivity. *Statistics in Medicine*, 17:2723–2732.

Kenward, M. G. and Jones, B. (1992). Alternative approaches to the analysis of binary and categorical repeated measurements. *Journal of Biopharmaceutical Statistics*, 2:137–170.

Kenward, M. G., Lesaffre, E., and Molenberghs, G. (1994). An application of maximum likelihood and generalized estimating equations to the analysis of ordinal data from a longitudinal study with cases missing at random. *Biometrics*, 50:945–953.

Kenward, M. G. and Molenberghs, G. (1999). Parametric models for incomplete continuous and categorical longitudinal data. *Statistical Methods in Medical Research*, 8:51–83.

Kepner, J. L. and Robinson, D. H. (1988). Nonparametric methods for detecting treatment effects in repeated-measures designs. *Journal of the American Statistical Association*, 83:456–461.

Khatri, C. G. (1966). A note on a MANOVA model applied to problems in growth curves. *Annals of the Institute of Statistical Mathematics*, 18:75–86.

Kirby, A. J., Galai, N., and Muñoz, A. (1994). Sample size estimation using repeated measurements on biomarkers as outcomes. *Controlled Clinical Trials*, 15:165–172.

Kleinbaum, D. G. (1973). A generalization of the growth curve model which allows missing data. *Journal of Multivariate Analysis*, 3:117–124.

Knuth, D. E. (1986). *The TEXbook*. Addison-Wesley, Reading, MA.

Koch, G. G. (1969). Some aspects of the statistical analysis of "split plot" experiments in completely randomized layouts. *Journal of the American Statistical Association*, 64:485–505.

Koch, G. G. (1970). The use of non-parametric methods in the statistical analysis of a complex split plot experiment. *Biometrics*, 26:105–128.

Koch, G. G., Amara, I. A., Stokes, M. E., and Gillings, D. B. (1980). Some views on parametric and non-parametric analysis for repeated measurements and selected bibliography. *International Statistical Review*, 48:249–265.

Koch, G. G., Landis, J. R., Freeman, J. L., Freeman, Jr., D. H., and Lehnen, R. G. (1977). A general methodology for the analysis of experiments with repeated measurement of categorical data. *Biometrics*, 33:133–158.

Koch, G. G. and Reinfurt, D. W. (1971). The analysis of categorical data from mixed models. *Biometrics*, 27:157–173.

Koch, G. G. and Sen, P. K. (1968). Some aspects of the statistical analysis of the mixed model. *Biometrics*, 24:27–48.

Korn, E. L. and Whittemore, A. S. (1979). Methods for analyzing panel studies of acute health effects of air pollution. *Biometrics*, 35:795–802.

Koziol, J. A., Maxwell, D. A., Fukushima, M., Colmerauer, M. E. M., and Pilch, Y. H. (1981). A distribution-free test for tumor-growth curve analyses with application to an animal tumor immunotherapy experiment. *Biometrics*, 37:383–390.

Kruskal, W. H. and Wallis, W. A. (1952). Use of ranks in one-criterion variance analysis. *Journal of the American Statistical Association*, 47:583–621.

Kshirsagar, A. M. and Smith, W. B. (1995). *Growth Curves*. Marcel Dekker, New York.

Kuk, A. Y. C. (1995). Asymptotically unbiased estimation in generalized linear models with random effects. *Journal of the Royal Statistical Society, Series B*, 57:395–407.

Lachin, J. M. (1992). Some large-sample distribution-free estimators and tests for multivariate partially incomplete data from two populations. *Statistics in Medicine*, 11:1151–1170.

Laird, N. M. (1988). Missing data in longitudinal studies. *Statistics in Medicine*, 7:305–315.

Laird, N. M. and Lange, N. (1987). Comments on "Prediction of future observations in growth curve models". *Statistical Science*, 2:451–454.

Laird, N. M., Lange, N., and Stram, D. (1987). Maximum likelihood computations with repeated measures: Application of the EM algorithm. *Journal of the American Statistical Association*, 82:97–105.

Laird, N. M. and Ware, J. H. (1982). Random-effects models for longitudinal data. *Biometrics*, 38:963–974.

Landis, J. R., Heyman, E. R., and Koch, G. G. (1978). Average partial association in three-way contingency tables: A review and discussion of alternative tests. *International Statistical Review*, 46:237–254.

Landis, J. R., Miller, M. E., Davis, C. S., and Koch, G. G. (1988). Some general methods for the analysis of categorical data in longitudinal studies. *Statistics in Medicine*, 7:233–261.

LaVange, L. M., Koch, G. G., and Schwartz, T. A. (2001). Applying sample survey methods to clinical trials data. *Statistics in Medicine*, 20:2609–2623.

Lawley, D. N. (1938). A generalization of Fisher's z test. *Biometrika*, 30:180–187.

Lee, E. W. and Dubin, N. (1994). Estimation and sample size considerations for clustered binary responses. *Statistics in Medicine*, 13:1241–1252.

Lee, Y. S. (1971). Asymptotic formulae for the distribution of a multivariate test statistic: Power comparisons of certain multivariate tests. *Biometrika*, 58:647–651.

Lefante, J. J. (1990). The power to detect differences in average rates of change in longitudinal studies. *Statistics in Medicine*, 9:437–446.

Lehmann, E. L. (1951). Consistency and unbiasedness of certain nonparametric tests. *Annals of Mathematical Statistics*, 22:165–179.

Lehmann, E. L. (1963). Robust estimation in analysis of variance. *Annals of Mathematical Statistics*, 34:957–966.

Lehmann, E. L. (1998). *Nonparametrics: Statistical Methods Based on Ranks.* Prentice-Hall, Upper Saddle River, NJ.

Leppik, I. E., Dreifuss, F. E., Porter, R., Bowman, T., Santilli, N., Jacobs, M., Crosby, C., Cloyd, J., Stackman, J., Graves, N., Sutula, T., Welty, T., Vickery, J., Brundage, R., Gates, J., Gumnit, R. J., and Gutierrez, A. (1987). A controlled study of progabide in partial seizures: Methodology and results. *Neurology*, 37:963–968.

Lesaffre, E., Molenberghs, G., and DeWulf, L. (1996). Effect of dropouts in a longitudinal study: An application of a repeated ordinal model. *Statistics in Medicine*, 15:1123–1141.

Li, N. (1994). *Analysis of Longitudinal Data Using Weighted Least Squares and Generalized Estimating Equations.* PhD thesis, University of Iowa, Iowa City, IA.

Liang, K. Y. and Zeger, S. L. (1986). Longitudinal data analysis using generalized linear models. *Biometrika*, 73:13–22.

Liang, K. Y. and Zeger, S. L. (1993). Regression analysis for correlated data. *Annual Review of Public Health*, 14:43–68.

Liang, K. Y., Zeger, S. L., and Qaqish, B. (1992). Multivariate regression analyses for categorical data (with discussion). *Journal of the Royal Statistical Society, Series B*, 54:3–40.

Lindsey, J. K. (1999). *Models for Repeated Measurements.* Oxford University Press, New York.

Lindsey, J. K. and Lambert, P. (1998). On the appropriateness of marginal models for repeated measurements in clinical trials. *Statistics in Medicine*, 17:447–469.

Lindsey, P. J. (2001). Adapting sample size calculations to repeated measurements in clinical trials. *Journal of Applied Statistics*, 28:81–89.

Lindstrom, M. J. and Bates, D. M. (1988). Newton-Raphson and EM algorithms for linear mixed-effects models for repeated-measures data. *Journal of the American Statistical Association*, 83:1014–1022.

Lipsitz, S. R. and Fitzmaurice, G. M. (1994). Sample size for repeated measures studies with binary responses. *Statistics in Medicine*, 13:1233–1239.

Lipsitz, S. R., Fitzmaurice, G. M., Orav, E. J., and Laird, N. M. (1994a). Performance of generalized estimating equations in practical situations. *Biometrics*, 50:270–278.

Lipsitz, S. R. and Harrington, D. P. (1990). Analyzing correlated binary data using SAS. *Computers and Biomedical Research*, 23:268–282.

Lipsitz, S. R., Kim, K., and Zhao, L. (1994b). Analysis of repeated categorical data using generalized estimating equations. *Statistics in Medicine*, 13:1149–1163.

Lipsitz, S. R., Laird, N. M., and Harrington, D. P. (1991). Generalized estimating equations for correlated binary data: Using the odds ratio as a measure of association. *Biometrika*, 78:153–160.

Lipsitz, S. R., Molenberghs, G., Fitzmaurice, G. M., and Ibrahim, J. G. (2000). GEE with Gaussian estimation of the correlations when data are incomplete. *Biometrics*, 56:528–536.

Little, R. J. A. (1995). Modeling the drop-out mechanism in repeated-measures studies. *Journal of the American Statistical Association*, 90:1112–1121.

Little, R. J. A. and Rubin, D. B. (1987). *Statistical Analysis with Missing Data.* John Wiley and Sons, New York.

Liu, G. and Liang, K. Y. (1997). Sample size calculations for studies with correlated observations. *Biometrics*, 53:937–947.

Longford, N. T. (1994). Logistic regression with random coefficients. *Computational Statistics and Data Analysis*, 17:1–15.

Lui, K. J. (1991). Sample sizes for repeated measurements in dichotomous data. *Statistics in Medicine*, 10:463–472.

Lui, K. J. and Cumberland, W. G. (1992). Sample size requirement for repeated measurements in continuous data. *Statistics in Medicine*, 11:633–641.

Macknin, M. L., Mathew, S., and Medendorp, S. V. (1990). Effect of inhaling heated vapor on symptoms of the common cold. *Journal of the American Medical Association*, 264:989–991.

MacMillan, J., Becker, C., Koch, G. G., Stokes, M., and Vandivire, H. M. (1981). An application of weighted least squares methods to the analysis of measurement process components of variability in an observational study. In *American Statistical Association Proceedings of Survey Research Methods*, pages 680–685, Alexandria, VA. American Statistical Association.

Madansky, A. (1963). Test of homogeneity for correlated samples. *Journal of the American Statistical Association*, 58:97–119.

Makuch, R. W., Escobar, M., and Merrill, III, S. (1991). Algorithm AS 262: A two-sample test for incomplete multivariate data. *Applied Statistics*, 40:202–212.

Mann, H. B. and Whitney, D. R. (1947). On a test of whether one of two random variables is stochastically larger than the other. *Annals of Mathematical Statistics*, 18:50–60.

Mantel, N. and Fleiss, J. L. (1980). Minimum expected cell size requirements for the Mantel-Haenszel one-degree-of-freedom chi-square test and a related rapid procedure. *American Journal of Epidemiology*, 112:129–134.

Mantel, N. and Haenszel, W. (1959). Statistical aspects of the analysis of data from retrospective studies of disease. *Journal of the National Cancer Institute*, 22:719–748.

Matthews, J. N. S. (1993). A refinement to the analysis of serial data using summary measures. *Statistics in Medicine*, 12:27–37.

Matthews, J. N. S., Altman, D. G., Campbell, M. J., and Royston, P. (1990). Analysis of serial measurements in medical research. *British Medical Journal*, 300:230–235.

Mauchly, J. W. (1940). Significance test for sphericity of a normal n-variate distribution. *Annals of Mathematical Statistics*, 29:204–209.

Mauger, J. W., Chilko, D., and Howard, S. (1986). On the analysis of dissolution data. *Drug Development and Industrial Pharmacy*, 12:969–992.

Mauritsen, R. H. (1984). *Logistic Regression with Random Effects*. PhD thesis, University of Washington, Seattle, WA.

McCullagh, P. (1980). Regression models for ordinal data. *Journal of the Royal Statistical Society, Series B*, 42:109–142.

McCullagh, P. (1983). Quasi-likelihood functions. *Annals of Statistics*, 11:59–67.

McCullagh, P. and Nelder, J. A. (1989). *Generalized Linear Models*. Chapman and Hall, London.

McCulloch, C. E. and Searle, S. R. (2000). *Generalized, Linear, and Mixed Models*. John Wiley and Sons, New York.

McGilchrist, C. A. (1994). Estimation in generalized mixed models. *Journal of the Royal Statistical Society, Series B*, 56:61–69.

McLean, R. A., Sanders, W. L., and Stroup, W. W. (1991). A unified approach to mixed linear models. *The American Statistician*, 45:54–64.

McNemar, Q. (1947). Note on the sampling error of the difference between correlated proportions or percentages. *Psychometrika*, 12:153–157.

Michiels, B. and Molenberghs, G. (1997). Protective estimation of longitudinal categorical data with nonrandom dropout. *Communications in Statistics—Theory and Methods*, 26:65–94.

Mikhail, N. N. (1965). A comparison of tests of the Wilks-Lawley hypothesis in multivariate analysis. *Biometrika*, 52:149–156.

Miller, M. E., Davis, C. S., and Landis, J. R. (1993). The analysis of longitudinal polytomous data: Generalized estimating equations and connections with weighted least squares. *Biometrics*, 49:1033–1044.

Mislevy, R. J. (1985). Estimation of latent group effects. *Journal of the American Statistical Association*, 80:993–997.

Molenberghs, G., Kenward, M. G., and Lesaffre, E. (1997). The analysis of longitudinal ordinal data with nonrandom drop-out. *Biometrika*, 84:33–44.

Molenberghs, G. and Lesaffre, E. (1994). Marginal modeling of correlated ordinal data using a multivariate Plackett distribution. *Journal of the American Statistical Association*, 89:633–644.

Moore, D. S. and McCabe, G. P. (1993). *Introduction to the Practice of Statistics*. W.H. Freeman and Company, New York.

Mori, M., Woodworth, G. G., and Woolson, R. F. (1992). Application of empirical Bayes inference to estimation of rate of change in the presence of informative right censoring. *Statistics in Medicine*, 11:621–631.

Mori, M., Woolson, R. F., and Woodworth, G. G. (1994). Slope estimation in the presence of informative right censoring: Modeling the number of observations as a geometric random variable. *Biometrics*, 50:39–50.

Morrison, D. F. (1976). *Multivariate Statistical Methods*. McGraw-Hill, New York.

Moulton, L. H. and Zeger, S. L. (1989). Analyzing repeated measures on generalized linear models via the bootstrap. *Biometrics*, 45:381–394.

Muñoz, A., Carey, V., Schouten, J. P., Segal, M., and Rosner, B. (1992). A parametric family of correlation structures for the analysis of longitudinal data. *Biometrics*, 48:733–742.

Muenz, R. and Rubinstein, L. V. (1985). Markov models for covariate dependence of binary sequences. *Biometrics*, 41:91–101.

Müller, H. G. (1988). *Nonparametric Regression Analysis of Longitudinal Data*. Springer-Verlag, Berlin.

Muller, K. E. and Barton, C. N. (1989). Approximate power for repeated-measures ANOVA lacking sphericity. *Journal of the American Statistical Association*, 84:549–555.

Muller, K. E., LaVange, L. M., Ramey, S. L., and Ramey, C. T. (1992). Power calculations for general linear multivariate models including repeated measures applications. *Journal of the American Statistical Association*, 87:1209–1226.

Nanda, D. N. (1950). Distribution of the sum of roots of a determinantal equation. *Annals of Mathematical Statistics*, 21:432–439.

Nelder, J. A. and Pregibon, D. (1987). An extended quasi-likelihood function. *Biometrika*, 74:221–232.

Nelder, J. A. and Wedderburn, R. W. M. (1972). Generalized linear models. *Journal of the Royal Statistical Society, Series A*, 135:370–384.

Nesselroade, J. R. and Baltes, P. B. (1980). *Longitudinal Methodology in the Study of Behavior and Development*. Academic Press, New York.

Neter, J., Wasserman, W., and Kutner, M. H. (1985). *Applied Linear Statistical Models: Regression, Analysis of Variance, and Experimental Designs*. R.D. Irwin, Homewood, IL.

Neuhaus, J. M. (1992). Statistical methods for longitudinal and clustered designs with binary responses. *Statistical Methods in Medical Research*, 1:249–273.

Neuhaus, J. M. and Jewell, N. P. (1990). Some comments on Rosner's multiple logistic model for clustered data. *Biometrics*, 46:523–531.

Neuhaus, J. M., Kalbfleisch, J. D., and Hauck, W. W. (1991). A comparison of cluster-specific and population-averaged approaches for analyzing correlated binary data. *International Statistical Review*, 59:25–35.

Núñez Antón, V. A. (1993). *Analysis of Longitudinal Data with Unequally Spaced Observations and Time Dependent Correlated Errors*. PhD thesis, University of Iowa, Iowa City, IA.

Núñez Antón, V. A. and Zimmerman, D. L. (2000). Modelling nonstationary longitudinal data. *Biometrics*, 56:699–705.

O'Brien, P. C. (1984). Procedures for comparing samples with multiple endpoints. *Biometrics*, 40:1079–1087.

Olson, C. L. (1974). Comparative robustness of six tests in multivariate analysis of variance. *Journal of the American Statistical Association*, 69:894–908.

Omar, R. Z., Wright, E. M., Turner, R. M., and Thompson, S. G. (1999). Analyzing repeated measurements data: A practical comparison of methods. *Statistics in Medicine*, 18:1587–1603.

Overall, J. E., Ahn, C., Shivakumar, C., and Kalburgi, Y. (1999). Problematic formulations of SAS PROC.MIXED models for repeated measurements. *Journal of Biopharmaceutical Statistics*, 9:189–216.

Overall, J. E. and Doyle, S. R. (1994). Estimating sample sizes for repeated measurement designs. *Controlled Clinical Trials*, 15:100–123.

Overall, J. E., Shobaki, G., and Anderson, C. B. (1998). Comparative evaluation of two models for estimating sample sizes for tests on trends across repeated measurements. *Controlled Clinical Trials*, 19:188–197.

Page, E. B. (1963). Ordered hypotheses for multiple treatments: A significance test for linear ranks. *Journal of the American Statistical Association*, 58:216–230.

Paik, M. C. (1988). Repeated measurement analysis for nonnormal data in small samples. *Communications in Statistics—Simulation and Computation*, 17:1155–1171.

Paik, M. C. (1997). The generalized estimating equation approach when data are not missing completely at random. *Journal of the American Statistical Association*, 92:1320–1329.

Palesch, Y. Y. and Lachin, J. M. (1994). Asymptotically distribution-free multivariate rank tests for multiple samples with partially incomplete observations. *Statistica Sinica*, 4:373–387.

Pan, J. X. and Fang, K. T. (2001). *Growth Curve Models with Statistical Diagnostics*. Springer-Verlag, New York.

Pan, W. (2001a). Akaike's information criterion in generalized estimating equations. *Biometrics*, 57:120–125.

Pan, W. (2001b). Sample size and power calculations with correlated binary data. *Controlled Clinical Trials*, 22:211–227.

Pandit, S. M. and Wu, S. M. (1983). *Time Series and System Analysis with Applications*. John Wiley and Sons, New York.

Parhizgari, A. M. and Prakash, A. J. (1989). Algorithm AS 250: Tests of the equality of dispersion matrices. *Applied Statistics*, 38:553–564.

Park, T. (1993). A comparison of the generalized estimating equation approach with the maximum likelihood approach for repeated measurements. *Statistics in Medicine*, 12:1723–1732.

Park, T. and Davis, C. S. (1993). A test of the missing data mechanism for repeated categorical data. *Biometrics*, 49:631–638.

Park, T., Davis, C. S., and Li, N. (1998). Alternative GEE estimation procedures for discrete longitudinal data. *Computational Statistics and Data Analysis*, 28:243–256.

Park, T., Park, J. K., and Davis, C. S. (2001). Effects of covariance model assumptions on hypothesis tests for repeated measurements: Analysis of ovarian hormone data and pituitary-pteryomaxillary distance data. *Statistics in Medicine*, 20:2441–2453.

Park, T. and Woolson, R. F. (1992). Generalized multivariate models for longitudinal data. *Communications in Statistics—Simulation and Computation*, 21:925–946.

Patel, H. I. (1986). Analysis of repeated measures designs with changing covariates in clinical trials. *Biometrika*, 73:707–715.

Patel, H. I. (1991). Analysis of incomplete data from a clinical trial with repeated measurements. *Biometrika*, 78:609–619.

Patterson, H. D. and Thompson, R. (1971). Recovery of inter-block information when block sizes are unequal. *Biometrika*, 58:545–554.

Pearson, E. S. and Hartley, H. O. (1966). *Biometrika Tables for Statisticians, Volume I.* Cambridge University Press, Cambridge.

Pendergast, J. F., Gange, S. J., Newton, M. A., Lindstrom, M. J., Palta, M., and Fisher, M. R. (1996). A survey of methods for analyzing clustered binary response data. *International Statistical Review*, 64:89–118.

Pepe, M. S. and Anderson, G. L. (1994). A cautionary note on inference for marginal regression models with longitudinal data and general correlated response data. *Communications in Statistics—Simulation and Computation*, 23:939–951.

Peterson, B. and Harrell, Jr., F. E. (1990). Partial proportional odds models for ordinal response variables. *Applied Statistics*, 39:205–217.

Pickles, A. (1990). *Longitudinal Data and the Analysis of Change.* Oxford University Press, New York.

Pillai, K. C. S. (1955). Some new test criteria in multivariate analysis. *Annals of Mathematical Statistics*, 26:117–121.

Pillai, K. C. S. and Jayachandran, K. (1967). Power comparisons of tests of two multivariate hypotheses based on four criteria. *Biometrika*, 54:195–210.

Plewis, I. (1985). *Analysing Change: Measurement and Explanation Using Longitudinal Data.* John Wiley and Sons, New York.

Pocock, S. J. (1983). *Clinical Trials: A Practical Approach.* John Wiley and Sons, New York.

Potthoff, R. F. and Roy, S. N. (1964). A generalized multivariate analysis of variance model useful especially for growth curve problems. *Biometrika*, 51:313–326.

Pourahmadi, M. (1999). Joint mean-covariance models with applications to longitudinal data: Unconstrained parameterisation. *Biometrika*, 86:677–690.

Preisser, J. S. and Qaqish, B. F. (1996). Deletion diagnostics for generalised estimating equations. *Biometrika*, 83:551–562.

Prentice, R. L. (1988). Correlated binary regression with covariates specific to each binary observation. *Biometrics*, 44:1033–1048.

Prentice, R. L. and Zhao, L. P. (1991). Estimating equations for parameters in means and covariances of multivariate discrete and continuous responses. *Biometrics*, 47:825–839.

Pulkstenis, E., Ten Have, T. R., and Landis, J. R. (1998). Model for the analysis of binary longitudinal pain data subject to informative dropout through remedication. *Journal of the American Statistical Association*, 93:438–450.

Pulkstenis, E., Ten Have, T. R., and Landis, J. R. (2001). A mixed effects model for the analysis of ordinal longitudinal pain data subject to informative drop-out. *Statistics in Medicine*, 20:601–622.

Puri, M. L. and Sen, P. K. (1971). *Nonparametric Methods in Multivariate Analysis*. John Wiley and Sons, New York.

Randles, R. H. and Wolfe, D. A. (1979). *Introduction to the Theory of Nonparametric Statistics*. John Wiley and Sons, New York.

Rao, C. R. (1965). The theory of least squares when the parameters are stochastic and its application to the analysis of growth curves. *Biometrika*, 52:447–458.

Rao, C. R. (1966). Covariance adjustment and related problems in multivariate analysis. In Krishnaiah, P. R., editor, *Multivariate Analysis*, pages 87–103. Academic Press, New York.

Rao, C. R. (1967). Least squares theory using an estimated dispersion matrix and its application to measurement of signals. In *Proceedings of the Fifth Berkeley Symposium on Mathematical Statistics and Probability, Volume I*, pages 355–372, Berkeley, CA. University of California.

Rao, C. R. (1973). *Linear Statistical Inference and Its Applications*. John Wiley and Sons, New York.

Rao, C. R. (1987). Prediction of future observations in growth curve models. *Statistical Science*, 2:434–447.

Raz, J. (1989). Analysis of repeated measurements using nonparametric smoothers and randomization tests. *Biometrics*, 45:851–871.

Reiczigel, J. (1999). Analysis of experimental data with repeated measurements. *Biometrics*, 55:1059–1063.

Robins, J. M., Rotnitzky, A., and Zhao, L. P. (1995). Analysis of semiparametric regression models for repeated outcomes in the presence of missing data. *Journal of the American Statistical Association*, 90:106–121.

Rochon, J. (1989). The application of the GSK method to the determination of minimum sample sizes. *Biometrics*, 45:193–205.

Rochon, J. (1991). Sample size calculations for two-group repeated-measures experiments. *Biometrics*, 47:1383–1398.

Rochon, J. (1998). Application of GEE procedures for sample size calculations in repeated measures experiments. *Statistics in Medicine*, 17:1643–1658.

Rosner, B. (1984). Multivariate methods in ophthalmology with application to other paired-data situations. *Biometrics*, 40:1025–1035.

Rothenberg, T. J. (1977). Edgeworth expansions for multivariate test statistics. Technical Report IP-255, Center for Research in Management Science, University of California, Berkeley.

Rotnitzky, A. and Jewell, N. P. (1990). Hypothesis testing of regression parameters in semiparametric generalized linear models for cluster correlated data. *Biometrika*, 77:485–497.

Rotnitzky, A., Robins, J. M., and Scharfstein, D. O. (1998). Semiparametric regression for repeated outcomes with nonignorable nonresponse. *Journal of the American Statistical Association*, 93:1321–1339.

Rotnitzky, A. and Wypij, D. (1994). A note on the bias of estimators with missing data. *Biometrics*, 50:1163–1170.

Roy, S. N. (1957). *Some Aspects of Multivariate Analysis*. John Wiley and Sons, New York.

Roy, S. N. and Bargmann, R. E. (1958). Tests of multiple independence and the associated confidence bounds. *Annals of Mathematical Statistics*, 29:491–503.

Roy, S. N., Gnanadesikan, R., and Srivastava, J. N. (1971). *Analysis and Design of Certain Quantitative Multiresponse Experiments*. Pergamon Press, Oxford.

Royall, R. M. (1986). Model robust confidence intervals using maximum likelihood estimators. *International Statistical Review*, 54:221–226.

Russell, T. S. and Bradley, R. A. (1958). One-way variances in a two-way classification. *Biometrika*, 45:111–129.

SAS Institute (1999). *SAS/STAT User's Guide, Version 8*. SAS Institute, Cary, NC.

Schafer, J. L. (1997). *Analysis of Incomplete Multivariate Data*. Chapman and Hall, London.

Schall, R. (1991). Estimation in generalized linear models with random effects. *Biometrika*, 78:719–727.

Schatzoff, M. (1966). Sensitivity comparisons among tests of the general linear hypothesis. *Journal of the American Statistical Association*, 61:415–435.

Scheffé, H. (1959). *The Analysis of Variance*. John Wiley and Sons, New York.

Schwarz, G. (1978). Estimating the dimension of a model. *Annals of Statistics*, 6:461–464.

Schwertman, N. C. (1982). Algorithm AS 174: Multivariate multisample non-parametric tests. *Applied Statistics*, 31:80–85.

Schwertman, N. C. (1985). Multivariate median and rank sum tests. In Kotz, S., Johnson, N. L., and Read, C. B., editors, *Encyclopedia of Statistical Sciences, Volume 6*, pages 85–88. John Wiley and Sons, New York.

Searle, S. R. (1982). *Matrix Algebra Useful for Statistics*. John Wiley and Sons, New York.

Self, S. G. and Mauritsen, R. H. (1988). Power/sample size calculations for generalized linear models. *Biometrics*, 44:79–86.

Self, S. G., Mauritsen, R. H., and Ohara, J. (1992). Power calculations for likelihood ratio tests in generalized linear models. *Biometrics*, 48:31–39.

Sen, P. K. (1984). Nonparametric procedures for some miscellaneous problems. In Krishnaiah, P. R. and Sen, P. K., editors, *Handbook of Statistics, Volume 4: Nonparametric Methods*, pages 699–739. Elsevier Science Publishers, Amsterdam.

Shah, B. V., Holt, M. M., and Folsom, R. E. (1977). Inference about regression models from sample survey data. *Bulletin of the International Statistical Institute*, 47:43–57.

Shapiro, S. S. and Wilk, M. B. (1965). An analysis of variance test for normality (complete samples). *Biometrika*, 52:591–611.

Sharples, K. and Breslow, N. (1992). Regression analysis of correlated binary data: Some small sample results for the estimating equation approach. *Journal of Statistical Computation and Simulation*, 42:1–20.

Shaw, D., Bijnens, L., and Senden, J. (1994). Generalised estimating equations for repeated measures designs resulting in categorical data. Unpublished SAS macro.

Sheiner, L. B., Beal, S. L., and Dunne, A. (1997). Analysis of nonrandomly censored ordered categorical longitudinal data from analgesic trials. *Journal of the American Statistical Association*, 92:1235–1244.

Shih, W. J. (1997). Sample size and power calculations for periodontal and other studies with clustered samples using the method of generalized estimating equations. *Biometrical Journal*, 39:899–908.

Shoukri, M. M. and Martin, S. W. (1992). Estimating the number of clusters for the analysis of correlated binary response variables from unbalanced data. *Statistics in Medicine*, 11:751–760.

Shults, J. and Chaganty, N. R. (1998). Analysis of serially-correlated data using quasi-least squares. *Biometrics*, 54:1622–1630.

Simpson, G. M. and Angus, J. W. (1970). A rating scale for extrapyramidal side effects. *Acta Psychiatrica Scandinavica, Supplementum*, 212:11–19.

Stanek, III, E. J. and Diehl, S. R. (1988). Growth curve models of repeated binary response. *Biometrics*, 44:973–983.

Stanek, III, E. J. and Koch, G. G. (1985). The equivalence of parameter estimates from growth curve models and seemingly unrelated regression models. *The American Statistician*, 39:149–152.

Stanish, W. M. (1986). Categorical data analysis strategies using SAS software. In Allen, D. M., editor, *Computer Science and Statistics: Proceedings of the 17th Symposium on the Interface*, pages 239–256, New York. Elsevier Science Publishers.

Stanish, W. M., Gillings, D. B., and Koch, G. G. (1978). An application of multivariate ratio methods for the analysis of a longitudinal clinical trial with missing data. *Biometrics*, 34:305–317.

Stanish, W. M. and Koch, G. G. (1984). The use of CATMOD for repeated measurement analysis of categorical data. In *Proceedings of the 9th Annual SAS Users Group International Conference*, pages 761–770, Cary, NC. SAS Institute Inc.

Stasny, E. A. (1987). Some Markov-chain models for nonresponse in estimating gross labor force flows. *Journal of Official Statistics*, 3:359–373.

Stata Corporation (2001). *Stata Reference Manual.* Stata Press, College Station, TX.

Sterczer, A., Vörös, K., and Karsai, F. (1996). Effect of cholagogues on the volume of the gallbladder of dogs. *Research in Veterinary Science*, 60:44–47.

Stiratelli, R., Laird, N. M., and Ware, J. H. (1984). Random-effects models for serial observations with binary response. *Biometrics*, 40:961–971.

Stock, J. R., Weaver, J. K., Ray, H. W., Brink, J. R., and Sadoff, M. G. (1983). *Evaluation of Safe Performance Secondary School Driver Education Curriculum Demonstration Project.* U.S. Department of Transportation, National Highway Traffic Safety Administration, Washington, DC.

Stram, D. O., Wei, L. J., and Ware, J. H. (1988). Analysis of repeated ordered categorical outcomes with possibly missing observations and time-dependent covariates. *Journal of the American Statistical Association*, 83:631–637.

SUDAAN (2001). *SUDAAN User Manual, Release 8.0.* Research Triangle Institute, Research Triangle Park, NC.

Ten Have, T. R. (1996). A mixed effects model for multivariate ordinal response data including correlated discrete failure times with ordinal responses. *Biometrics*, 52:473–491.

Ten Have, T. R., Kunselman, A. R., Pulkstenis, E. P., and Landis, J. R. (1998). Mixed effects logistic regression models for longitudinal binary response data with informative drop-out. *Biometrics*, 54:367–383.

Ten Have, T. R., Landis, J. R., and Hartzel, J. (1996). Population-averaged and cluster-specific models for clustered ordinal response data. *Statistics in Medicine*, 15:2573–2588.

Thall, P. F. and Lachin, J. M. (1988). Analysis of recurrent events: Nonparametric methods for random-interval count data. *Journal of the American Statistical Association*, 83:339–347.

Thall, P. F. and Vail, S. C. (1990). Some covariance models for longitudinal count data with overdispersion. *Biometrics*, 46:657–671.

Thompson, G. L. (1991). A unified approach to rank tests for multivariate and repeated measures designs. *Journal of the American Statistical Association*, 86:410–419.

Thompson, Jr., W. A. (1962). The problem of negative estimates of variance components. *Annals of Mathematical Statistics*, 33:273–289.

Timm, N. H. (1980). Multivariate analysis of variance of repeated measurements. In Krishnaiah, P. R. and Sen, P. K., editors, *Handbook of Statistics, Volume 1: Analysis of Variance*, pages 41–87. Elsevier Science Publishers, Amsterdam.

van Elteren, P. H. (1960). On the combination of independent two-sample tests of Wilcoxon. *Bulletin de l'Institut Internationale de Statistique*, 37:351–361.

Vasey, M. W. and Thayer, J. F. (1987). The continuing problem of false positives in repeated measures ANOVA in psychophysiology: A multivariate solution. *Psychophysiology*, 24:479–486.

Verbeke, G. and Molenberghs, G. (1997). *Linear Mixed Models in Practice.* Springer-Verlag, New York.

Verbeke, G. and Molenberghs, G. (2000). *Linear Mixed Models for Longitudinal Data.* Springer-Verlag, New York.

Verbeke, G., Molenberghs, G., Thijs, H., Lesaffre, E., and Kenward, M. G. (2001). Sensitivity analysis for non-random dropout: A local influence approach. *Biometrics*, 57:7–14.

Verbyla, A. P. (1988). Analysis of repeated measures designs with changing covariates. *Biometrika*, 75:172–174.

Verbyla, A. P. and Venables, W. N. (1988). An extension of the growth curve model. *Biometrika*, 75:129–138.

Volberding, P. A., Lagakos, S. W., Koch, M. A., Pettinelli, C., Myers, M. W., Booth, D. K., Balfour, Jr., H. H., Reichman, R. C., Bartlett, J. A., Hirsch, M. S., Murphy, M., Hardy, W. D., Soeiro, R., Fischl, M. A., Bartlett, J. G., Merigan, T. C., Hyslop, N. E., Richman, D. D., Valentine, F. T., and Corey, L. (1990). Zidovudine in asymptomatic human immunodeficiency virus infection: A controlled trial in persons with fewer than 500 CD4-positive cells per cubic millimeter. *The New England Journal of Medicine*, 322:941–949.

von Eye, A. (1990a). *Statistical Methods in Longitudinal Research. Volume 1. Principles and Structuring Change.* Academic Press, New York.

von Eye, A. (1990b). *Statistical Methods in Longitudinal Research. Volume 2. Time Series and Categorical Longitudinal Data.* Academic Press, New York.

Vonesh, E. F. and Carter, R. L. (1987). Efficient inference for random-coefficient growth curve models with unbalanced data. *Biometrics*, 43:617–628.

Vonesh, E. F. and Chinchilli, V. M. (1996). *Linear and Nonlinear Models for the Analysis of Repeated Measurements*. Marcel Dekker, New York.

Vonesh, E. F. and Schork, M. A. (1986). Sample sizes in the multivariate analysis of repeated measurements. *Biometrics*, 42:601–610.

Waclawiw, M. A. and Liang, K. Y. (1993). Prediction of random effects in the generalized linear model. *Journal of the American Statistical Association*, 88:171–178.

Walker, S. H. and Duncan, D. B. (1967). Estimation of the probability of an event as a function of several independent variables. *Biometrika*, 54:167–179.

Wallenstein, S. (1982). Regression models for repeated measurements. *Biometrics*, 38:849–853.

Ware, J. H. (1985). Linear models for the analysis of longitudinal studies. *The American Statistician*, 39:95–101.

Ware, J. H., Lipsitz, S. R., and Speizer, F. E. (1988). Issues in the analysis of repeated categorical outcomes. *Statistics in Medicine*, 7:95–107.

Wedderburn, R. W. M. (1974). Quasilikelihood functions, generalized linear models and the Gauss-Newton method. *Biometrika*, 61:439–447.

Wegman, E. J. (1990). Hyperdimensional data analysis using parallel coordinates. *Journal of the American Statistical Association*, 85:664–675.

Wei, L. J. and Johnson, W. E. (1985). Combining dependent tests with incomplete repeated measurements. *Biometrika*, 72:359–364.

Wei, L. J. and Lachin, J. M. (1984). Two-sample asymptotically distribution-free tests for incomplete multivariate observations. *Journal of the American Statistical Association*, 79:653–661.

Wei, L. J. and Stram, D. O. (1988). Analysing repeated measurements with possibly missing observations by modelling marginal distributions. *Statistics in Medicine*, 7:139–148.

Weiss, R. E. and Lazaro, C. G. (1992). Residual plots for repeated measures. *Statistics in Medicine*, 11:115–124.

Weissfeld, L. A. and Kshirsagar, A. M. (1992). A modified growth curve model and its application to clinical studies. *Australian Journal of Statistics*, 34:161–168.

Wilcoxon, F. (1945). Individual comparison by ranking methods. *Biometrics*, 1:80–83.

Wilks, S. S. (1932). Certain generalizations in the analysis of variance. *Biometrika*, 24:471–494.

Williamson, J. M., Kim, K., and Lipsitz, S. R. (1995). Analyzing bivariate ordinal data using a global odds ratio. *Journal of the American Statistical Association*, 90:1432–1437.

Wishart, J. (1938). Growth rate determination in nutrition studies with the bacon pig, and their analysis. *Biometrika*, 30:16–28.

Wolfinger, R. and O'Connell, M. (1993). Generalized linear mixed models: A pseudo-likelihood approach. *Journal of Statistical Computation and Simulation*, 48:233–243.

Wong, W. H. (1986). Theory of partial likelihood. *Annals of Statistics*, 14:88–123.

Woolson, R. F. and Clarke, W. R. (1984). Analysis of categorical incomplete longitudinal data. *Journal of the Royal Statistical Society, Series A*, 147:87–99.

Wu, C., Gumpertz, M. L., and Boos, D. D. (2001). Comparison of GEE, MINQUE, ML, and REML estimating equations for normally distributed data. *The American Statistician*, 55:125–130.

Wu, M. and Bailey, K. R. (1989). Estimation and comparison of changes in the presence of informative right censoring: Conditional linear model. *Biometrics*, 45:939–955.

Wu, M. and Carroll, R. J. (1988). Estimation and comparison of changes in the presence of informative right censoring by modeling the censoring process. *Biometrics*, 44:175–188.

Xie, F. and Paik, M. C. (1997a). Generalized estimating equation model for binary outcomes with missing covariates. *Biometrics*, 53:1458–1466.

Xie, F. and Paik, M. C. (1997b). Multiple imputation methods for the missing covariates in generalized estimating equation. *Biometrics*, 53:1538–1546.

Zeger, S. L. (1988). Commentary. *Statistics in Medicine*, 7:161–168.

Zeger, S. L. and Karim, M. R. (1991). Generalized linear models with random effects: A Gibbs sampling approach. *Journal of the American Statistical Association*, 86:79–86.

Zeger, S. L. and Liang, K. Y. (1986). Longitudinal data analysis for discrete and continuous outcomes. *Biometrics*, 42:121–130.

Zeger, S. L. and Liang, K. Y. (1992). An overview of methods for the analysis of longitudinal data. *Statistics in Medicine*, 11:1825–1839.

Zeger, S. L., Liang, K. Y., and Albert, P. S. (1988). Models for longitudinal data: A generalized estimating equation approach. *Biometrics*, 44:1049–1060.

Zeger, S. L. and Qaqish, B. (1988). Markov regression models for time series: A quasi-likelihood approach. *Biometrics*, 44:1019–1031.

Zellner, A. (1962). An efficient method of estimating seemingly unrelated regressions and tests for aggregation bias. *Journal of the American Statistical Association*, 57:348–368.

Zerbe, G. O. (1979a). Randomization analysis of randomized blocks extended to growth and response curves. *Communications in Statistics—Theory and Methods*, 8:191–205.

Zerbe, G. O. (1979b). Randomization analysis of the completely randomized design extended to growth and response curves. *Journal of the American Statistical Association*, 74:215–221.

Zerbe, G. O. and Murphy, J. R. (1986). On multiple comparisons in the randomization analysis of growth and response curves. *Biometrics*, 42:795–804.

Zerbe, G. O. and Walker, S. H. (1977). A randomization test for comparison of groups of growth curves with different polynomial design matrices. *Biometrics*, 33:653–657.

Zhao, L. P. and Prentice, R. L. (1990). Correlated binary regression using a quadratic exponential model. *Biometrika*, 77:642–648.

Zhaorong, J., McGilchrist, C. A., and Jorgensen, M. A. (1992). Mixed model discrete regression. *Biometrical Journal*, 34:691–700.

Zimmerman, D. L. (2000). Viewing the correlation structure of longitudinal data through a PRISM. *The American Statistician*, 54:310–318.

Zimmerman, D. L. and Núñez Antón, V. A. (1997). Structured antedependence models for longitudinal data. In Gregoire, T. G., Brillinger, D. R., Diggle, P. J., Russek-Cohen, E., Warren, W. G., and Wolfinger, R., editors, *Modelling Longitudinal and Spatially Correlated Data. Methods, Applications, and Future Directions*, pages 63–76. Springer-Verlag, New York.

Author Index

Subject Index

Springer Texts in Statistics *(continued from page ii)*

Lehmann: Testing Statistical Hypotheses, Second Edition
Lehmann and Casella: Theory of Point Estimation, Second Edition
Lindman: Analysis of Variance in Experimental Design
Lindsey: Applying Generalized Linear Models
Madansky: Prescriptions for Working Statisticians
McPherson: Applying and Interpreting Statistics: A Comprehensive Guide, Second Edition
Mueller: Basic Principles of Structural Equation Modeling: An Introduction to LISREL and EQS
Nguyen and Rogers: Fundamentals of Mathematical Statistics: Volume I: Probability for Statistics
Nguyen and Rogers: Fundamentals of Mathematical Statistics: Volume II: Statistical Inference
Noether: Introduction to Statistics: The Nonparametric Way
Nolan and Speed: Stat Labs: Mathematical Statistics Through Applications
Peters: Counting for Something: Statistical Principles and Personalities
Pfeiffer: Probability for Applications
Pitman: Probability
Rawlings, Pantula and Dickey: Applied Regression Analysis
Robert: The Bayesian Choice: From Decision-Theoretic Foundations to Computational Implementation, Second Edition
Robert and Casella: Monte Carlo Statistical Methods, Second Edition
Rose and Smith: Mathematical Statistics with *Mathematica*
Ruppert: Statistics and Finance: An Introduction
Santner and Duffy: The Statistical Analysis of Discrete Data
Saville and Wood: Statistical Methods: The Geometric Approach
Sen and Srivastava: Regression Analysis: Theory, Methods, and Applications
Shao: Mathematical Statistics, Second Edition
Shorack: Probability for Statisticians
Shumway and Stoffer: Time Series Analysis and Its Applications
Simonoff: Analyzing Categorical Data
Terrell: Mathematical Statistics: A Unified Introduction
Timm: Applied Multivariate Analysis
Toutenburg: Statistical Analysis of Designed Experiments, Second Edition
Wasserman: All of Statistics: A Concise Course in Statistical Inference
Whittle: Probability via Expectation, Fourth Edition
Zacks: Introduction to Reliability Analysis: Probability Models and Statistical Methods

Printed in the United States
by Baker & Taylor Publisher Services

Printed in the United States
by Baker & Taylor Publisher Services